T0258157

Current Progress in Biomaterials

Current Progress in Biomaterials

Edited by **Ralph Seguin**

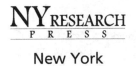

New York

Published by NY Research Press,
23 West, 55th Street, Suite 816,
New York, NY 10019, USA
www.nyresearchpress.com

Current Progress in Biomaterials
Edited by Ralph Seguin

International Standard Book Number: 978-1-63238-110-1 (Hardback)

Printed in the United States of America.

Contents

Preface   VII

Section 1   Biomaterials for Tissue Engineering and Regeneration   1

Chapter 1   Innovative Strategies for Tissue Engineering   3
Juliana Lott Carvalho, Pablo Herthel de Carvalho, Dawidson Assis
Gomes and Alfredo Miranda de Goes

Chapter 2   Biomaterials and Stem Cell Therapies for Injuries Associated to
Skeletal Muscular Tissues   22
Tiago Pereira, Andrea Gärtner, Irina Amorim, Paulo Armada-da-
Silva, Raquel Gomes, Cátia Pereira, Miguel L. França, Diana M.
Morais, Miguel A. Rodrigues, Maria A. Lopes, José D. Santos, Ana
Lúcia Luís and Ana Colette Maurício

Chapter 3   Biofabrication of Tissue Scaffolds   57
Ning Zhu and Xiongbiao Chen

Chapter 4   Alignment of Cells and Extracellular Matrix Within Tissue-
Engineered Substitutes   71
Jean-Michel Bourget, Maxime Guillemette, Teodor Veres, François
A. Auger and Lucie Germain

Chapter 5   Autograft of Dentin Materials for Bone Regeneration   97
Masaru Murata, Toshiyuki Akazawa, Masaharu Mitsugi, Md Arafat
Kabir, In-Woong Um, Yasuhito Minamida, Kyung-Wook Kim,
Young-Kyun Kim, Yao Sun and Chunlin Qin

Chapter 6   The Integrations of Biomaterials and Rapid Prototyping
Techniques for Intelligent Manufacturing of
Complex Organs   110
Xiaohong Wang, Jukka Tuomi, Antti A. Mäkitie, Kaija-Stiina
Paloheimo, Jouni Partanen and Marjo Yliperttula

Chapter 7   **Healing Mechanism and Clinical Application of Autogenous**
             Tooth Bone Graft Material   137
             Young-Kyun Kim, Jeong Keun Lee, Kyung-Wook Kim, In-Woong
             Um and Masaru Murata

Chapter 8   **Mesenchymal Stem Cells from Extra-Embryonic Tissues for**
             Tissue Engineering – Regeneration of the
             Peripheral Nerve   168
             Andrea Gärtner, Tiago Pereira, Raquel Gomes, Ana Lúcia Luís,
             Miguel Lacueva França, Stefano Geuna, Paulo Armada-da-Silva and
             Ana Colette Maurício

Section 2   **Special Applications of Biomaterials**   202

Chapter 9   **Dental Materials**   204
             Junko Hieda, Mitsuo Niinomi, Masaaki Nakai and Ken Cho

Chapter 10   **Hydroxylapatite (HA) Powder for Autovaccination Against**
             Canine Non Hodgkin's Lymphoma   228
             Michel Simonet, Nicole Rouquet and Patrick Frayssinet

Chapter 11   **Ceramic-On-Ceramic Joints: A Suitable Alternative Material**
             Combination?   241
             Susan C. Scholes and Thomas J. Joyce

Permissions

List of Contributors

Preface

Over the recent decade, advancements and applications have progressed exponentially. This has led to the increased interest in this field and projects are being conducted to enhance knowledge. The main objective of this book is to present some of the critical challenges and provide insights into possible solutions. This book will answer the varied questions that arise in the field and also provide an increased scope for furthering studies.

This book compiles reviews and original researches conducted by experts and scientists working in the field of biomaterials, covering a broad range from design to new applications. This book elucidates different features of biomaterials and examines techniques used to produce biomaterials with the specific properties required for certain clinical and medical functions. It covers various topics like latest methods for characterization and evaluation of new materials, traditional applications in nanotechnology and tissue engineering, and new applications of these products.

I hope that this book, with its visionary approach, will be a valuable addition and will promote interest among readers. Each of the authors has provided their extraordinary competence in their specific fields by providing different perspectives as they come from diverse nations and regions. I thank them for their contributions.

Editor

Biomaterials for Tissue Engineering and Regeneration

Innovative Strategies for Tissue Engineering

Juliana Lott Carvalho, Pablo Herthel de Carvalho,
Dawidson Assis Gomes and
Alfredo Miranda de Goes

Additional information is available at the end of the chapter

1. Introduction

Unmet need. It is beyond dispute that human population is ageing. For the first time in history, people age 65 and over will outnumber children under age 5. This trend is emerging around the globe, and will bring several challenges for health technologies. For instance, in a few decades, the loss of health and life worldwide will be greater from chronic diseases than from infectious diseases and accidents [4].

The report made by the National Institute of Health and the National Institute of Aging (NIH/ NIA) underscores the unmet needs lying ahead for regenerative medicine. Chronic diseases, in opposition to infectious diseases, are mainly treated by regenerative approaches, instead of immunization and antibiotics.

Actually, many of those challenges are already present in our daily living: malformations [9,14], accidents [16], chronic infections [9,15], and end-organ failure [17] (usually occurs during the final stages of degenerative and other diseases), may, in some cases, only be treated by organ replacement. In fact, end-organ failure alone already affects millions of Americans. More specifically, nearly six million Americans suffer from heart failure with approximately 550,000 new cases diagnosed annually, 530,000 Americans suffer from end-stage renal disease and nearly 25 million Americans suffer from chronic obstructive pulmonary disease with an estimated 12 million new annual diagnoses [5]. As already stated, for many of those patients, organ transplantation is their only treatment option. Currently, organ transplantation is considered the best option for some patients and achieves up to 98,5% of patient 1-year survival rates [18]. Unfortunately, though, current organ shortage/recovering engenders waiting lines of up to three or more years [5]. During 2008, for instance, the number of heart transplantations decreased 2,67%, even though waiting lines increased during the same year. Such decrease occurred mainly due to a reduction in number of recovered organs [18].

It is clear that alternatives to organ transplantation need to be developed as soon as possible. That's where tissue engineering comes into picture.

Tissue engineering. Tissue engineering refers to an "interdisciplinary field that applies the principles of engineering and the life sciences toward the development of biological substitutes that restore, maintain, or improve tissue function" [3]. The term was first coined by Dr. Fung, from California University, which suggested this name during the National Science Foundation Meeting, in 1987 [2]. The first official definition dates to 1988, though, when Skalak and Fox published it after the "Tissue engineering Meeting" held in Lake Tahoe, USA during that year [1].

In 1993, Langer and Vacanti described three strategies for the creation of new tissue in vitro [3].

1. *Isolated cells or substitutes.* The concept of treating injured tissues with isolated cells is currently regarded as cell therapy. Infusion of cells, e.g. stem cells, has presented several promising results, and have already been approved for human use for specific applications [21] but in some cases, is hindered by the lack of fixation of cells in the site of lesion. When injected systemically, stem cells are attracted to injured tissues, but are also found in several organs such as lungs, liver and spleen [56].

2. *Tissue inducing substances.* At the time, tissue inducing substances included growth factors, small molecules, and other classes of molecules which, if delivered in the organism, would promote several effects on cells, such as growth [58], survival [58], migration [57] and neo tissue formation.

3. *Cells placed on or within matrices.* Associated cells and substrates provide the injured tissue with continuity, and promotes cell attachment and fixation. In this context, scaffolds may be associated with inducing substances, providing means to combine all the aforementioned strategies. The combination of cells and matrices, in addition to inducing substances or not, is currently the main strategy for tissue engineering, as depicted in Figure 1.

Currently, tissue engineering focuses mainly of associating cells with supports (also called biomaterials or scaffolds), in order to: i. promote cell attachment and restrict their distribution in the tissue, ii. direct cell distribution and differentiation, iii. sustain large tissue losses while new tissue is formed, and ultimately, to iv. lead to new tissue formation.

Since its early days, tissue engineering has significantly evolved in each of its pillars – Cells, signaling molecules and scaffolds. This evolution covered both conceptual aspects - as evidenced above – as well as practical aspects, mainly reflected in the achievements of the field (for more information, go to conclusion section). Unfortunately, even though cells and signaling molecules platforms have evolved during the past decades, leading to major field evolution, the degree of success of tissue engineering methods is still highly dependent on the properties of the scaffold. Therefore, this study focuses on the main Achille's Hill of tissue engineering: production of scaffolds for biological applications.

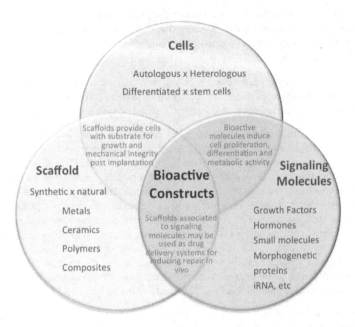

Figure 1. Tissue engineering strategies. Based on [59]. Tissue engineering may be performed by several different approaches, as proposed by Langer and Vancanti. In order to obtain tissue regeneration, cells, scaffolds and signaling molecules may be introduced into the body alone or in association. Currently, the association of all three elements, composing bioactive constructs, is proposed to be the best option for tissue engineering.

In the present chapter, we present the current status of tissue engineering. First, we present a comprehensive picture of classical tissue engineering approaches, as well as an analytic view of its main achievements and limitations. Secondly, we present innovative and paradigm breaking strategies for successful tissue engineering, accompanied by the history and rationale behind each of them. Finally, we analyze the next steps of tissue engineering translation into the clinic.

2. Classical tissue engineering approaches

Association of cells to classic biodegradable solid/porous biomaterial represents a dominating conceptual framework in tissue engineering. Actually, men have used biomaterials (alone, not associated to cells) in order to substitute eventual tissue loss since ancient civilizations [11]. In the early days, all kinds of materials derived from natural and manufactured sources were used as biomaterials. Natural materials included wood and shells, and manufactured materials comprised metals such as iron, gold and zinc. The host responses to these materials were extremely varied, and only after the concept of sterility, biomaterial implants began to achieve consistent safety. During the last 30 years, further progress has been made in understanding the interactions between the tissues and the materials.

Since then, tissue reconstitution evolved to a more sophisticated approach, in which the regeneration of the tissue/organ was clearly viewed as the ideal way of treating injuries, compared to biomaterial science, which simply reconstitutes tissue structure, without restoring tissue function in most situations. This paradigm evolution led to the emergence of tissue engineering.

Tissue engineering based on biomaterials relies on four main classes of materials: i. Polymers, ii. Ceramics, iii. Metals and iv. Composites (blends and combinations of the aforementioned materials). Biomaterials may derive from natural or synthetic sources [12].

The association of cells to biomaterials is called construct and is the base of current tissue engineering, as already stated. Construct-based classic tissue engineering platform derives from several basic assumptions, as described by Mironov et al., 2009 [31]: "1) cell growth is substrate attachment-dependent; cells need a solid substrate for attachment and proliferation; 2) tissue constructs must have an organo-specific shape; a solid scaffold is essential to keep the desired shape; a tissue construct could not maintain its shape without a solid rigid scaffold; 3) the scaffold serves not only as an attachment substrate, but also as a source of inductive and instructive signals for cell differentiation, migration, proliferation and orientation; 4) the porous structure of a solid scaffold will allow optimal cell seeding, tissue construct viability, and vascularization; and 5) mechanical properties initially provided by the rigid solid scaffold after its biodegradation will be maintained by controlled neomorphogenesis of parenchymal and stromal tissue synthesized *in vitro* or *in vivo* in the tissue construct".

Considering these basic assumptions, currently, classic tissue engineering is made taking several aspects into account, which will be highlighted below.

1. *Construct design.* Currently, scaffold design is a complex science, in which several aspects are carefully addressed in order to produce successful constructs. Those aspects include, but are not restricted to:

i.   *Choosing the most suitable biomaterial for the envisioned application.* Organs and tissues in the human body present different characteristics, therefore, the ideal biomaterial must reproduce as many as those features as possible. Such aspects include tissue resistance, elasticity, resilience, and chemical composition, among others, in addition to biocompatibility. For instance, a biomaterial designed to be used in a skin construct must be thin and elastic. A biomaterial for application in corneas, on the other hand, must also be thin, but most importantly, it must be transparent.

ii.   *Customizing the material in order to promote cell colonization.* The ideal construct must promote rapid and equal cell adhesion and colonization, therefore scaffolds are usually porous and present a surface which is recognized directly or indirectly (by promoting protein adsorption) by the cell as a substrate for attachment. Usually, materials such as chitosan and collagen are used as biomaterials, due to their resemblance to the extracellular matrix and their efficacy in promoting cell adhesion [26,27]. In case of other materials, such as metals and ceramics, biomaterial surface may not be easily recognized by cells. In order to improve cell contact and adhesion by cells, many strategies have been developed, such as blending biomaterials, recovering them with other substances or still covering them with protein residues recognized by cells, such as isoleucine-lysine-valine-alanine-valine (IKVAV) residue, derived from Laminin [28,29].

iii. *Studying material tribology and surface topography* [19]. For several tissues, such as muscles and tendons, cell organization is paramount for optimal tissue function. The heart, for instance, works as a pumping organ, and needs to contract in a specific, synchronized way in order to actually eject blood into body and lungs. If muscle fibers are not synchronized, no pumping force is generated, and great deficit of function is witnessed by the patient [60]. Tendon is a specific connective tissue composed of parallel collagen fibers. Along with the heart, tendon constitutes another of several tissues which depend on specific cell organization for proper function. It has been thoroughly described in literature that tendon strength is directly linked to cell orientation, and, following injuries, the lack of orientation of scar tissue promotes tendon weakness, leading to repetitive lesion [61]. Tissue engineering approaches for tendon must promote cell alignment in order to achieve significant benefit for patients. cell alignment has been shown to be achievable and effective in promoting tissue organization and maturation [30], as shown in Figure 2.

iv. *Optimizing biomaterial degradation rate.* Tissue engineering has been envisioned to promote tissue regeneration, therefore in this context, biomaterials should be biodegradable. Ideally, biomaterial should gradually degrade, at the same rate as neotissue is formed.

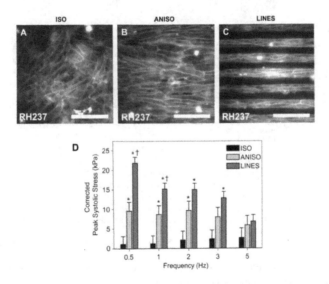

Figure 2. Cell orientation promotes major contractile strength of construct. In order to assess cell orientation importance for construct function, Dr. Parker`s group engineered bidimensional cardiac muscles with different micropatterned surfaces in order to promote degrees of cell orientation. Confluent unaligned isotropic (A), aligned anisotropic (B) and non confluent, 20µm spaced, parallel arrays of myocardial fibers (C) were build and studied *in vitro*. The cited work showed that contractile force increases with major sarcomere alignment, as measured by peak systolic stress in kPa (D). This panel was based on [60] and was kindly provided by Dr. Kevin Kit Parker, from Harvard University.

2. *Cell seeding.* Cell seeding is paramount for construct optimization, and must be carefully planned. Usually, most cells have low capacity of invasion, therefore, cell seeding must be optimized to promote an equal distribution of cells along construct surface and interior [62].

3. *Construct maintenance in vitro.* The maintenance of small constructs may be achievable in static cultures, but when it comes to larger constructs, static culture is hindered by the limitation of nutrient diffusion. Several strategies have been developed for large construct maintenance *in vitro*, represented mainly by bioreactors, as depicted in Figure 3.

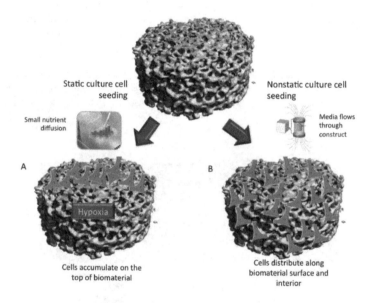

Figure 3. Importance of non-static cell seeding and culture for construct equal distribution of cell elements and viability of construct. As depicted, static culture seeding promotes cell accumulation in specific regions of the construct. As no media is perfused through the construct, nutrient distribution along the biomaterial depends on diffusion only, which leads to normoxic construct edges, colonized with cells and hypoxic center, which is not feasible to be colonized by cells. Nonstatic culture strategies, on the other hand, promote equal cell seeding and colonization of the construct, as it enhances nutrient diffusion. Even though nonstatic culture is not sufficient to promote viability of large constructs, it increases maximum size of constructs and is more adequate for tissue engineering purposes.

4. *Construct implant.* The ultimate function of a construct built *in vitro* is to be implanted and substitute/regenerate an injured organ or tissue. Construct implant must be performed in order to promote construct integration and viability. Several techniques have already been applied to promote construct long term viability, such as designing VEGF (vascular endothelial growth factor) releasing constructs; previously implanting the construct in an ectopic site, in order to promote *in vivo* vascularization, prior to implantation; and reducing the size of implants, among others.

In spite of its major advances, scaffold-based tissue engineering suffers from several limitations, as explored by Mironov et al., 2009 [31], and further explained here:

1. Vascularization of thick tissue constructs

Cell survival requires continuous supply of nutrients and oxygen, as well as the removal of metabolites, which, if accumulated, might be toxic. Such demand is addressed mainly by osmosis, therefore, to facilitate nutrient and metabolite flow, cells must be kept near vessels and capilars. Actually, few cells are able to survive at more than 200um distance from the nearest blood vessel [8]. Cells cultured in tridimensional scaffolds also need to be maintained in homeostasis in order to survive. *In vitro*, several strategies have been developed in order to maintain construct viability prior to implantation, mainly through the development of bioreactors, as reviewed by Rauh et. *al.* [10]. *In vivo*, however, none of those strategies are applicable, and only through vascularization cells are kept alive, especially for modular organs, such as heart, kidney and liver, which are organized in functioning units and require their own vascular supply [9]. Studies indicate that vessels grow at a rate of <1mm a day [6], and although the effectiveness of an enhanced angiogenic response using various growth factors has been demonstrated in many tissue systems, the rate of angiogenesis hasn`t been accelerated so far [7]. Considering the relatively large sizes of constructs for humans, it is clear the urgent need to promote faster vascularization of tissue constructs, or to improve cell survival in scaffolds.

Actually, several attempts of increasing tissue vascularization are underway.

As previously mentioned, increasing cell survival is also an interesting strategy. Actually, recently, oxygen generating scaffolds have been developed and tested with encouraging results, even though no *in vivo* tests were performed [7].

2. Precise placing of different multiple cell types inside 3D porous scaffolds is technologically challenging.

Modular organs, such as the heart, liver, kidneys and others, are complex structures of several types of cells, including stromal and parenchymal cells. They function as working units, such as muscle fibers, liver lobules and kidney nephrons. Modular organs also count on intrinsic vascular system for cell survival, constituting incredibly difficult organs to build *in vitro*, even though many papers have shown a significant capacity of self-organization of several cells [22,23,24]. For such organs, whole organ approaches are more suitable then partial reconstitution of those structures.

On the other hand, non-modular organs have witnessed several successful strategies, such as the construction of bladders [44] and the recellularization of tracheas [15], both of which have already been translated to the clinic.

3. Achieving organo-specific level of cell density in tissue constructs remains a big challenge

Currently, porous matrices are paramount to allow cell invasion and colonization of the matrix. Porous present in the matrices are usually optimized to have specific sizes and to be interconnected, in order to permit cell invasion. The size of the produced porous is usually large, though, and cells within the scaffold are not able to fully fill it and achieve cell density similar to natural tissues. Therefore, it is almost as if cells were still in two-dimensional surfaces [31]. Actually, extracellular matrix molecules can be washed out from 3D porous scaffolds in the same way as in 2D cultures, and may not provide means for real tridimensional tissue formation.

4.   Recent reports on the effect of matrix rigidity on (stem) cell differentiation can undermine the value of solid rigid biodegradable scaffolds at least for certain tissue applications [35-37]

Stem cell differentiation has traditionally employed cocktails of various growth factors, but recently, mechanobiological concepts have been described as important to cell fate decision. The mechanism underlying cellular response to tension comprises the force generated by myosin bundles sliding along actin filaments and transmission to the ECM. Transduction of these signals link the extracellular and intracellular worlds, ultimately affected by proteins such as Rho GTPases, which not only regulate contraction of stress fibers, but also regulate gene expression by acting over their effector target proteins, [45].

Actually, matrix rigidity has been involved in embryonic development, as well as adult stem cell differentiation. As expected, rigid surfaces facilitates adult stem cell differentiation into bone, and soft surfaces lead to differentiation of adult stem cells into soft tissues, such as fat or central nervous system (brain) [45].

5.   Biodegradability of constructs

Even though it makes sense that biomaterials should be absorbed by the body in order to give space to neotissue formation, the same is not true when whole tissue engineering is planned. There is no use in spending efforts in order to build a construct, which will be invaded by inflammatory cells and vessels and disorganized, previously to being substituted by neotissue.

Therefore, even though current tissue engineering techniques are fairly successful in treating bone, skin and cartilage loss, they are extremely limited in treating large tissue loss, as well as in regenerating complex tissues, such as heart annd kidneys, among several other tissues and organs.

3. Innovative tissue engineering approaches

3.1. Decellularized matrices

The Extracellular Matrix (ECM) represents the three-dimensional fibrilar protein scaffold, produced by cells of each tissue and organ, which surrounds and anchors them. It is kept in a state of dynamic reciprocity with those cells, in response to changes in the microenvironment. ECM has been shown to provide cues that affect cell migration, proliferation, gene expression and differentiation [32, 37].

The ECM is obviously the optimal support for tissue engineering, as it provides the perfect chemical composition, surface topology and physical properties experienced by cells *in vivo in their niche* [32]. Even though sometimes that's exactly what is needed to be avoided (e.g. Central Nervous System ECM has been shown to contain molecules which inhibit axonal growth and hinders tissue regeneration [33,34]), ECM has been considered a great option for tissue engineering.

Recently, it has been shown that cell sensibility towards ECM chemical composition is higher than previously expected. For instance, Tsai et al. showed that MG63, an osteoblast like cell lineage, behaves differently when grown in collagen or gelatin electrospun matrices. When grown in electrospun collagen, MG63 did not show variation on cell attachment or proliferation rates. On the other hand, cells seeded on electrospun collagen showed increased expression of osteogenic genes such as Osteopontin and alkaline phosphatase. Collagen and gelatin present high chemical composition similarity, varying mainly in secondary and tertiary structure. Such fact underscores the strikingly cell sensitivity to all aspects of ECM chemical and physical composition [62]. It also underscores the potential of decellularized matrices on tissue engineering.

Decellularized tissues have been used in regenerative medicine approaches since the early eighties [38], specially focused on treating cardiovascular diseases by engineering vascular grafts. Most of the grafts produced, derived from synthetic and natural sources suffered from several limitations. When the issue of natural graft calcification and immunological recognition were related to residual cellular components of unmodified biological materials, decellularization techniques began to be developed [38,39].

Initially, decellularization was considered for tissue grafts. Developed techniques are continuously evolving, as every cell removal agent and method currently available alters ECM composition and cause some degree of ultrastructure disruption. Decellularization agents include chemical, biological and physical agents, each of them with different mechanisms of action.

More specifically: acids and bases promote hydrolytic degradation of biomolecules; hypotonic solutions lyses cells through osmosis with minimal changes in matrix molecules and tissue architecture; hypertonic solutions dissociates DNA from proteins; ionic, non-ionic, and zwitterionic detergents solubilize cell membranes leading to effective removal of cellular material from tissue; solvents, such as alcohol and acetone, promote either cell lysis by dehydration or solubilization and removal of lipids and biological agents, such as enzymes, and chelating agents act through protein cleavage and disrupting cell adhesion to ECM. Finally, physical agents promote cell lysis through freezing and thawing cycles, electroporation or pressure [32].

The most effective agents for decellularization of each tissue and organ will depend upon many factors, including the tissue's cellularity, density, lipid content, and thickness [32].

Lately, whole organ decellularization began to be performed, offering an interesting option for modular organs such as the heart, lung and kidneys. In 2008, Ott et al. not only performed whole heart decellularization, but also recellularized the organ with neonatal cardiomyocytes and obtained organ function [17]. This groundbreaking work highlighted the possibilities of decellularized matrix-based whole organ tissue engineering.

The major breakthrough of organ decellularization is to obtain scaffolds with perfect (or very similar) chemical composition and tridimensional structure, compared to natural organs. In addition, the vascular bed is completely preserved, facilitating *in vitro* maintenance of the construct via perfusion bioreactors, as well as *in vivo* viability of the construct, which may be reconnected to the circulatory system of host, also shown by Ott et al [17]. As decellularization is performed making use of vascular system of organs, virtually any vascularized organ may be decellularized, disregarding its size, as depicted in Figure 4. Acellular organs, such as tracheas, may also be decellularized through different protocols [15].

Perfusion Decellularization Results in Exquisite Retention of Structure

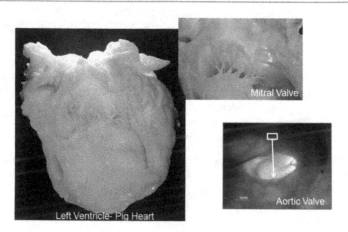

Figure 4. Decellularized pig heart. As published by Ott et al., perfusion decellularization is feasible in small rat organs, but also in bigger size organs, such as the pig heart. Illustration owned by Miromatrix Medical Inc., available at http://miromatrix.com/technology/perfusion-decellularization-recellularization/, accessed on September 2012.

3.2. Biomimetic scaffolds

As already mentioned, an optimal scaffold attempts to mimic the function of the natural extracellular matrix [52]. The functionality of most tissues is related to their complex architecture, therefore mimicking and recapitulating this complexity *in vitro* is paramount for successful tissue engineering. In the *in vivo* condition, cells are surrounded by other cells and by the extracellular matrix (ECM), whose components, such as collagen, elastin, and laminin, are organized in nanostructures (i.e., fibers, triple helixes, etc) with specific bioactive motifs that regulate cell homeostasis [42].

Following the initial concept of mimicking the ECM chemical composition, it has been shown that the structure of the cell-surrounding niche is also paramount for optimal cell function. In accordance, modulating the scaffold microarchitecture is one of the most potent ways of achieving biomimetic tissues. Advances in microfabrication technologies have been exploited by an increasing number of research groups. Often technologies from other engineering disciplines have been translated and used in creating microfeatures in engineered scaffolds in a controlled manner. These include photolithographic approach of the electrical engineering, electrospinning tools of the textile industry, emulsification and fluid dynamics principles of chemical engineering and rapid prototyping methods of mechanical engineering. The latter will be covered in further detail in the next section [40].

Vacanti and coworkers pioneered the concept of engineering a vasculature using photolithographic techniques (which use light, e.g. UV, to selectively remove parts of a thin film or the bulk of a substrate), literally generating channels within biomaterials [43].

Electrospining techniques have also been considered and tested for tissue engineering application, due to their potential of producing polymer fibers with nano to micrometer diameter scale that are physically and topographically comparable to the collagen fibers, commonly found in the natural ECM, as shown in Figure 5. It has been extensively employed in tissue engineering strategies, including vascularization strategies [41].

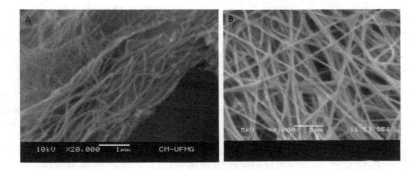

Figure 5. Similarity between ultrastructure of natural collagen fibers (A) and electrospun biomaterials (B). Source: A – author`s unpublished data; B - http://en.wikipedia.org/wiki/Electrospinning, accessed on September 2012.

Electrospun biomaterials must also be carefully fabricated, as even fiber diameter variation results in different cell behavior, as observed in endothelial cells cultured on electrospun poly(l-lactide-co-ε-caprolactone) with different fiber diameters. In contrast to cells cultured on fibers of 0.3 or 1.2μm, cells cultured on 7μm presented lower cell adhesion, spreading and proliferation [63].

Even though electrospining has presented promising results, it also suffers from some limitations, such as poor cell invasion, as usually the electrospun biomaterials are highly compacted, impeding cell migration towards the inner side of the scaffold. The search for different solvents and electrospining conditions may solve this issue, promoting less fiber compactation.

Still, as cited, many excellent constructs have been built using those techniques, and in association with the other tissue engineering strategies presented in the present chapter, strongly contribute to novel advances in the field.

Another exciting tissue engineering strategy, which have gained growing interest since the nineties, has been the hydrogel approach. Hydrogels are 3D cross-linked insoluble, hydrophilic networks of polymers that partially resemble the physical characteristics of native ECM. The biocompatibility of various hydrogels (e.g., collagen, agarose and polyethylene glycol) is well characterized, and the possibility of optimizing their physico-chemical and mechanical properties to levels that are desirable for tissue scaffolds, in order to achieve cell encapsulation, immobilization, and drug delivery turn hydrogels into an extremely promising technique [64].

Hydrogels have been successfully used in mimicking ECM of simple tissues, composed of one cell type. In many cases, hydrogels provide means for nutrient diffusion, facilitating cell maintenance *in vitro* and *in vivo*. Still, maintaining the viability of high cell density constructs remains a challenge as well as promoting cell organization within the scaffold. In many cases, construct implantation near host rich vascularization sites may be an effective strategy to promote construct viability *in vivo*.

In the cell's point of view, hydrogels possess the advantage of completely surround encapsulated cells, and providing tridimensional substrate for cell interaction. This strategy prevents cell polarization which is common to regular scaffolds. Usually, as already stated, even though most scaffolds may be tridimensional macroscopically, they are commonly seen as bidimensional surfaces by cells.

As expected, truly tridimensional environments promote several effects over cultured cells. Some of them include, but are not limited to: cell morphology/spreading [65], cell motility and proliferation [66], and metabolic rate [67]. Obviously, all of those cell behaviors reflect differential gene expression.

Even though cell gene expression is a paramount factor to be evaluated in tissue engineering, it must be clearly noted that an exact gene expression profile is not essential for tissue engineering effectiveness. Cells will always interact with their microenvironment. What is important for tissue engineering is to maintain cell plasticity in a manner that, once in vivo, implanted cells start to behave as host cells would.

Finally, a third highly modern and innovative approach for tissue engineering, which shares the truly tridimensional environment for cells as provided by hydrogels, but which doesn't suffer from vascularization and cell organization limitations presented by the latter, is the organ printing tissue engineering technique, which will be more thoroughly described in the next section.

3.3. Organ printing

As listed before, the main limitations of the solid scaffold approach include the low level of precision in cell placement, especially when engineering multicellular constructs, considering the intrinsic problem of vascularization of thick tissue constructs [53]. Ideally, a possible way to solve many of those aforementioned problems would be to assemble cells and ECM elements at the same time and in an organized way, in order to obtain the most similar structure found in a functional organ as possible. Over the years, technology evolution turned tissue engineers unreachable dream into a feasible objective to be fulfilled in the next years or decades. This strategy is known as organ printing and/or robotic biofabrication, and offer interesting alternatives to solid scaffold-based tissue engineering.

According to the First International Workshop on Bioprinting and Biopatterning, organ printing was defined as "The use of material transfer processes for patterning and assembling biologically relevant materials (molecules, cells, tissues, and biodegradable biomaterials) with a prescribed organization to accomplish one or more biological functions" [45]. In fact, this technology could be defined as computer-aided, layer-by-layer deposition of biologically relevant materials [53].

The ultimate goal of organ-printing technology is to fabricate 3D vascularized functional living human organs suitable for clinical implantation in reasonable time scales. Other applications of this technology are in histogenesis and organogenesis, pharmacological tests and disease research [45, 46, 47, 48].

Wilson and Boland (2003) showed protein and cell printing using a commercial ink-jet device can be possible. In this technology, either individual cells or small clusters are printed over ECM hydrogels, designed for involve printed cells and to provide them with desired signals. Therefore, organ printing has derived from hydrogel classical approach, described in the previous section. The method is rapid, versatile and cheap. Its disadvantage is that it is difficult to assure high cell density needed for the fabrication of solid organ structures. Furthermore, due to the high speed of cell deposition, considerable damage is caused to cells, although the latest developments in the field have led to considerable improvement in cell survival [54, 55]. In the other approach, mechanical extruders are used to place 'bio-ink' particles, multicellular aggregates of definite composition into a supporting environment, the 'bio-paper', according to computer-generated templates consistent with the topology of the desired biological structure. Organoids are formed by postprinting fusion of the bio-ink particles and the sorting of cells within the bio-ink particles. The advantage of this technology is that the bio-ink particles represent small 3D tissue fragments. Thus, cells in them are in a more physiologically relevant arrangement, with adhesive contacts with their neighbors, which may assure the transmission of vital molecular signals. Both inkjet and extruder bioprinting are compatible with rapid prototyping [55].

In this biomanufacturing a precise layer-by-layer placement of self-assembled tissue spheroids in sprayed tissue fusion permissive hydrogels is used to obtain an organ or tissue. The hydrogels work as "biopapers" and cell blocks or tissue spheroids work as a "bioink". Both biopaper and bioink must be optimized in order to obtain viable tissues. For instance, biopapers vary according to each "printed" organ, and cell spheroids vary in properties according to their composition. Cell viability during and after printing is an obvious goal for bioprinting [45]. Preliminary studies of both ink-jet and laser forward transfer indicated that cells can survive deposition condition forces. Problems associated with ink-jet delivery of cell suspensions may also come about from the high shear stresses observed during ejection and impact of a fluid drop [50, 51, 52].

In many cases, the bioprinting process requires that before and during printing, cells and molecules must be carried in a fluid vehicle that shortly after printing requires consolidation and should consequently behave as a viscoelastic solid. This phase change must occur without damage to the biochemical, cells, or more complex units within the fluid, which presents a considerable challenge. Concurrently, tissue printed mustn't be too solid, or cell spheroids won`t interact and form a continued tissue.

Organ printing is a technology that promises to transform tissue engineering into a commercially successful biomedical industry. Unlike other tissue engineered approaches, organ printing involves the high throughput generation of organs, relying on automated cell sorters, cell and organ bioreactors and robotic bioprinters, most of them which are already commercially available [46]. However, much research is necessary to turn this technology into reality of clinical application.

4. Conclusion: Tissue engineering — From the bench to the bedside

It is known that any technology takes about 20 years to reach the market, and despite progress in many fields, this timeframe has yet to shorten [20]. Accordingly, tissue engineering, which has officially given its first steps during the late eighties, hasn`t brought many products to the bedside [20].

In contrast to biomaterials - which are readily available as hip implants, contact lenses, silicon breast prosthesis, among others –, and cell therapy – which is also available for bone marrow transplants, as well as its first allogeneic stem cell therapy products [21] -, constructs have been successfully produced for only few applications, largely limited to non-modular organs such as skin epidermis, corneal epithelium and cartilage [40]. Indeed, Apligraf - a bilayered skin substitute - was the first allogeneic cell based therapy to be approved by the US Food and Drug Administration (FDA), receiving permission for sale as a treatment for venous leg ulcers13.

Apligraf is constructed by culturing human foreskin-derived neonatal fibroblasts in a bovine type I collagen matrix over which human foreskin-derived neonatal epidermal keratinocytes are then cultured and allowed to stratify [68]. Even though it is considered one of the first tissue engineering products ever approved for commercialization, Apligraf doesn`t directly restore skin, but transiently protects and provides injured skin with scaffold and signaling molecules (produced by the cells within the construct) which fosters and accelerate skin regeneration.

Engineered bladders and airways have also been built and implanted *in vivo*, but as they require highly customized and complex approaches, they are available to a small number of patients, and are not considered products to be sold, such as Apligraf and other similar products.

Therefore, it is clear that, in spite of recent advances, tissue engineering has much to deliver. Innovative strategies, such as the presented in this chapter, present out of the box solutions for some of the present challenges in the field, and may one day constitute the major breakthroughs to finally catalyze translating tissue engineering from bench to bedside.

Author details

Juliana Lott Carvalho[1], Pablo Herthel de Carvalho[2], Dawidson Assis Gomes[1] and Alfredo Miranda de Goes[1]

*Address all correspondence to: julianalott@gmail.com

1 Department of Biochemistry and Immunology, Federal University of Minas Gerais, Belo Horizonte, Brazil

2 Department of Veterinary Clinicals and Surgery of the Federal University of Minas Gerais, Belo Horizonte, Brazil

References

[1] Skalak R, Fox CF. Tissue engineering. New York: Liss; 1988.

[2] Lanza RP, Langer R, Vacanti J. Principles of tissue engineering. 3rd edition. Elsevier Inc; 2007

[3] Langer RL, Vacanti JP. Tissue Engineering. Science 1993; 260(5110) 920-926.

[4] National Institutes of Aging. Why population aging matters – A global perspective. http://www.nia.nih.gov/research/publication/why-population-aging-matters-global-perspective (accessed 18 july 2012).

[5] Song JJ, Ott HC. Organ engineering based on decellularized matrix scaffolds. Trends in Molecular Medicine 2011. Article in press. doi:10.1016/j.molmed.2011.03.005.

[6] Mikos AG, Sarakinos G, Ingber DE, Vacanti J, Langer R. Prevascularization of porous biodegradable polymers. Biotech Bioengineering 1993; 42(6) 716-23.

[7] Oh SH, Ward CL, Atala A, Yoo JJ, Harrison BS. Oxygen generating scaffolds for enhancing engineered tissue survival. Biomaterials 2009; 30(5) 757-762).

[8] Kaully T, Kaufman-Francis K, Lesman A, Levenberg S. Vascularization--the conduit to viable engineered tissues. Tissue Eng Part B Rev. 2009; 15(2) 159-69.

[9] Alberti C. Hollow organ tissue engineering: short updating about current approaches and forecast for major research advances. Giornal e Chirurgia 2011; 32(8-9) 345-351.

[10] Rauh J, Milan F, Günther KP, Stiehler M. Bioreactor systems for bone tissue engineering. Tissue Eng Part B Rev. 2011; 17(4) 263-80.

[11] Williams DF, Cunningham J. Materials in Clinical Dentistry. Oxford; Oxford University Press, 1979.

[12] Ratner BD. Biomaterials Science: An Introduction to Materials in Medicine. London: Elsevier Academic Press, 2004

[13] Pham C, Greenwood J, Cleland H, Woodruff P, Maddern G. Bioengineered skin substitutes for the management of burns: a systematic review. Burns 2007; 33(8) 946-57

[14] Burchill LJ, Ross HJ. Heart transplantation in adults with end-stage congenital heart disease. Future Cardiol. 2012; 8(2) 329-42.

[15] Macchiarini P, Jungebluth P, Go T, Asnaghi MA, Rees LE, Cogan TA, Dodson A, Martorell J, Bellini S, Parnigotto PP, Dickinson SC, Hollander AP, Mantero S, Conconi MT, Birchall MA. Clinical transplantation of a tissue-engineered airway. The Lancet 2008; 372: 2023–30.

[16] Molzahn AE, Starzomski R, McCormick J. The supply of organs for transplantation: issues and challenges. Nephrol Nurs J. 2003;30(1) 17-26.

[17] Ott HC, Matthiesen TS, Goh SK, Black LD, Kren SM, Netoff TI, Taylor DA. Perfusion-decellularized matrix: using nature's platform to engineer a bioartificial heart. Nat Med. 2008; 14(2) 213-21.

[18] U.S. Organ Procurement and Transplantation Network and the Scientific Registry of Transplant Recipients. 2009 OPTN / SRTR Annual Report: Transplant Data 1999-2008. http://www.ustransplant.org/annual_Reports/current/default.html (accessed 2 august 2012).

[19] Chaureya V, Blocka F, Sua YH, Chiang PC, Botchweyc E, Choub CF, Swamia NS. Nanofiber size-dependent sensitivity of fibroblast directionality to the method of alignment of the scaffold. Acta Biomaterialia 2012. Epub ahead of print.

[20] Future Directions in Regenerative Medicine. Business Insights, February 2012.

[21] Osiris therapeutics, Press release: Osiris Therapeutics Reports Second Quarter 2012 Financial Results. http://investor.osiris.com/ (accessed 6 august 2012).

[22] Wei C, Larsen M, Hoffman MP, Yamada KM. Self-organization and branching morphogenesis of primary salivary epithelial cells. Tissue Eng. 2007;13(4) 721-35.

[23] Takebe T, Sekine K, Suzuki Y, Enomura M, Tanaka S, Ueno Y, Zheng YW, Taniguchi H. Self-organization of human hepatic organoid by recapitulating organogenesis *in vitro*. Transplant Proc. 2012; 44(4) 1018-20.

[24] Takebe T, Koike N, Sekine K, Enomura M, Chiba Y, Ueno Y, Zheng YW, Taniguchi H. Generation of functional human vascular network. Transplant Proc. 2012; 44(4) 1130-3.

[25] Green JB, Dominguez I, Davidson LA. Self-organization of vertebrate mesoderm based on simple boundary conditions. Dev Dyn. 2004; 231(3) 576-81.

[26] Miranda SC, Silva GA, Mendes RM, Abreu FA, Caliari MV, Alves JB, Goes AM. Mesenchymal stem cells associated with porous chitosan-gelatin scaffold: A potential strategy for alveolar bone regeneration. J Biomed Mater Res A. 2012. doi: 10.1002/jbm.a. 34214. [Epub ahead of print]

[27] Miranda SC, Silva GA, Hell RC, Martins MD, Alves JB, Goes AM. Three-dimensional culture of rat BMMSCs in a porous chitosan-gelatin scaffold: A promising association for bone tissue engineering in oral reconstruction. Arch Oral Biol. 2011; 56(1) 1-15.

[28] Ding T, Luo ZJ, Zheng Y, Hu XY, Ye ZX. Rapid repair and regeneration of damaged rabbit sciatic nerves by tissue-engineered scaffold made from nano-silver and collagen type I. Injury. 2010; 41(5) 522-7.

[29] X. Lin, K. Takahashi, Y. Liu, P.O. Zamora. Enhancement of cell attachment and tissue integration by a IKVAV containing multi-domain peptide. Biochimica et Biophysica Acta 2006; 1760(9) 1403–1410.

[30] Choi JS, Lee SJ, Christ GJ, Atala A, Yoo JY. The influence of electrospun aligned poly(ε-caprolactone)/collagen nanofiber meshes on the formation of self-aligned skeletal muscle myotubes. Biomaterials 2008; 29(19), 2899–2906.

[31] Mironov V, Visconti RP, Kasyanov V, Forgacs G, Drake CJ, Markwald RR. Organ printing: tissue spheroids as building blocks. Biomaterials 2009; 30(12) 2164-74.

[32] Crapo PM, Gilbert TW, Badylak SF. An overview of tissue and whole organ decellularization processes. Biomaterials 2011; 32(12) 3233–3243.

[33] Giger RJ, Hollis ER, Tuszynski MH. Guidance molecules in axon regeneration. Cold Spring Harb Perspect Biol. 2010; 2(7) a001867.

[34] Sharma K, Selzer ME, Li S. Scar-mediated inhibition and CSPG receptors in the CNS. Exp Neurol. 2012. [Epub ahead of print]

[35] Parka JS, Chua JS, Tsou AD, Diopa R, Tanga Z, Wang A, Li S. The effect of matrix stiffness on the differentiation of mesenchymal stem cells in response to TGF-b. Biomaterials 2011; 32 3921-3930.

[36] Chaudhuri O, David J. Mooney. Stem-cell differentiation: Anchoring cell-fate cues. Nature Materials 2012; 11 568–569.

[37] Reilly GC, Engler AJ, Intrinsic extracellular matrix properties regulate stem cell differentiation. Journal of Biomechanics 2010; 43(1) 55-62.

[38] Malone JM, Brendel K, Duhamel RC, Reinert RL. Detergent-extracted small-diameter vascular prostheses. Journal of Vascular Surgery 1984. 1(1) 181-194.

[39] Schmidt CE, Baier JM. Acellular vascular tissues: natural biomaterials for tissue repair and tissue engineering. Biomaterials 2000; 21(22) 2215-31.

[40] Zorlutuna P, Annabi N, Camci-Unal G, Nikkhah M, Cha JM, Nichol JW, Manbachi A, Bae H, Chen S, Khademhosseini A. Microfabricated Biomaterials for Engineering 3D Tissues. Advanced Biomaterials 2012; 4 1782–1804.

[41] Zonari A, Novikoff S, Electo NRP, Breyner NM, Gomes DA, et al. Endothelial Differentiation of Human Stem Cells Seeded onto Electrospun Polyhydroxybutyrate/ Polyhydroxybutyrate-Co-Hydroxyvalerate Fiber Mesh. PLoS ONE 2012; 7(4) e35422. doi:10.1371/journal.pone.0035422

[42] Perán M, García MA, López-Ruiz E, Bustamante M, Jiménez G, Madeddu R, Marchal JA. Functionalized Nanostructures with Application in Regenerative Medicine. Int. J. Mol. Sci. 2012; 13 3847-3886.

[43] Kaully T, Kaufman-Francis K, Lesman A, Levenberg S. Vascularization: The Conduit to Viable Engineered Tissues. Tissue Eng Part B Rev. 2009; 15(2) 159-169.

[44] Atala A, Bauer SB, Soker S, Yoo JJ, Retik AB. Tissue-engineered autologous bladders for patients needing cystoplasty. Lancet 2006; 367(9518) 1241-1246.

[45] Mironov V, Reis N, Derby B. Bioprinting: A Beginning. Tissue Engineering 2006; 12(4) 631-634.

[46] Mironov V, Kasyanov, V, Markwald RR. Organ printing: from bioprinter to organ biofabrication line. Current Opinion in Biotechnology 2011; 22 667-673.

[47] Mironov V, Trusk T, Kasyanov, Little S, Swaja R, Markwald RR. Biofabrication: a 21st century manufacturing paradigm. Biofabrication 2009; 1 1-16.

[48] Partridge R, Conlisk N, Davies JA. In-lab three-dimensional printing. An inexpensive tool for experimentation and visualization for the field of organogenesis. Organogenesis 2012; 8(1) 22-27.

[49] Lalan S, Pomerantseva I, Vacanti JP. Tissue engineering and its potential impact on surgery. World Journal of Surgery 2001; 25 1458-1466.

[50] Mironov V, Boland T, Trusk T, Forgacs G, Markwald RR. Organ printing: computer-aided jet-based 3D tissue engineering. TRENDS in Biotechnology 2003; 21(4) 157-161.

[51] Mironov V, Visconti RP, Kasyanov V, Forgacs G, Drake CJ, Markwald RR. Organ printing: tissue spheroids as building blocks. Biomaterials 2009; 30 2164-2174.

[52] Yeong WY, Chua CK, Leong KF, Chandrasekaran M. Rapid prototyping in tissue engineering: challenges and potential. TRENDS in Biotechnology, 22(12) 663–662.

[53] Mirononv V, Kasyanov V, Drake C, Markwald RR. Organ printing: promises and challenges. Regenerative Medicine 2008; 3(1) 93-103.

[54] Wilson WC, Boland T. Cell and organ printing 1: protein and cell printers. The Anatomical Record Part A 2003; 272 491-496.

[55] Jakab K, Norotte C, Marga F, Murphy K, Vunjak-Novakovic G, Forgacs G. Tissue engineering by self-assembly and bio-printing of living cells. Biofabrications 2010; 2 1-14.

[56] Assis AC, Carvalho JL, Jacoby BA, Ferreira RL, Castanheira P, Diniz SO, Cardoso VN, Goes AM, Ferreira AJ. Time-dependent migration of systemically delivered bone marrow mesenchymal stem cells to the infarcted heart. Cell Transplantation 2010;19(2) 219-30.

[57] Kumar S, Ponnazhagan S. Mobilization of bone marrow mesenchymal stem cells *in vivo* augments bone healing in a mouse model of segmental bone defect. Bone 2012; 50(4) 1012-8.

[58] Liu Z, Yang D, Xie P, Ren G, Sun G, Zeng X, Sun X. MiR-106b and MiR-15b modulate apoptosis and angiogenesis in myocardial infarction. Cell Physiol Biochem 2012; 29(5-6) 851-62.

[59] Daher JD, Chahine NO, Greenberg AS, Sgaglione NA, Grande DA. New methods to diagnose and treat cartilage degeneration. Nature Reviews Rheumatology 2009; 5 599-607.

[60] Feinberg AW, Alford PW, Jin H, Ripplinger CM, Werdich AA, Sheehy SP, Grosberg A, Parker KK. Controlling the contractile strength of engineered cardiac muscle by hierarchal tissue architecture. Biomaterials 2009; 33(23) 5732-5741.

[61] Wang JH, Jia F, Gilbert TW, Woo SL. Cell orientation determines the alignment of cell-produced collagenous matrix. J Biomech. 2003; 36(1) 97-102.

[62] Tsai SW, Liou HM, Lin CJ, Kuo KL, Hung YS, Weng RC, Hsu FY. MG63 osteoblast-like cells exhibit different behavior when grown on electrospun collagen matrix versus electrospun gelatin matrix. PLoS One 2012; 7(2) e31200.

[63] Kwon IK, Kidoaki S, Matsuda T. Electrospun nano- to microfiber fabrics made of biodegradable copolyesters: structural characteristics, mechanical properties and cell adhesion potential. Biomaterials 2005; 26(18) 3929-39.

[64] Geckil H, Xu F, Zhang X, Moon S, Demirci U. Engineering hydrogels as extracellular matrix mimics. Nanomedicine 2010; 5(3) 469–484.

[65] Burdick JA, Vunjak-Novakovic G. Engineered microenvironments for controlled stem cell differentiation. Tissue Eng Part A. 2009; 15(2) 205-19.

[66] Tibbitt MW, Anseth KS. Hydrogels as extracellular matrix mimics for 3D cell culture. Biotechnol Bioeng. 2009; 103(4) 655-63.

[67] Zahir N, Weaver VM. Death in the third dimension: apoptosis regulation and tissue architecture. Current Opinion in Genetics and Development 2004; 14(1) 71-80.

[68] Zaulyanov L, Kirsner RS. A review of a bi-layered living cell treatment (Apligraf) in the treatment of venous leg ulcers and diabetic foot ulcers. Clin Interv Aging 2007; 2(1) 93-8.

Chapter 2

Biomaterials and Stem Cell Therapies for Injuries Associated to Skeletal Muscular Tissues

Tiago Pereira, Andrea Gärtner, Irina Amorim,
Paulo Armada-da-Silva, Raquel Gomes,
Cátia Pereira, Miguel L. França, Diana M. Morais,
Miguel A. Rodrigues, Maria A. Lopes, José D. Santos,
Ana Lúcia Luís and Ana Colette Maurício

Additional information is available at the end of the chapter

1. Introduction

Skeletal muscle injuries are common in humans, particularly in athletes and it is important to develop new methods to improve muscle regeneration. Skeletal muscle has good regenerative ability, but the extent of muscle injury might prevent complete regeneration, especially in terms of functional recovery. Severe lesions, like those originated by trauma associated with loss of healthy muscular tissue and development of fibrous tissue scar and irreversible muscular atrophy after long-term peripheral nervous injuries are examples of those situations where regeneration is limited. An alternative approach for the restoration of the damaged skeletal muscular tissue, considered to be an ultimate treatment of some traumatic or degenerative diseases, is the transplantation of stem cells that limit the fibrosis and the atrophy of the involved muscle masses, and even imply the myocytes regeneration and local revascularization [1]. Stem cells and regenerative medicine is a fast emerging field with rapid strides of progress and focus on human health. Successful clinical use of stem cells in regenerative medicine depends on 3 important features:

i.   stem cells can grow and divide indefinitely,

ii.   stem cells can differentiate into specialized cell types, like skeletal muscle; and

iii.   the stem cells can be delivered to the site of lesion associated to biomaterials, nowadays available with excellent characteristics concerning biocompatibility.

The purpose of this review is to describe the current research lines in the skeletal muscle regeneration field, with special emphasis to the work performed by our research group in testing different biomaterials and cellular therapies, emphasizing the use of mesenchymal stem cells (MSCs) isolated from the Wharton's jelly of the umbilical cord. We also focused our research in developing skeletal muscular lesion models which could be reproducible. It is important to state, that a multidisciplinary team has a crucial role in the development of these biomaterials associated to cellular systems, and in pre-clinical tests. MSCs comprise a rare population of multipotent progenitor cells with a great therapeutic potential since they are capable of self-renewal and multi-lineage differentiation. Due to this ability, MSCs appear to be an attractive tool in the context of Tissue Engineering and cell-based therapy concerning skeletal muscle regeneration. Several biomaterials associated to MSCs from the Wharton's jelly of the umbilical cord have been tested in standard lesions of the rat muscle and the results of these tests will be discussed here. The umbilical cord matrix is an important and safe source of MSCs with positive effects in nerve and skeletal muscle regeneration, with no ethical or technical issues.

2. Skeletal muscle tissue

2.1. Basic structure and terminology

The muscle fibers are the basic contractile units of skeletal muscles. They are individually surrounded by a connective tissue layer and grouped into bundles to form a skeletal muscle [1]. Each muscle is surrounded by a layer of dense connective tissue - the epimysium - which is continuous with the tendon. The muscle is composed of numerous bundles of muscle fibers – fascicles - which are separated from each other by another connective tissue layer named perimysium. The endomysium is the connective tissue that separates individual muscle fibers from each other. Mature muscle cells are termed muscle fibers or myofibers. Each myofiber is a multinucleate syncytium formed by fusion of immature muscle cells termed myoblasts. In the cytoplasm of each myofiber – the sarcoplasm - lays the contractile apparatus of the cell which is composed of sarcomeres arranged in series to form myofibrils, which give myofibers their striated appearance. The sarcomeres contain a number of proteins, including alpha-actinin — which is the major constituent of the Z band — and actin and myosin, which are the major components of the thin and thick filaments, respectively. The sarcoplasm, located between the myofibrils, is called the intermyofibrillar network and contains the mitochondria, lipid, glycogen, T-tubules, and sarcoplasmic reticulum [1-3]. Skeletal muscles are highly vascularized to provide essential nutrients for muscle function. As the myofiber matures, it is contacted by a single motoneuron and expresses characteristic molecules for contractile function, principally different myosin heavy chain isoforms and metabolic enzymes. Both the motoneuron and the myoblast origin have been implicated to play a role in specifying the myofiber contractile properties, although the precise mechanisms remain to be defined [1].

2.1.1. Fiber type

Individual adult skeletal muscles are composed of a mixture of myofibers with different physiological properties, ranging from a slow-contracting/fatigue-resistant type to a fast-contracting/non-fatigue-resistant type. The proportion of each fiber type within a muscle determines its overall contractile properties [1]. The slow contracting *soleus* muscle is rich in myofibers expressing the slow type I myosin heavy chain isoform, whereas the fast contracting plantaris muscle is devoid of slow type I myofibers [1-3]. The most informative methods to delineate muscle fiber types are based on specific myosin profiles, specially the myosin heavy chain (MHC) isoform complement. According to the major MHC isoforms found in adult mammalian skeletal muscles, the following pure fiber types exist: slow type I with MHCIb, and three fast types, namely type IIA with MHCIIa, type IID with MHCIId and type IIB with MHCIIb [4]. Despite having different physiological properties, the basic mechanism of muscle contraction is similar in all myofiber types and is the result of a "sliding mechanism" of the myosin-rich thick filament over the actin-rich thin filament after neuronal activation [5]. The connective tissue framework in skeletal muscle combines the contractile myofibers into a functional unit, in which the contraction of myofibers is transformed into movement via myotendinous junctions at their ends, where myofibers attach to the skeleton by tendons. Thus the functional properties of skeletal muscle depend on the maintenance of a complex framework of myofibers, motor neurons, blood vessels, and extracellular connective tissue matrix [1].

2.2. Regeneration of the skeletal muscle

Regeneration is a unique adaptation of skeletal muscle that occurs in response to injury. Following direct trauma or disease, the regeneration of skeletal muscle results in restoration, to some degree, of the original structure and function of the muscle tissue [6]. Skeletal muscle regeneration is a physiological response of the tissue to traumatic or pathological injuries and its progress depends on the type of damaged muscle and the extent of the injury. Under normal conditions, the regenerated muscle is morphologically and functionally indistinguishable from undamaged muscle [1]. Regeneration resembles the process of formation of skeletal muscle during embryogenesis. Skeletal myogenesis begins in the somites where multipotencial mesodermal cells commit to the myogenic lineage. These mononucleated myoblasts then fuse and form multinucleated cells (myotubes) that ultimately develop into mature myofibers [1, 7]. During the course of muscle development, a distinct subpopulation of myoblasts fails to differentiate and remains associated with the surface of the developing myofiber as quiescent muscle satellite cells (SCs) in fully developed mature skeletal tissue [1, 7].

2.2.1. Satellite Cells and other cells involved in regeneration of skeletal muscle tissue

During regeneration and muscle repair, SCs fuse together or to the existing fibers to form new muscle fibers [8]. Although the number of SCs is greatly reduced in aged muscle, those remaining maintain an intrinsic capacity to regenerate the muscle tissue as efficiently as in younger muscles. A vital condition for successful regeneration is the presence of SCs in the uninjured portions of the basal membrane of the myofiber, along with its ability for reinnervation and revascularization. After a skeletal muscle injury, myofibers become completely desintegrated via myolysis and the SCs are realeased from the basal membrane. From this point SCs start to divide and are capable of differentiating into muscle fibers, reestablishing myofiber's architecture and restoring the muscle function [9, 10]. In post-natal skeletal muscle, PW1 expression is detected in SCs and a subset of interstitial cells and is markedly up-regulated during muscle regeneration [11]. These interstitial multipotent stem cells are extralaminal and exhibit fibroblastic morphology but do not express the same myogenic markers such as Pax7 [10]. PW1$^+$/Pax7$^-$ interstitial cells (PICs) are myogenic *in vitro* and efficiently contribute to skeletal muscle regeneration *in vivo* as well as generating satellite cells and PICs. PICs show bipotential behavior *in vitro*, generating both smooth and skeletal muscle. Isolated PICs do not express Pax7 or MyoD, but they convert to a Pax7$^+$/MyoD$^+$ state before forming skeletal muscle *in vitro*. PICs are not derived from a Pax3-expressing parental cell and thus do not share a satellite cell lineage; however, PICs do express Pax3 upon conversion to skeletal muscle. PICs are a key cell population that cannot be recruited into the skeletal muscle lineage in the absence of Pax7 function and is likely to contribute to the Pax7 muscle phenotype during postnatal growth. PICs are as abundant as SCs in muscle tissue and correspond to the only population of PW1+/Pax7– cells *in vivo*, requiring Pax7 for their myogenic capacity [11]. PDGFRα+ mesenchymal progenitor cells located in the muscle *interstitium* were also identified as being distinct from SCs. Of the muscle-derived cell populations, only PDGFRα+ cells show efficient adipogenic differentiation both *in vitro* and *in vivo*, being strongly inhibited by the presence of satellite cell-derived myofibres. These results suggest that PDGFRα+ mesenchymal progenitors are the major contributor to ectopic fat cell formation in skeletal muscle that is more conspicuous in perimysium and particularly in perivascular space. The balance between satellite cell-dependent myogenesis and PDGFRα+ cell-dependent adipogenesis, rather than multipotency of satellite cells, has a considerable impact on muscle homeostasis [12]. Hematopoietic and dendritic cells are also present in the perimysium of the skeletal tissue, as well as some lymphocytes and macrophages [10].

2.2.2. Myogenic differentiation

Cells derived from Pax3-expressing cells are myofibres and SCs [11]. Once activated, SCs express factors involved in the specification of the myogenic program, such as Pax-7, desmin, MNFα, Myf5, MRF4 and MyoD. Activated SCs enter the cell cycle and proliferate as indicated by the expression of factors involved in cell cycle progression, such as PCNA and by the incorporation of BrDU. Recently, miRNAs have also been reported to regulate gene expression in skeletal muscle. Upon activation, SCs generate fusion-competent myoblasts and can self-renew at least to a limited extent. Any interruption in the proliferation or fusion of myoblasts, or any alterations in the extracellular matrix leads to the development of fibrosis, compromising the establishment of the correct muscular function [8, 10]. Proliferative MyoD and/or Myf5 positive myogenic cells are termed myoblasts. Both SCs and myoblasts increase their cytoplasmic-nuclear ratio and can migrate along myofibers. Proliferating myoblasts withdraw from the cell cycle to become terminally differentiated myocytes that express the "late" myogenic regulatory factors (MRFs), Myogenin and MRF4, and subsequently muscle-specific genes such as MHC and muscle creatine kinase (CK$_M$), and stopping Pax7 expression. Myogenic subpopulations have also been identified by their enriched M-cadherin and CD34 expression. M-cadherin can be considered to be a reliable marker for both quiescent and activated SCs. Once fusion of myogenic cells is completed, newly formed myofibers increase in size and myonuclei move to the periphery of the muscle fiber [1, 10, 13].

2.2.3. Degeneration

This scenario changes dramatically when the muscle is damaged, in which muscle degeneration after acute injury is characterized by myofiber necrosis and is followed by inflammation, tissue reconstruction and remodeling [10]. The necrosis is triggered by disruption of the myofiber sarcolemma resulting in increased myofiber permeability. The disruption of myofiber integrity is reflected by increased serum levels of muscle proteins, such as CK (usually restricted to the myofiber cytosol) [1]. It has been hypothesized that increased Ca^{2+} influx after sarcolemmal or sarcoplasmic reticulum damage results in a loss of Ca^{2+} homeostasis and increased Ca^{2+}-dependent proteolysis that drives tissue degeneration resulting in focal or total autolysis depending on the extent of the injury [1].

2.2.4. Inflammation

The early regenerative response in skeletal muscle is similar to that in other tissues and requires the coordinated regulation of inflammation, extracellular matrix remodeling, and myofiber growth [14]. The early phase of muscle injury is usually accompanied by the activation of mononucleated cells, mainly inflammatory cells and myogenic cells. Factors released by the injured muscle activate inflammatory cells residing within the muscle, which in turn provide the chemotactic signals to circulating immune cells. Neutrophils are the first immune cells to invade the injured muscle, with a significant increase in their number being observed as early as 1–6h after myotoxin or exercise-induced muscle damage. After neutrophil infiltration and 48h post-injury, macrophages become the predominant inflammatory cell type within the site of injury. Macrophages infiltrate the injured site and through phagocytosis remove cellular debris and may affect other aspects of muscle regeneration by activating myogenic cells [1]. Testosterone has a documented ability to modulate the activity of immune, fibroblast, and myogenic precursor cells, which are all components of regeneration [14].

3. Skeletal muscle injury models

In order to study the process of muscle regeneration in a controlled and reproducible way, it was necessary to develop experimental models of muscle injury [1]. In this sense, a variety of experimental models that compromise skeletal muscle function or destroy this tissue is available. Each of the injury models can potentially have a different effect on the fate of resident cells and circulating cells within the muscle bed after the trauma [10]. A large number of studies, involving a variety of experimental injuries, such as injection of myotoxic agents, crush, ischemia, denervation and muscular dystrophies, demonstrate the unique ability of skeletal muscle for regeneration, irrespectively the precise method used to induce the initial injury [15]. In this review we will focus on chemical and mechanical models of skeletal muscle injury, adding a new model of muscle injury based on surgical myectomy, developed in order to mimic severe losses of skeletal muscle mass. Other models, like exercise and denervation, will also be outlined. The latter is not a model of injury but else of skeletal muscle disuse but that also can be used to investigate skeletal muscle remodeling. There is a variety of other genetic models that are essential in studying diseases like Duchenne muscle dystrophy (Mdx mouse is currently the most widely used in this case) but will not be discussed in this review.

3.1. Chemical methods of skeletal muscle injury

The use of myotoxins, such as bupivacaine (Marcaine), cardiotoxin (CTX), and notexin (NTX) is perhaps the easiest and most reproducible way to induce muscle injury and regeneration. Myotoxins are also widely used to induce skeletal muscle injury because their inoculation by intramuscular injection does not require complex surgery. Several chemical agents are known to produce skeletal muscle damage. Severe muscle fiber damage, like breakdown of sarcolemma and myofibrils, has been described after intramuscular injections of 0.75% bupivacaine, 2% mepivacaine, or 2% lidocaine associated to epinephrine [18]. While lidocaine can cause rapid destruction of skeletal muscle fibers, long-acting anesthetics, like bupivacaine, are more often used to cause skeletal muscle injury in rodents [19].

3.1.1. Bupivacaine

The bupivacaine injection procedure is simple and quick, does not involve extensive surgery, and induces a regeneration process which is qualitatively similar to that observed in other model systems. Doses of 1.5 and 1% wt/vol produce significant levels of muscle injury and subsequent regeneration, but these doses also produce large regions of ischemic muscle tissue. Doses of 0.75 and 0.5% bupivacaine are also effective in inducing regeneration and produce little or no ischemia [16]. Muscle fiber necrosis is extremely rapid after induced bupivacaine injury [14]. Injection of the drug into small skeletal muscles of rat or mouse leads to immediate and massive myonecrosis followed by phagocytosis of necrotic debris and a rapid and apparently complete regeneration of muscle fibers 3-4 wk after injection. The peak isometric twitch and tetanic tensions produced by rat fast-twitch *extensor digitorum longus* muscle injected with bupivacaine returns to normal values by 21 d after injection [17]. Morphological analysis has shown that many indexes of successful regeneration in healthy muscle can be completed within 2–3 weeks of recovery from injury [14]. The sequence of fiber breakdown induced by bupivacaine is similar to that of progressive muscular dystrophy [18] and it is also striking that the same types of muscle fibers are spared by both Duchenne's muscular dystrophy and bupivacaine toxicity. It has been suggested that bupivacaine may disrupt Ca^{2+} homeostasis *in vivo*, triggering Ca^{2+}-activated cellular death pathways that include proteolysis. This suggestion is supported by the findings that

i.   bupivacaine affects sarcoplasmic reticulum function *in vitro*,

ii.   extracellular Ca^{2+} omission delays the morphological changes and decreases the protein degradation rate that are observed in isolated rat soleus muscle exposed to bupivacaine, and

iii.   bupivacaine uncouples isolated rat liver and heart mitochondria and decreases mitochondrial membrane potential and oxygen consumption both in cultured fibroblasts and Ehrlich tumor cells [19].

Extracellular Ca^{2+} plays a part in mediating the muscle damage caused by bupivacaine but other factors must also be involved [20]. For example macrophage invasion is necessary for complete degeneration of myofibrillar components [21]. Saito and Nonaka [22] injected 0,5ml of 0,5% bupivacaine after *soleus* muscle exposure of Wistar rats, and observed that SCs proliferation began at almost the same time as following muscle crush injuries. Bupivacaine is still commonly used for the purpose of studying the mechanisms of skeletal muscle regeneration following injury [7, 14, 15, 22].

3.1.2. Cardiotoxin and Notexin

Snake venom is known for a long time to directly affect the skeletal muscle, producing fibrillation, contractures and depolarization of the sarcolemma. Although initially ascribed to the phospholipase A content of this venom, muscle contracture and depolarization seem to be related to the cardiotoxic action of cobra venom [23]. Notexin (NTX) is a phospholipase A2 neurotoxin peptide extracted from snake venoms that blocks neuromuscular transmission by inhibition of acetylcholine release. Cardiotoxin (CTX) is also a peptide isolated from snake venoms, but it is a protein kinase C-specific inhibitor that appears to induce the depolarization and contraction of muscle cells, disruption of membrane structure, and lysis of various cell types [1]. CTX is postulated to be neurotoxic as its injection destroys neuromuscular junctions [24]. However, CTX might cause direct destruction of muscle tissues [25]. Snake CTX polypeptide is now known to be a potent inducer of muscle contracture with phospholipase A likely acting in accelerating the action of CTX rather than in augmenting it [23, 26]. Dantrolene antagonizes CTX-induced contractures, suggesting a role for Ca^{2+} derived from the sarcoplasmic reticulum in CTX action. CTX rapidly lowers the threshold for Ca^{2+}-induced Ca^{2+} release in heavy sarcoplasmic reticulum fractions. The mechanism of action involved in contractures of skeletal muscle appears to be related to the immediate and specific effect of CTX (Ca^{2+} release by the sarcoplasmic reticulum) [27, 28].

A more recent study by Gutiérrez and Ownby [25] focused on the role of PLA_2 as important myotoxic components in these venoms suggesting that myotoxic PLA_2s binds to acceptors in the plasma membrane leading to its disruption and pronounced Ca^{2+} influx which, in turn, initiates a complex series of degenerative events associated with contracture, activation of calpains and cytosolic Ca^{2+}-dependent PLA_2s, and mitochondrial Ca^{2+} overload. Fourie et al. [30] already had suggested that the biological effects of CTX could be a consequence of inhibition of plasma membrane ($Ca^{2+} + Mg^{2+}$)-ATPases. The local myonecrosis is often associated with other effects, such as hemorrhage, blistering and edema, in a complex pattern of local tissue damage. Apart from membrane-active CTXs, snake venom hemorrhagic metalloproteinases also cause myonecrosis, but the mechanism involved is likely to be an indirect one, probably related to ischemia [25]. CTX is a useful model for muscle regeneration that does not influence muscle architecture like basal lamina or microvasculature, making the regeneration process less complicated than other models like crush, where for example, inadequate blood supply might result in an increase of fibrosis. CTX injection also results in faster and more extensive muscle degeneration, and an earlier start of the reconstruction phase, than muscle crushing [24].

3.2. Mechanical methods of skeletal muscle injury

Crush injuries of the skeletal muscle can occur in considerable numbers following natural disasters or acts of war and terrorism. They can also occur sporadically after industrial accidents or following periods of unconsciousness from drug intoxication, anesthesia, trauma or cerebral events [31]. Crushing as a method of inducing muscle injury and regeneration was first described by Bassaglia and Gautron [32], and has since been used in several published research studies [24]. Muscle damage occurs at three distinct stages: at the time of the initial mechanical crushing force, during the period of ischemia and during the period of reperfusion [31]. It has been hypothesized that ischemia is the primary instigator of local muscle damage following crush injuries [33]. However, studies have shown that although skeletal muscle tissue can survive circulatory ischemia for 4h, the mechanical force sustained in crushing, along with ischemia, causes skeletal muscle death in only 1 h. Studies of enzyme release suggest that most damage to myocytes occurs during the reperfusion stage rather than the ischemic stage [31]. Animal models of muscle injury should closely mimic the clinical situation. Among these models open crush lesion have been used frequently, allowing standardized evaluation of regeneration in a selected muscle. For application of the trauma, either forceps or custom-made devices have been used. There are two types of muscle-crush models described in the literature: the segmental crush and the complete crush, where only 4-6% of the fibers remain intact [34]. There are different forms to accomplish the segmental crush model but most of them include the use of a surgical instrument (hemostatic clamp e.g.) to produce a standardized closing force in a specific area of a muscle causing a compression contusion injury [35]. One of the important steps of this procedure is denervation, which makes the initial steps of regeneration less painful for the animal. Skeletal muscle contusion can also be performed without skin incision by dropping a mass over a selected muscle. This technique was used by Iwata, Fuchioka [36] employing a 640g mass dropped from a 25 cm height onto an impactor (diameter 10 mm) placed on the belly of the rat medial *gastrocnemius*. This procedure damaged around 47% of the entire cross-sectional area of both medial and lateral *gastrocnemius*. At day 2 post-injury, an intense inflammatory response and necrotized myofibers with infiltrated mononuclear cells were observed. No myotubes were found at this stage. However, a number of regenerative myotubes were detected at days 7, 14, and 21 days post-injury. This study also showed that normal locomotion recovers prior to isometric force and complete regeneration of the injured muscle [36]. The main disadvantage of the complete muscle crush is the potential damaging of myoneural junctions which triggers not only regeneration of muscle substance but also initial innervation deficits. These deficits always lead to impaired healing [34]. Histological analysis of muscle regeneration after crush injury shows an initial phase of inflammation followed by SCs activation, myotube regeneration and fibrosis of the muscle. It has been shown that development of fibrotic tissue is one of the main factors affecting the recovery of muscle function after traumatic muscle injury [34]. In a qualitative assessment performed by our group we tested the open crush lesion in the *tibialis anterior* (TA) muscle of adult Sasco Sprague rats. Different standardized force intensities, durations of muscle compression (30 seconds and 1 minute) and time points (3, 8, 15 and 21 days post-surgery) were considered for the histological evaluation of skeletal muscle injury. Hematoxilin-eosin (HE) and Masson's trichrome staining were employed in this preliminary study. At day 3 post-surgery, myofiber damage was evident and the lymph nodes were reactive due to the active inflammatory process. The presence of fibrosis was evident only following 15 days from the initial injury. This evaluation revealed that the crush model was not the most appropriate for *in vivo* evaluation of cellular therapies for skeletal muscle regeneration aid, since the extent of this injury type did not present the magnitude required to accurately appreciate the biological effects of MSCs utilization [38].

3.3. Myectomy and myotomy

The loss of a portion of a skeletal muscle poses a unique challenge for regeneration of muscle tissue and restoration of its normal structure and function [39]. In the event of large-scale soft tissue traumas, extensive loss of full-thickness native tissue architecture renders the wound site unable to support normal regeneration process. In severe tissue injuries the acute inflammatory response is followed by formation of a provisional fibrin matrix derived from trauma-associated blood clotting and this matrix is then infiltrated by type I collagen-producing fibroblasts [40]. In order to mimic those situations, new experimental models have been developed in which a defined portion of the muscle tissue is removed, creating a myectomy defect within the muscle. For example, Merrit et al. [39] removed a 0.5 x 1.0 cm or a 1.0 x 1.0 cm fraction of the *gastrocnemius* muscle of rats, creating a small and large defect respectively. This was accomplished lacerating the lateral side of the muscle with a #9 scalpel blade. We have recently developed a novel experimental muscle injury model in the TA muscle of adult Sasco Sprague rat, by using a biopsy punch to create a standardized myectomy defect. Sasco Sprague male rats with 250-300g were used and after a standardized 5 mm diameter myectomy lesion in the mid-belly of the *tibialis anterior* muscle, the defect was completely filled with different vehicles and/or biomaterials, cellular suspensions containing 1×10^6 human MSCs isolated from Wharton's jelly and conditioned media (Figure 1). This concentrated media contains trophic factors secreted by MSCs during cell culture. In our research work, the myectomy model proved to be the most appropriate for a comprehensive and standard evaluation of the rat skeletal muscular regeneration ability. The regeneration process in other models of lesion, like simple muscle crush, did not present the magnitude required to accurately appreciate the biological effects of MSCs [38].

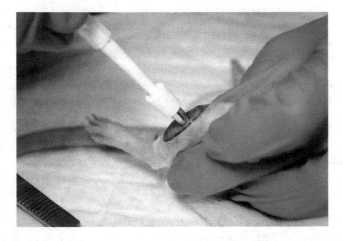

Figure 1. Biopsy punch for myectomy lesion creating a 5 mm Ø defect in the rat *tibialis anterior* (TA) muscle.

Another less invasive model of muscle injury has been used in a number of studies by producing a laceration injury (myotomy) [42-44]. In some cases this was obtained by a partial thickness (50%) cut of gastrocnemius muscles in mice at 60% of their length from their distal insertion, through 75% of their width and then sutured with a modified Kessler stitch and simple sutures using a PDS 7.0 wire (Ethicon, Somerville, New Jersey) [43]. Other studies used a full-thickness (100%) cut though 50% of the *gastrocnemius* muscle width [44]. The advantages of this model are its reproducibility and the ability to apply consistently precise injections into the laceration site [43].

3.4. Denervation (indirect model)

Innervation regulates skeletal muscle mass and muscle phenotype and peripheral nerve injury in the rat is a widely used model to investigate nerve regeneration and can also be employed as a model of muscle inactivity and muscle atrophy. Changes in the muscles may contribute to functional deficit after nerve injury [47]. Denervation induces muscle atrophy and 25 months post denervation muscle fibers cross sectional area of the *extensor digitorium longus* (EDL) muscle diminish to only 2.5% of control animals although their fascicular organization is maintained [47]. The effect of denervation on muscle atrophy is both activity-dependent and activity-independent since the degree of hindlimb muscle atrophy after spinal isolation (activity-independent nerve influence) is less when compared to the atrophy caused by removal of all nerve influences by transecting the sciatic nerve [9]. Two basic mechanisms are responsible for denervation-induced muscle atrophy. First, there is augmented activity of the ubiquitin-proteasome pathway and proteolysis [48]. Second, there is cell death and myonuclei apoptosis conjugated with decreased capacity of satellite cell-dependent reparative myogenesis [49]. Together with atrophy, denervated/reinnervated muscles undergo phenotypical changes and conversion between muscle fiber types [50]. The relative increase in type I or type II muscle fibers following denervation seems to depend on the type of muscle fibers predominant in the muscle, with type II muscle fibers (fast fibers) increasing in proportion in *soleus* (considered a slow muscle) and type I muscle fiber number increasing in *gastrocnemius* and TA muscles [51]. Likewise, the degree of muscle fiber atrophy in short-term denervation (4 weeks) has been noticed to be greater in the muscle fiber type that is more abundant in the affected muscles [52]. Earlier studies suggested that it was possible that denervated muscles could have increased muscle plasticity due to acceleration in the early myoblastic stages of muscle regeneration. Nevertheless McGeachie and Grounds [53] data proved that very few precursors were proliferating in denervated muscle within 30 h after injury, and the onset of myogenesis at 30 h was essentially the same in denervated and innervated muscle. They compared the onset of DNA synthesis in muscle precursors in denervated and innervated muscle of adult BALBc mice regenerating after a simple cut injury. This study concluded that although denervation of skeletal muscles causes an increase in SCs and connective tissue cell turnover, it does not "prime" the general population of muscle precursors to start synthesizing DNA more rapidly after injury than in innervated muscle [53]. After sciatic nerve transection at an adult age, electromyography (EMG) patterns in hindlimb muscles during locomotion remained highly abnormal even after recovery periods lasting 15 or 21 weeks [54]. This may be a limitation when using denervated muscles as a model of muscle injury since regeneration might be affected for a very prolonged period. Like already mentioned, other models of skeletal muscle injury, like complete crush or myectomy, can be accompanied by denervation since these traumatic models may possibly damage peripheral nerves or myoneural junctions. This might also be an undesirable occurrence in the standardization of these models of muscle injury. In fact, our preliminary work using TA myectomy showed that few animals developed severe muscle force deficit after 4 weeks recovery, suggesting that damaged of the supplying nerve occurred in these animals subset.

In our research group, standard peripheral nerve injuries in the rat sciatic nerve model have been performed [57-63] in order to evaluate different therapeutic approaches including several biomaterials and cellular systems to promote sensitive and functional recovery of the nerve. A standard crush injury is performed by a non-serrated clamp (Institute of Industrial Electronic and Material Sciences, University of Technology, Vienna, Austria), exerting a constant force of 54 N for a period of 30s, 10mm above the bifurcation into tibial and common peroneal nerves, inducing a 3mm axonotmesis lesion [57-63]. In order to induce a standard neurotmesis lesion in the rat sciatic nerve model, considered a more serious lesion, under deep anaesthesia, the right sciatic nerve is exposed through a skin incision extending from the greater trochanter to the distal mid-half followed by a muscle splitting incision. After nerve mobilisation, a transection injury is performed (neurotmesis) using straight microsurgical scissors. The nerve is injured at a level as low as possible, in general, immediately above the terminal nerve ramification. To prevent autotomy, a deterrent substance should be daily applied to rat right foot [57-63]. Both experimental injuries induce severe motor deficit and loss of sensory function, evaluated by measuring extensor postural thrust (EPT) and withdrawal reflex latency (WRL), respectively [57-63]. Sensory and motor deficit then progressively decreased along the post-operative, depending on the therapeutic approach used.

Very promising results were obtained with chitosan type III membranes and MSCs isolated from the umbilical cord matrix. In addition, we also perform kinematic analysis of the rat walk which is a more sensitive behavioral test. This analysis is increasingly being used to assess functional recovery in peripheral nerve research because of its higher accuracy and better relationship with histological outcome [57-63]. We should bare in mind that locomotion is also of higher functional relevance since it involves integrated function of both the motor and sensory systems and their respective components, such as skeletal muscles, sensory endings, efferent and afferent nerve fibers and integrative centers within the central nervous system. Muscles innervated by sciatic nerve branches include both dorsiflexors and plantarflexors and, although in our published studies we focused our kinematic analysis only in the stance phase, we now prefer to include analysis of the ankle joint motion also during the swing phase in order to provide additional information [59]. Denervation can be a very useful model of skeletal muscle injury for some experimental studies but some limitations might be pointed out in studies that attempt to focus exclusively on the muscular regeneration process. Nevertheless and as demonstrated by several studies, this muscular regeneration process is highly dependent of the neural supply and the nerve regeneration itself can be influenced by the damaged muscle tissue.

4. Tissue engineering and regenerative medicine

Every day thousands of clinical procedures are performed to replace or repair tissues in the human body that have been damaged through disease or trauma that use tissue engineering technology. The use of constructs for tissue engineering (TE) and regenerative medicine are promising innovative therapies that can address several clinical situations. These constructs are often combination of cells, scaffolds and biological factors. Although there are only a few commercial products currently in the market for cell/drug delivery, probably because each type of cell requires its own specific encapsulating microenvironment with cell-specific material properties and spatially controlled bioactive features, a vast amount of research is being performed worldwide on all aspects of tissue engineering/regenerative medicine exploring polymer materials. To implant cells into defective skeletal muscles, there are two main techniques. The cellular system may be directly injected into the scaffold which is localized in the injury site. It can also be performed by pre-adding the cells to the scaffold via injection or co-culture (in most of the cellular systems, cells are allowed to form a monolayer) and then the biomaterial with the cellular system is implanted in the injured muscle. In case of multiple sites of injury, the systemic administration of cells capable of reaching damaged tissues would be an interesting alternative [64].

4.1. – Scaffolds and Biomaterials

Scaffolds, which are used to deliver cells, drugs, and genes into the body, can take on various forms from porous solid devices to injectable networks, such as a typical three-dimensional porous matrix, a nanofibrous matrix, a hydrogel, and microspheres. Although solid scaffold provide a mechanically strong matrix for seeded cells, hydrogel scaffolds and microspheres are becoming increasingly popular in TE. The spherical nature maximizes the surface area, and the small volume of beads facilitating biomolecular transport. Regarding hydrogels, they have a similar microstructure to the extracellular matrix (ECM) and allow good physical integration into the defect by the use of minimally invasive approaches for material and cell/drug delivery. The biological, chemical, topography features and mechanical properties, as well as the degradation kinetics of hydrogels, can be tailored depending on the application [65-68]. Aligned nanoscale and microscale topographic features in scaffolds have been also reported to influence the alignment of cells. For example, this alignment is an important requirement of functional skeletal muscle since it leads to alignment of myoblasts and cytoskeletal proteins and promote myotube assembly along the nanofibres and microgrooves to mimic the myotube organization in muscle fibres [65, 68-70]. Scaffolds are used successfully in various fields of tissue engineering such as bone formation, periodontal regeneration, cartilage development, as artificial corneas, in tendon repair and in ligament replacement. In addition, the incorporation of drugs (i.e., inflammatory inhibitors and/or antibiotics) into scaffolds or specific molecules to provide adequate signals to the cells is also possible [71] Depending on the medical applications, scaffolds requirements will depend on its function. Hydrogels can be used as a physical barrier to protect the cells from hostile extrinsic factors before delivery, or be used as a matrix to drug controlled release or cell adhesion, growth and differentiation to further improve the secretion of therapeutic proteins from cells. In fact cells are capable of delivering drugs in response to an external stimulus, which is highly advantageous to maintain homeostasis for patients suffering from chronic diseases. For the first application, the scaffold needs:

i.   to be biocompatible, by minimizing the patients' immune response, which is detrimental to cell viability, hydrogel stability, and mass transport. Ideally, the scaffold should evoke no or only minimal fibrous tissue reaction, macrophage activation, and cytokine and cytotoxic agent release

ii.   to have controllable degradability, being the degradation products not toxic and eliminated easily from the implantation site by the body, and

iii.   to have mechanical properties that are sufficient to shield cells from tensile forces without inhibiting biomechanical cues to cells through mechanotransduction pathways that mediate tissue homeostasis, morphogenesis, cell growth, contractility, differentiation, and pathophysiology [70-72].

For the second applications further requirements are needed, mainly:

i.   a microstructure that allows for the influx of nutrients and oxygen toward the encapsulated cells and prevents the efflux of therapeutic molecules and cellular wastes away from the scaffold; this is assured through adequate pore size distribution and its interconnectivity. A high surface:volume ratio should be suitable for cell/drug attachment;

ii.   adequate drug binding affinity to allow a controllable drug released to be stable when incorporated in the scaffold at a physiological conditions;

iii.   bioadhesion, to allows cells and tissues to adhere to scaffolds. Some hydrogels such as fibrin or collagen inherently exhibit bioadhesive properties, but others do not and therefore linker molecules that enable covalent or non-covalent molecular interactions between the scaffold and its surroundings are incorporated;

iv.   the mechanical properties of the scaffold, commonly controlled with the polymer concentration and molar ratio between polymers and cross-linking molecules, should match those of the tissue at the implantation site as well as the degradation rate that should match the rate of tissue regeneration [73-77].

4.1.1. Hydrogel scaffolds

Hydrogels, three-dimensional (3D) networks of hydrophilic polymers, are appealing for biological applications because of their high water content, high permeability, biocompatibility, and the ability of be placed into critical defects in a minimally invasive manner [78]. They are being used in a wide range of tissues, including cartilage, bone, muscle, fat, liver, and neurons. For use in drug/cell delivery, hydrogels should be low-viscosity solutions prior to gelling, which is crucial to maintain cell viability during the encapsulation process, and should rapidly gel in the human body. These properties can be fine-tuned through variations in the chemical structure and cross-linking density in hydrogels. Injectable hydrogels can be formed *in situ* by either chemical or physical cross-linking methods [79, 80]. Physical cross-linked hydrogels are capable of phase transition in response to external stimuli such as temperature, pH or both [81]. Chemically cross-linked hydrogels are prepared through photopolymerization, disulfide bond formation, or reaction between thiols and acrylate or sulfone. The latter hydrogels undergo significant volume changes compared to the first ones [81-83]. The pH/temperature-sensitive hydrogels show several advantages over thermo-sensitive ones, such as the absence of clogging during injection and avoidance of pH decreased caused by degradation. The pH/temperature-sensitive copolymer hydrogels can be prepared by combining a pH-sensitive moiety with a temperature-sensitive block. For example, if acidic sulfamethazine oligomers (OSMs) are coupled with thermosensitive poly(e-CL-co-LA)-PEG-poly-(e-CL-co-LA) triblock copolymers a pH/temperature-sensitive hydrogels (OSM-PCLA-PEG-PCLA-OSM) is produced. Photopolymerized hydrogel systems have been reported to provide better temporal and spatial control over the gelation process [79, 81, 84].

4.1.2. Biomaterials for scaffold fabrication

A wide variety of natural and synthetic materials have been used to prepare injectable hydrogels. Natural polymers, which are either components of or have macromolecular properties similar to the natural ECMs, are known to often undergo rapid degradation upon contact with body fluids or medium and show batch-to-batch variation. Synthetic hydrogels offer improved control of the matrix architecture and chemical composition, no immunogenicity, consistent supply of large quantities, but tend to have lower biological activity. Therefore, modification of natural and synthetic derived hydrogels is usually required [79]. A natural biodegradable 3D scaffold can be made of acellular muscle ECM but it's fragile and difficult to handle [85]. Another natural biodegradable scaffold can be created by using fibrin, which leads to a process much similar to wound healing, in which fibrin forms a temporary scaffold to serve tissue regeneration and then is replaced by the physiological ECM. Fibrin has the additional advantage that it binds growth factors [70].

Fibrin hydrogels are made from commercially purified allogeneic fibrinogen and purified thrombin, and have been used in a variety of tissue engineering applications. Its main disadvantages reported to be shrinkage of the gel, low mechanical stiffness and its rapid degradation can be overcome by incorporating other polymers such as gelatin, hyaluronic acid, and chondroitin-6-sulfate. Fibrin glue is clearly distinguished from fibrin hydrogels that are prepared from purified fibrinogen and thrombin. Despite the commercial fibrin glue is available in standardized quality; autologous fibrin glue is cheaper and has no viral transmission and prion infection [86]. Tisseel® VH, is a fibrin glue commercialized by Baxter, and consists of a two-component fibrin biomatrix with highly concentrated human fibrinogen to produce fibrin gel from a blood sample and is safe to be used in TE. FloSeal® is another commercial hemostatic matrix with potential in TE, and consists of a cross-linked bovine-derived Gelatin Matrix component and a human-derived Thrombin component. Literature reports that myoblasts seeded on fibrin gels have been shown to differentiate into contracting muscle fibres and to demonstrate a normal length–tension and force–frequency relationship [87, 88].

Alginate is the designation given to a natural family of biodegradable, biocompatible, hydrophilic and non-toxic polysaccharides extracted from some marine algae and some microorganisms. Alginates are linear block co-polymers composed of two different monomers, β-D-mannuronic acid (M) and α-L-glucuronic acid (G), which are linked by (1-4) glycosidic bonds. The main property of alginate that potentiates its use in different areas, it is its ability to bind some divalent cations such as Ca^{2+} in the carboxylic groups which provides the gelation of the alginate solution. The properties of the gel are dependent of the ratio between M and G monomers (M:G ratio); if the proportion of the G monomer is predominant, a strong brittle gel it obtained, whereas if the proportion of the M monomer is predominant, the formed gel will be weaker, but more flexible, because there are less junction zones between the polymer chains. As alginate is a polyelectrolyte, more specifically a polyanion, it can be ionically associated with a polycation existent in the same solution through hydrogen bonding or electrostatic interactions, forming a polyelectrolyte complex [89, 90]. Cell-encapsulating calcium cross-linked alginate hydrogels have been extensively studied because alginate molecules are anionic polysaccharides and do not associate with many proteins. Since alginate itself is inert for cell attachment and spreading, the cell adhesion properties can be tailored by linking molecules such as RGD peptides to its backbone [91].

Chitosan is a natural and hydrophilic copolymer, and it is composed by two monomeric units, D-glucosamine and N-acetyl-D-glucosamine linked by β(1–4)-glycosidic bond. This linear polysaccharide has been widely studied in medical applications due to its biocompatibility, biodegradability, non-toxicity, fungistaticity, antimicrobial activity, non-carcinogenicity, notable affinity to proteins, promotion of cell adhesion as well as proliferation and differentiation [67]. Chitosan results from the alkaline deacetylation of the chitin and its solubility is mainly influenced by its molecular weight and degree of deacetylation. Some methods have been developed to lower the molecular weight of chitosan by hydrolysis of the polymeric chains, in order to produce chitosan salts which are soluble in water. Chitosan-based hydrogels have been gelled via glutaraldehyde cross-linking, UV irradiation, and thermal variations [81].

Hyaluronic Acid (HA) is a natural, hydrophilic and non-sulfated glycosaminoglycan. This polymer is a linear polysaccharide, in which the repeating unity is a disaccharide composed by two monomers, D-glucuronic acid and N-acetyl-D-glucosamine, linked through alternating β1,3 and β1,4 glycosidic bonds. HA has been used as a biomaterial in various medical applications, due to its biocompatibility, biodegradability, and non-immunogenicity. HA is the main component existent in the extracellular matrix (ECM) of living tissues, namely in the connective, epithelial and neural. This polymer, due to its structural and biological properties, has the ability of mediate the cell signalling and behaviour, and the matrix organization. HA is able of interact with some cell surface receptors, being involved in the tissue hydrodynamics, cell migration and proliferation. Several strategies have been reported to prepare HA-based hydrogels [92, 93].

Among the most widely used synthetic polymers for scaffolds, either alone or copolymerized with synthetic or natural polymers, as biodegradable polymers are polyglycolide, polylactide and its copolymer poly(lactide-co-glycolide), polyphosphazene, polyanhydride, poly(propylene fumarate), polycyanoacrylate, polycaprolactone, polydioxanone, and polyurethanes, and as non-biodegradeable polymers are included polyvinyl alcohol (PVA), polyhydroxyethymethacrylate, and poly(N-isopropylacrylamide) [71, 94].

The majority of natural biomaterials used in clinical applications are derived from animal or human cadavers' sources. In spite of thorough purification methods, these materials bear the inherent risk of transfer viral diseases and may cause immunological body reactions while synthetic biomaterials are not associated with these risks. So, a critical issue in this type of cellular transplants is the search for an optimal vehicle to provide the ideal environment for cell hosting and for the release and conduction of molecules to the site of injury for cell-host interaction. Taking this into account we evaluated different biomaterials as vehicles for the cellular system intended to be tested for skeletal muscle regeneration using our myectomy injury model in the rat. Plasma derived substances, hemostatic matrix solutions and hydrogels (Figure 2 and Figure 3) were tested and the in vivo response was compared histologically according to the International Standard ISO 10993-6 (see 5.1.3). The following procedure was done under sterile conditions. For preparation of the spherical hydrogel, the polymer solution is prepared by adding in a ratio of 1:1 (V/V), a sodium alginate aqueous solution 7% (m/V) to a sodium hyaluronate aqueous solution 0.5% (m/V), under magnetic stirring. Afterwards the polymer solution is inserted into an insulin syringe and a droplet is released into an excess of cerium nitrate solution 135mM, in order to obtain a cross-linked polymer sphere of approximately 60 μl of volume. Cerium nitrate and sodium hyaluronate solution were sterilized by microfiltration (0.22 μm membrane) and sodium alginate powder is sterilized in an autoclave (120ºC for 15 minutes) previous to the solution preparation (Figure 2 and Figure 3). These tested biomaterials including the spherical hydrogel were not only used as vehicles but their properties were also evaluated and optimized to find a suitable matrix for the cellular implants.

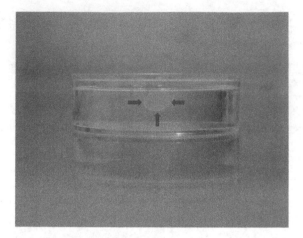

Figure 2. Hydrogel preparation (alginate, hyaluronic acid and cerium).

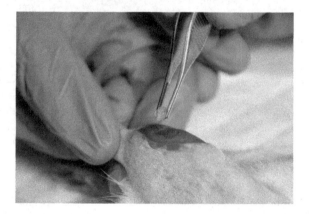

Figure 3. Application of a spherical hydrogel containing 1x10⁶ MSCs from the Wharton's jelly, in the 5 mm Ø TA myectomy defect.

4.2. Cells

There is evidence both from animal studies and clinical investigations that cell therapy involving different types of stem cells application is promising as means to promote regeneration of skeletal muscles following severe injuries. Technical or/and ethical difficulties in obtaining sufficient and appropriate stem cells from the bone marrow or from embryos (obtained from assisted reproduction techniques or somatic nuclear transfer - cloning) have limited the application of this type of therapy. Stem cells are known as an undifferentiated population, with endless self-renewal and sustained proliferation *in vitro* and multilineage differentiation ability [95]. The *in vitro* multilineage differentiation is the concept that gives these cells an extreme priority for use in tissue and cell-based therapies. Stem cells can be loosely classified into 3 categories based on their functional role: hematopoietic stem cells, mesenchymal stem cells (MSCs) and embryonic stem cells [95].

MSCs have become one of the most exciting targets for tissue regeneration due to their high plasticity, proliferative and multilineage differentiation capacity. These cells are capable of differentiating into adipose, bone cartilage and muscle. Among all this notable characteristics, MSCs reveal other properties of great importance, they present low immunogenicity and high immunosuppressive properties due to a decreased or even absence HLA Class II expression [96]. Differentiation potential of MSCs in multilineage end-stage cells has been proven, so as the treatment potential in musculoskeletal disorders [97, 98]. Since their first isolation in 1968, from rat bone marrow [99], MSCs have been isolated with success from almost all tissue sources: skeletal muscle, adipose tissues, synovial membranes, umbilical cord matrix and blood, placental tissue, amniotic fluid among others. Along with differentiation capacity, an increasing amount of data has demonstrated that the MSCs have the capacity of modulating the surrounding environment, by secretion of multiple factors and activation of endogenous progenitor cells [100, 101].

4.2.1. Umbilical cord

From our data and from previously published experimental work, the development of cell therapies associated to biomaterials is a promising tool for increase skeletal muscle regeneration, avoiding the irreversible loss of function and limit the fibrous scar tissue presence [57-59]. Recent years have witnessed an explosion in the number of adult stem cells populations isolated and characterized. While still multipotent, adult stem cells have long been considered restricted, giving rise only to progeny of their resident tissues. Recently, and currently controversial studies have challenged this dogma, suggesting that adult stem cells may be far more plastic than previously appreciated [102, 103]. Extra-embryonic tissues as stem cell reservoirs offer many advantages over both embryonic and adult stem cell sources. The umbilical cord matrix is an important and safe source of MSCs with positive effects in nerve and skeletal muscle regeneration, with no ethical or technical issues. MSC isolated from umbilical cord matrix (Wharton's jelly), as well as embryonic stem cells (ESCs) are originated from inner cell mass of blastocyst [104]. Comparing with ESCs, MSCs have shorter population doubling time; can be easily cultured in plastic flasks, are well tolerated by immune system; therefore transplantation of these cells into non-immune-suppressed animals does not induce acute rejection. Most important, these cells do not originate teratomas [104]. Like bone marrow stromal cells and other MSCs, the MSCs from the Wharton's jelly are plastic adherent, stain positively for markers of the mesenchymal lineage (CD10, CD13, CD29, CD44, CD90, and CD105) and negatively for markers of the hematopoietic lineage. These MSCs are capable of self-renewal with sustained proliferation *in vitro* and can differentiate into multiple mesodermal cells. The high plasticity and low immunogenicity of these cells turn them into a desirable form of cell therapy for the injured musculoskeletal tissue without requiring the use of immunosuppressive drugs during the treatments. Interestingly, these cells, which are HLA class II negative, not only express both an immuno-privileged and immuno-modulatory phenotype, but their HLA complex class I expression levels can also be manipulated, making them a potential cell source for MSC-based therapies. In addition and as previously referred, these cells represent a non-controversial source of primitive mesenchymal progenitor cells that can be harvested after birth, cryogenically stored, thawed, and expanded for therapeutic uses. MSCs from the Wharton's jelly display a high proliferative rate and plasticity, being able to differentiate into adipocytes, osteoblasts, chondrocytes, cardiomyocites, neurons, and glia. More recently, Conconi et al. [105] demonstrated that CD105(+)/CD31(-)/KDR(-) cells are able not only to differentiate *in vivo* towards the myogenic lineage as demonstrated by the co-localization of HLA 1 and sarcomeric tropomyosine antigens, but also to contribute to the muscle regenerative process. These cells were found to differentiate *in vitro* into myoblast-like cells, expressing Myf5 and MyoD after 7 and 11 days of myogenic induction, respectively. The timing of expression of Myf5 and MyoD in CD105(+)/CD31(-)/KDR(-) cells is similar to that described during embryonic development and in myoblast cultures [105].

Using the myectomy model we tested the use of Human MSCs isolated from the Wharton's jelly in order to improve skeletal muscle regeneration. The cells were directly infiltrated into the lesion or delivered by different vehicles including Floseal®, Tisseel®, carboximetilcellulose (Sigma) and spherical hydrogel (own fabrication). MSC from Wharton's jelly were purchased from PromoCell GmbH (C-12971, lot-number: 8082606.7). The MSCs are cultured and maintained in a humidified atmosphere with 5% CO_2 at 37°C. Mesenchymal Stem Cell Medium, PromoCell (C-28010) is replaced every 48 hours. At 90% confluence, cells are harvested with 0.25% trypsin with EDTA (GIBCO) and passed into a new flask for further expansion. MSCs at a concentration of 2 x 10^5cells are cultured exhibiting a 90% confluence after 3-4 days. The application of human MSCs in rats is possible without inducing any immunossupression in the experimental animals. The MSCs exhibited a normal star-like shape with a flat morphology in culture (Figure 4). A total of 20 Giemsa-stained metaphases of these cells, were analyzed for numerical aberrations. Sporadic, non-clonal aneuploidy was found in 3 cells (41-45 chromosomes) the other 17 metaphases had 46 chromosomes. The karyotype was determined in a completely analyzed G-banding metaphase and no structural alterations were found [57]. The karyotype analysis to the MSCs cell line derived from Human Wharton jelly demonstrated that this cell line hasn't neoplasic characteristics and is stable during the cell culture procedures in terms of number and structure of the somatic and sexual chromosomes. Also, the morphologic characteristics of these cells in culture, observed in an inverted microscope, are normal. These cells presented a star-like shape with a flat morphology, characteristic of the MSCs been adequate to be used in *in vivo* rat experimental model [57]. The MSCs karyotype was studied in order to be sure that these cells did not present any number or structure chromosome abnormalities due to isolation and cell culture procedures before *in vivo* application. This concern was due to the negative effects that some cellular systems, like the ESCs present, inducing the production of teratomas. The cellular systems implanted into the injured skeletal muscle improved the skeletal muscle regeneration since these cells produce growth factors, ECM molecules, and even modulate the inflammatory process.

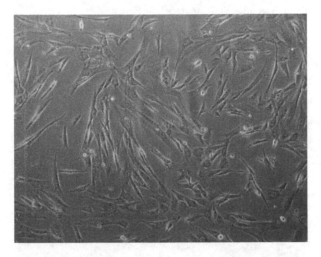

Figure 4. Undifferentiated MSCs from Wharton's jelly, exhibiting a star-like shape with a flat morphology (100x magnification).

5. Evaluation of muscle regeneration

Muscle biopsies should be considered in order to obtain careful clinical assessment or for investigation purposes. After the collection of the muscle samples, they should be immediately equally divided in three. One sample should be placed into formalin (for hematoxilin and eosin - HE), another sample should be fixed into 2.5% purified glutaraldehyde in 0.1M Sorensen phosphate buffer (for electron microscopy - EM) and the other sample should remain unfixed and refrigerated (for histochemistry, biochemistry/genetics analysis).

5.1. Routine histological evaluation

Routine evaluation of the muscle biopsy sample involves the examination of formalin-fixed, paraffin processed sections and unfixed frozen sections with standard histological and enzyme histochemical stains at the light microscopic level. HE is the routine histological stain used for evaluation of basic tissue organization and cellular structure. For HE, the whole piece of tissue should be fixed in a clamp and after the tissue is infiltrated with wax, both longitudinal and cross sections must be cut before embedding. Five levels should be obtained, especially in cases suspected of vasculitis. The parameters that can be evaluated are: the type of inflammatory infiltrate present; examination of the structure of vessels walls (vasculitis and/or fibrinoid necrosis); presence of endomysial and perimysial fibrosis/fatty infiltration; the range of fiber caliber; presence of angulated fibers; increase in number of centrally located nuclei; central capillary migration; split fiber; group atrophy; necrotic/ myopathic (degenerating) fibers; atrophic fibers; regenerating fibers; target fibers; whorl fibers and ring fibers. The rounding of fiber contour and the variation of fiber diameter should also be analyzed, however they are better evaluated with frozen sections (Figure 5).

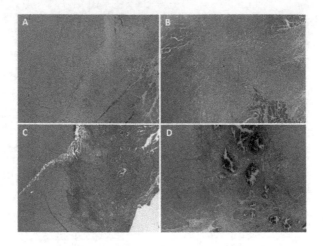

Figure 5. HE staining of TA muscles 15 days post myectomy (A - control) and application of fibrin (B), hydrogel (C), Floseal® (D).

5.1.1. Morphological analysis

Long-standing histological characteristics are still used to identify the mammalian skeletal muscle regeneration process. On muscle cross-sections, these fundamental morphological characteristics are newly formed myofibers of small caliber and with centrally located myonuclei. Newly formed myofibers are often basophilic (reflecting high protein synthesis) and express embryonic/developmental forms of MHC (reflecting *de novo* fiber formation). On muscle longitudinal sections and in isolated single muscle fibers, central myonuclei are observed in discrete portions of regenerating fibers or along the entire new fiber, suggesting that cell fusion is not diffuse during regeneration but rather focal to the site of injury [1]. Cross-sectional area (CSA) analysis is one of the features that can be assessed. This can be achieved with imaging software processing (Scio Image, ImageJ) of HE-stained muscle sections. A predefined number of fibers is traced per sample and should be determined as appropriate by the examination of no additional changes in standard deviation. The classification of small and large fibers can be determined for example by setting three standard deviations from the mean CSA for the uninjured group at different time points [14]. The CSA and number of myotubes can be used to estimate the development degree of muscle regeneration following injury [36].

5.1.2. Collagen quantification

Collagen content in the wound bed can be calculated by image analysis of Masson's Trichrome-stained histological images taken at a predefined image magnification. Color separations must be performed and an analysis threshold must be established for each image series collected using the same brightness and white balance settings. Output images showing only computed blue coverage must be compared to the color images to ensure the representation of truly blue color due to collagen staining. As a control the analysis must be performed on uninjured (control) skeletal muscle tissue sections stained with Masson's Trichrome and collected using the same camera and threshold settings to confirm a collagen content of zero for control tissue. The ratio of blue pixels above the threshold to total pixels in the image is used to calculate the collagen content for each image [40].

5.1.3. International Standard (ISO 10993-6)

The International Standard (ISO 10993-6) specifies test methods for the assessment of the local effects after implantation of biomaterials intended for use in medical devices. These implantation tests are not intended to evaluate or determine the performance of the test specimen in terms of mechanical or functional loading. The local effects are evaluated by a comparison of the tissue response caused by the tested implant to that caused by the control. The objective of the test methods is to characterize the history and evolution of the tissue response after implantation of a medical device/biomaterial including final integration or resorption/degradation of the material. The test sample shall be implanted into the tissues most relevant to the intended clinical use of the material. For short-term testing, animals such as rodents or rabbits are commonly used. During the first two weeks after implantation the reaction due to the surgical procedure itself may be difficult to distinguish from the tissue reaction evoked by the implant and for that reason in our study we collected the muscle samples 15 days after implantation. For degradable/resorbable materials the test period shall be related to the estimated degradation time of the test product. In our case the majority of the vehicles/matrices tested the degradation time is less than 4 days. In the absence of complete degradation, absorption, or restoration to normal tissue structure and function, the overall data collected may be sufficient to allow characterization of the local effects after implantation. A sufficient number of implants shall be inserted to ensure that the final number of specimens to be evaluated will give valid results. The evaluation of the biological response must be accomplished by documenting the macroscopic and histopathological responses as a function of time. The responses to the test sample must be compared to the responses obtained at the control sample or sham operated sites. The scoring system used for the histological evaluation shall take into account the extent of the area affected, either quantitatively (e.g. in micrometres) or semi-quantitatively (Annex E of this Standard) [44, 106]. The biological response parameters, which shall be assessed and recorded, include:

i.   the extent of fibrosis/fibrous capsule (layer in μm) and inflammation;

ii.   the degeneration as determined by changes in tissue morphology;

iii.   the number and distribution as a function of distance from the material/tissue in-
         terface of the inflammatory cell types, namely polymorph nuclear neutrophilic leu-
         cocytes, lymphocytes, plasma cells, eosinophils, macrophages and multinucleated
         cells;

iv.   the presence, extent and type of necrosis;

v.   other tissue alterations such as vascularization, fatty infiltration, granuloma forma-
         tion and bone formation;

vi.   the material parameters such as fragmentation and/or debris presence, form and lo-
         cation of remnants of degraded material;

vii.   the quality and quantity of tissue ingrowth, for porous and degradable implant
         materials [106].

Under the conditions of the study and following the results for the mentioned parameters in
the semi-quantitative scoring system (Annex E of this Sandard), the test sample is considered as non-irritant (0,0 up to 2,9), slight irritant (3,0 up to 8,9), moderate irritant (9,0 up to
15,0), severe irritant (> 15) to the tissue as compared to the negative control sample [106].
This test method is used for assessing the biological response of muscle tissue to an implanted material (Annex C of this Standard). As already mentioned, the method compares the biological response to implants of test specimens with the biological response to implants of
control specimens. The control materials are those used in medical devices of which the clinical acceptability and biocompatibility characteristics have been established [106]. In our
study we developed an adaptation of this Standard by considering the control as the group
where the surgical procedure (myectomy) was performed without any biomaterial or cell
implantation (Figure 6). Although the surgical technique may profoundly influence the result of any implantation procedure, we assumed that our standardized myectomy lesion
could be considered as the *Control* group since we were able to determine the local effects of
the different implants by their comparison to the minor effects of the surgical procedure.
The surgeries were executed under general anesthesia with a xylazine (1.25 mg/100 g BW
im) and ketamine (9 mg/100 g BW im) combination [38].

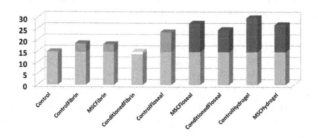

Figure 6. ISO 10993-6 scoring for the groups tested. The *Control* group obtained a score of 14.7 (in blue). Scorings above the *Control* group were considered as non-irritant (in yellow), slight irritant (in orange) and moderate irritant (in red).

5.2. Histochemistry

For histochemistry a basic panel should be performed, preferentially in frozen sections. Depending on the objectives, an extended panel can be done concerning the study of some molecules like the already mentioned Masson's Trichrome-stain or enzyme processes such as ATPase; NADH-TR or Esterase (Bancroft&Stevens). When necessary, other special stains can be performed on paraffin sections.

5.3. Immunohistochemistry

In general, the immunohistochemical stains are utilized for the diagnosis of various muscular dystrophies. They also may help to determine the subtypes of inflammatory cells within an infiltrate or for other investigation purposes. Specific skeletal muscle markers such as myosin heavy chain and desmin can be applied in order to clearly identify this tissue. The distinction of SCs, considered as the reservoir of myogenic precursor cells, from other cells must be made (like plasma cells, which may be occasionally seen under the basal lamina in pathologic conditions). SCs can be easily demonstrated by immunostaining for N-CAM; they also express vimentin. Activated SCs generally express Myo-D and myogenin [107]. The regenerating fibers express N-CAM, MyoD and myogenin, and also embryonic and neonatal isoforms of myosin heavy chain. In contrast to mature fibers, MCH class I histocompatibility complex is expressed in regenerating fibers.

5.4. Immunofluorescence

For the preparation of TA muscles for immunofluorescence they should be embedded in Tissue-Tek OCT compound. Sections are cut at 10 μm using a Leica CM1850 cryostat and placed onto Surgipath microscope slides. Laminin-α2 chain is detected with a 1:500 dilution of rabbit anti-laminin-α2 (2G) polyclonal antibody. The laminin-α1 chain is detected with a rat anti-laminin-α1 monoclonal antibody. Primary rabbit antibodies are detected with a 1:500 dilution of fluorescein isothiocyanate-conjugated anti-rabbit secondary antibody and the rat monoclonal antibody is detected with 1:500 dilution of fluorescein isothiocyanate-conjugated anti-rat secondary antibody. In all immunofluorescence experiments, secondary only antibody controls are included to test for specificity. For mouse monoclonal antibodies, endogenous mouse immunoglobulin is blocked with a mouse-on-mouse (MOM) kit. A 1-μg/ml concentration of tetramethylrhodamine-conjugated wheat germ agglutinin (WGA) is used to define muscle fibers. To examine immune response, cytotoxic T cells are detected with fluorescein isothiocyanate-labeled rat anti-mouse CD8a and macrophages are detected with fluorescein isothiocyanateconjugated anti-mouse F4/80 at 1:1000 (Figure 7 and Figure 8) [50].

Figure 7. Double imunofluorescence staining for laminin and CD31.

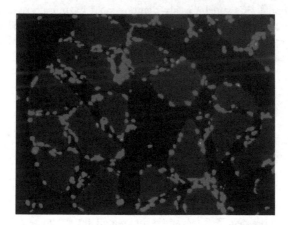

Figure 8. Pax7+ SC counterstained with DAPI.

5.5. Electron microscopy

Electron microscopic (EM) examination of the glutaraldehyde-fixed portion of the biopsy is performed when the light microscopic studies are inconclusive. Thus, it is reserved for selected circumstances in which the pathologist determines that EM has the potential of contributing significantly to determining a specific diagnosis. A specimen placed in glutaraldehyde must be small, approximately 1-2 mm in width and depth, allowing the complete tissue penetration by this fixative. Glutaraldehyde makes tissue brittle and interferes with immunohistochemical studies, so it is not appropriate for the paraffin specimen. With EM, other muscle cell parameters can be analyzed in detail: the myofibril architecture;

the plasma and sarcolemmal membrane; the mitochondria (size, density and shape); T-tubule; amount of lipid; nucleus; phagocytic granules and amount of glycogen. EM is extremely useful in some cases: to identify inclusions primarily found by light microscopy; to help in the characterization of stored material found on light microscopy and define its intracellular localization; to analyze structural abnormalities found by light microscopy; can assist in the diagnosis of mitochondrial myopathy or seeking evidence to support a diagnosis of dermatomyositis (EM can be used to look for tubuloreticular inclusion in endothelial cells when light microscopic fails to reveal it).

5.6. Contraction force measurement

To obtain an estimate of total TA muscle strength reduced by the injury and possibly recovered by the cell/vehicle implants, contractile force due to electrical stimulation can be measured before injury, after injury and at the time of sacrifice (at different time points) for non-implanted and implanted animals. This can be accomplished with the animals under general anesthesia and by anchoring the knee joint using a custom clamping system anchored to the floor of the surgical stereomicroscope stand and attaching a silk ligature to the cleft between digits 1 and 2 that must be anchored to a transducer at the other end. This can also be executed by cutting the TA tendon just before the insertion at the ankle and tying it with a 4.0 nylon suture attached to the isometric transducer. The exposed muscle is stimulated using 2 custom needle electrodes placed at the proximal muscle surface. Electrical stimulation of the TA muscle is applied at 5 volts, 4 ms pulse duration, at 500 ms intervals and the resultant tetanic force recorded (200 points(s) using a BioPac MP-100 (Harvard Apparatus) and accompanying software (Acknowledge™). The muscle must be kept hydrated during the procedure using sterile saline. Maximum tetanic force is measured by reducing the stimulation interval to 20 ms, generating continuous stimulation simulating tetanus condition. Another method of applying the electrical stimulation can be obtained by exposing the sciatic nerve with an incision in the hamstring region The tibial nerve is cut just after the sciatic nerve splits into the tibial and peroneal nerves to eliminate any contraction from the *gastrocnemius* muscle causing background in the force data. The exposed sciatic nerve is then laid over two electrodes with a small piece of parafilm and should also be kept moist with periodic treatment of mineral oil. Stimulation is made using a supra-maximal square-wave pulse of 0.1 ms duration. Measurements are performed at the length at which maximal extension is obtained during the twitch and the data should be recorded for sub-maximal and maximal isometric force. Specific maximal force should be quantified by correcting for muscle mass [40, 98].

Acknowledgements

The authors would like to thank the support by Dr. José Manuel Correia Costa, from INSRJ, Porto, Portugal; and Biosckin, Molecular and Cell Therapies SA for the umbilical cord units supply and access to the GMP cell culture room (Scientific Protocol between Porto University and Biosckin, Molecular and Cell Therapies SA). This work was supported by Fundação para a Ciência e Tecnologia (FCT), Ministério da Ciência e Ensino Superior (MCES), Portugal, through the financed research project PTDC/DES/104036/2008, and by QREN Nº 1372 para Criação de um Núcleo I&DT para Desenvolvimento de Produtos nas Áreas de Medicina Regenerativa e de Terapias Celulares – Núcleo Biomat & Cell. A Gärtner (SFRH/BD/ 70211/2010) and I Amorim (SFRH/BD/76237/2011) acknowledge FCT for financial support.

Author details

Tiago Pereira[1,3*], Andrea Gärtner[1,3], Irina Amorim[3], Paulo Armada-da-Silva[2], Raquel Gomes[1,3], Cátia Pereira[2], Miguel L. França[1,3], Diana M. Morais[4], Miguel A. Rodrigues[4], Maria A. Lopes[4], José D. Santos[4], Ana Lúcia Luís[1,3] and Ana Colette Maurício[1,3]

*Address all correspondence to: tiago.vet@gmail.com

1 Centro de Estudos de Ciência Animal (CECA), Instituto de Ciências e Tecnologias Agrárias e Agro - Alimentares (ICETA), Universidade do Porto (UP), Portugal

2 Faculdade de Motricidade Humana (FMH), Universidade Técnica de Lisboa (UTL), Portugal

3 Instituto de Ciências Biomédicas Abel Salazar (ICBAS), Universidade do Porto (UP), Portugal

4 CEMUC, Departamento de Engenharia Metalúrgica e Materiais, Faculdade de Engenharia, Universidade do Porto (FEUP), Portugal

References

[1] Charge, SBP, & Rudnicki, M. A. (2004). Cellular and molecular regulation of muscle regeneration. *Physiological Reviews*, 84(1), 209-38.

[2] Gibson, M. C., & Schultz, E. (1982). The distribution of satellite cells and their relationship to specific fiber types in soleus and extensor digitorum longus muscles. *Anat Rec*, 202(3), 329-37, Epub 1982/03/01.

[3] Snow, M. H. (1983). A quantitative ultrastructural analysis of satellite cells in denervated fast and slow muscles of the mouse. *Anat Rec*, 207(4), 593-604, Epub 1983/12/01.

[4] Pette, D., & Staron, R. S. (2000). Myosin isoforms, muscle fiber types, and transitions. *Microscopy research and technique*, 50(6), 500-9, Epub 2000/09/22.

[5] Huxley, A. F. (2000). Cross-bridge action: present views, prospects, and unknowns. *Journal of biomechanics*, 33(10), 1189-95, Epub 2000/07/19.

[6]   Carlson, B. M., & Faulkner, J. A. (1983). The regeneration of skeletal muscle fibers fol-
      lowing injury: a review. *Medicine and science in sports and exercise*, 15(3), 187-98.

[7]   Yamanouchi, K., Soeta, C., Naito, K., & Tojo, H. (2000). Expression of Myostatin Gene
      in Regenerating Skeletal Muscle of the Rat and Its Localization. *Biochemical and Bio-
      physical Research Communications*, 270(2), 510-6.

[8]   Musaro, A., Giacinti, C., Pelosi, L., Dobrowolny, G., Barberi, L., Nardis, C., et al.
      (2007). Stem cell-mediated muscle regeneration and repair in aging and neuromuscu-
      lar diseases. *European journal of histochemistry : EJH*, 51(1), 35-43, Epub 2007/08/21.

[9]   Hyatt, J. P., Roy, R. R., Baldwin, K. M., & Edgerton, V. R. (2003). Nerve activity-inde-
      pendent regulation of skeletal muscle atrophy: role of MyoD and myogenin in satel-
      lite cells and myonuclei. *American journal of physiology Cell physiology*, 285(5),
      C1161-73, Epub 2003/07/04.

[10] Gayraud-Morel, B., Chretien, F., & Tajbakhsh, S. (2009). Skeletal muscle as a para-
      digm for regenerative biology and medicine. *Regenerative medicine*, 4(2), 293-319,
      Epub 2009/03/26.

[11] Mitchell, K. J., Pannerec, A., Cadot, B., Parlakian, A., Besson, V., Gomes, E. R., et al.
      (2010). Identification and characterization of a non-satellite cell muscle resident pro-
      genitor during postnatal development. *Nat Cell Biol*, 12(3), 257-66, Epub 2010/02/02.

[12] Uezumi, A., Fukada, S-i., Yamamoto, N., Takeda, Si., & Tsuchida, K. (2010). Mesen-
      chymal progenitors distinct from satellite cells contribute to ectopic fat cell formation
      in skeletal muscle. *Nat Cell Biol*, 12(2), 143-52.

[13] Cooper, RN, Tajbakhsh, S., Mouly, V., Cossu, G., Buckingham, M., & Butler-Browne,
      G. S. (1999). In vivo satellite cell activation via Myf5 and MyoD in regenerating
      mouse skeletal muscle. *Journal of cell science*, 112(Pt 17), 289-901, Epub 1999/08/13.

[14] White, J. P., Baltgalvis, K. A., Sato, S., Wilson, L. B., & Carson, J. A. (2009). Effect of
      nandrolone decanoate administration on recovery from bupivacaine-induced muscle
      injury. *Journal of Applied Physiology*, 107(5), 1420-30.

[15] Politi, P. K., Havaki, S., Manta, P., & Lyritis, G. (2006). Bupivacaine-induced regener-
      ation of rat soleus muscle: ultrastructural and immunohistochemical aspects. *Ultra-
      structural Pathology*, 30(6), 461-9.

[16] Jones, GH. (1982). Protein synthesis in bupivacaine (Marcaine)-treated, regenerating
      skeletal muscle. *Muscle & nerve*, 5(4), 281-90.

[17] Rosenblatt, J., & Woods, R. (1992). Hypertrophy of rat extensor digitorum longus
      muscle injected with bupivacaine. A sequential histochemical, immunohistochemi-
      cal, histological and morphometric study. *Journal of Anatomy*, 181(Pt 1), 11.

[18] Nonaka, I., Takagi, A., Ishiura, S., Nakase, H., & Sugita, H. (1983). Pathophysiology
      of muscle fiber necrosis induced by bupivacaine hydrochloride (Marcaine). *Acta Neu-
      ropathologica*, 60(3), 167-74.

[19] Irwin, W., Fontaine, E., Agnolucci, L., Penzo, D., Betto, R., Bortolotto, S., et al. (2002). Bupivacaine Myotoxicity Is Mediated by Mitochondria. *Journal of Biological Chemistry*, 277(14), 12221-7.

[20] Steer, J. H., Mastaglia, F. L., Papadimitriou, J. M., & Van Bruggen, I. (1986). Bupivacaine-induced muscle injury: The role of extracellular calcium. *Journal of the Neurological Sciences*, 73(2), 205-17.

[21] Ishiura, S., Nonaka, I., & Sugita, H. (1986). Biochemical aspects of bupivacaine-induced acute muscle degradation. *Journal of cell science*, 83, 197-212, Epub 1986/07/01.

[22] Saito, Y., & Nonaka, I. (1994). Initiation of satellite cell replication in bupivacaine-induced myonecrosis. *Acta Neuropathologica*, 88(3), 252-7.

[23] Chang, C., Chuang, S. T., Lee, C., & Wei, J. (1972). Role of cardiotoxin and phospholipase A in the blockade of nerve conduction and depolarization of skeletal muscle induced by cobra venom. *British journal of pharmacology*, 44(4), 752.

[24] Czerwinska, A. M., Streminska, W., Ciemerych, M. A, & Grabowska, I. (2012). Mouse gastrocnemius muscle regeneration after mechanical or cardiotoxin injury. *Folia histochemica et cytobiologica/ Polish Academy of Sciences, Polish Histochemical and Cytochemical Society*, 50(1), 144-53, Epub 2012/04/26.

[25] Gutiérrez, J. Ma, & Ownby, C. L. (2003). Skeletal muscle degeneration induced by venom phospholipases A2: insights into the mechanisms of local and systemic myotoxicity. *Toxicon*, 42(8), 915-31.

[26] Lin Shiau, S. Y., Huang, M. C., & Lee, C. Y. (1976). Mechanism of action of cobra cardiotoxin in the skeletal muscle. *The Journal of pharmacology and experimental therapeutics*, 196(3), 758-70, Epub 1976/03/01.

[27] Fletcher, J. E., & Lizzo, F. H. (1987). Contracture induction by snake venom cardiotoxin in skeletal muscle from humans and rats. *Toxicon*, 25(9), 1003-10, Epub 1987/01/01.

[28] Fletcher, J. E., Jiang, S. M., Gong-H, Q., Yudkowsky, M. L., & Wieland, S. J. (1991). Effects of a cardiotoxin from Naja naja kaouthia venom on skeletal muscle: Involvement of calcium-induced calcium release, sodium ion currents and phospholipases A2 and C. *Toxicon*, 29(12), 1489-500.

[29] Ownby, C. L., Fletcher, J. E., & Colberg, T. R. (1993). Cardiotoxin 1 from cobra (Naja naja atra) venom causes necrosis of skeletal muscle in vivo. *Toxicon*, 31(6), 697-709.

[30] Fourie, A. M., Meltzer, S., Berman, M. C., & Louw, A. I. (1983). The effect of cardiotoxin on (Ca2+ + Mg2+)-ATPase of the erythrocyte and sarcoplasmic reticulum. *Biochemistry international*, 6(5), 581-91, Epub 1983/05/01.

[31] Jagodzinski, N. A., Weerasinghe, C., & Porter, K. (2010). Crush injuries and crush syndrome- a review. Part 2: the local injury. *Trauma*, 12(3), 133-48.

[32] Bassaglia, Y., & Gautron, J. (1995). Fast and slow rat muscles degenerate and regenerate differently after whole crush injury. *Journal of muscle research and cell motility,* 16(4), 420-9.

[33] Järvinen, T. A. H., Järvinen, T. L. N., Kääriäinen, M., Kalimo, H., & Järvinen, M. (2005). Muscle Injuries. *The American Journal of Sports Medicine,* 33(5), 745-64.

[34] Winkler, T., von Roth, P., Matziolis, G., Schumann, M. R., Hahn, S., Strube, P., et al. (2011). Time course of skeletal muscle regeneration after severe trauma. *Acta orthopaedica,* 82(1), 102-11, Epub 2010/12/15.

[35] Ghaly, A., & Marsh, D. R. (2010). Ischaemia-reperfusion modulates inflammation and fibrosis of skeletal muscle after contusion injury. *International journal of experimental pathology,* 91(3), 244-55, Epub 2010/04/01.

[36] Iwata, A., Fuchioka, S., Hiraoka, K., Masuhara, M., & Kami, K. (2010). Characteristics of locomotion, muscle strength, and muscle tissue in regenerating rat skeletal muscles. *Muscle & nerve,* 41(5), 694-701, Epub 2010/04/21.

[37] Zhang, L. Y., Ding, J. T., Wang, Y., Zhang, W. G., Deng, X. J., & Chen, J. H. (2011). MRI quantitative study and pathologic analysis of crush injury in rabbit hind limb muscles. *The Journal of surgical researche,* 357-63, Epub 2010/11/03.

[38] Pereira, T., Gärtner, A., Amorim, I., Ribeiro, J., França, M., Armada-da-Silva, P., et al. Development of a skeletal muscle injury model in the rat and in vivo evaluation of the use of Human Mesenchymal Stem Cells (HMSCs) from the umbilical cord matrix in myectomy injury treatment. *17th annual Congress of the European College of Sport Science,* Bruges- Belgium.

[39] Merritt, E. K., Hammers, D. W., Tierney, M., Suggs, L. J., Walters, T. J., & Farrar, R. P. (2010). Functional assessment of skeletal muscle regeneration utilizing homologous extracellular matrix as scaffolding. *Tissue Engineering Part A,* 16(4), 1395-405.

[40] Page, R. L., Malcuit, C., Vilner, L., Vojtic, I., Shaw, S., Hedblom, E., et al. (2011). Restoration of Skeletal Muscle Defects with Adult Human Cells Delivered on Fibrin Microthreads. *Tissue Engineering Part A,* 17(21-22), 2629-2640.

[41] Coppi, P. D., Bellini, S., Conconi, M. T., Sabatti, M., Simonato, E., Gamba, P. G., et al. (2006). Myoblast-acellular skeletal muscle matrix constructs guarantee a long-term repair of experimental full-thickness abdominal wall defects. *Tissue engineering,* 12(7), 1929-36.

[42] Sato, K., Li, Y., Foster, W., Fukushima, K., Badlani, N., Adachi, N., et al. (2003). Improvement of muscle healing through enhancement of muscle regeneration and prevention of fibrosis. *Muscle & nerve,* 28(3), 365-72, Epub 2003/08/21.

[43] Menetrey, J., Kasemkijwattana, C., Day, C., Bosch, P., Vogt, M., Fu, F., et al. (2000). Growth factors improve muscle healing in vivo. *Journal of Bone and Joint Surgery-British,* 82(1), 131-7.

[44] Li, Y., & Huard, J. (2002). Differentiation of Muscle-Derived Cells into Myofibroblasts in Injured Skeletal Muscle. *The American journal of pathology*, 161(3), 895-907.

[45] Valero, M. C., Huntsman, H. D., Liu, J., Zou, K., & Boppart, MD. (2012). Eccentric exercise facilitates mesenchymal stem cell appearance in skeletal muscle. *PloS one*, 7(1), e29760, Epub 2012/01/19.

[46] Boppart, MD, Volker, S. E., Alexander, N., Burkin, D. J., & Kaufman, S. J. (2008). Exercise promotes α7 integrin gene transcription and protection of skeletal muscle. *American Journal of Physiology-Regulatory, Integrative and Comparative Physiology*, 295(5), R1623.

[47] Dedkov, E. I., Kostrominova, T. Y., Borisov, A. B., & Carlson, B. M. (2001). Reparative myogenesis in long-term denervated skeletal muscles of adult rats results in a reduction of the satellite cell population. *Anat Rec*, 263(2), 139-54, Epub 2001/05/22.

[48] Bruusgaard, J. C., & Gundersen, K. (2008). In vivo time-lapse microscopy reveals no loss of murine myonuclei during weeks of muscle atrophy. *The Journal of clinical investigation*, 118(4), 1450-7, Epub 2008/03/05.

[49] IJ-P, J., Meek, M. F., & Gramsbergen, A. (2005). Long-term reinnervation effects after sciatic nerve lesions in adult rats. *Annals of anatomy = Anatomischer Anzeiger : official organ of the Anatomische Gesellschaft*, 187(2), 113-20, Epub 2005/05/20.

[50] Edgerton, V. R., & Roy, R. R. (2002). How selective is the reinnervation of skeletal muscle fibers? *Muscle & nerve*, 25(6), 765-7, 2002/07/13.

[51] Ijkema-Paassen, J., Meek, M. F., & Gramsbergen, A. (2001). Muscle differentiation after sciatic nerve transection and reinnervation in adult rats. *Annals of anatomy = Anatomischer Anzeiger : official organ of the Anatomische Gesellschaft*, 183(4), 369-77, 2001/08/18.

[52] Cebasek, V., Radochova, B., Ribaric, S., Kubinova, L., & Erzen, I. (2006). Nerve injury affects the capillary supply in rat slow and fast muscles differently. *Cell Tissue Res*, 323(2), 305-12, 2005/09/15.

[53] Mc Geachie, J., & Grounds, M. (1989). The onset of myogenesis in denervated mouse skeletal muscle regenerating after injury. *Neuroscience*, 28(2), 509-14.

[54] Gramsbergen, A., van Eykern, L. A., & Meek, M. F. (2001). Sciatic nerve transection in adult and young rats: abnormal EMG patterns during locomotion. *Equine veterinary journal*, 33(S33), 36-40.

[55] Siu, P. M., & Always, S. E. (2005). Mitochondria-associated apoptotic signalling in denervated rat skeletal muscle. *The Journal of physiology*, 565(Pt 1), 309-23, 2005/03/19.

[56] Bulken-Hoover, JD, Jackson, W. M., Ji, Y., Volger, J. A., Tuan, R. S., & Nesti, L. J. (2011). Inducible Expression of Neurotrophic Factors by Mesenchymal Progenitor Cells Derived from Traumatically Injured Human Muscle. *Molecular biotechnology*, 2011/09/10.

[57] Gärtner, A., Pereira, T., Simões, M. J., Armada-da-Silva, P., França, M. L., Sousa, R., et al. (2012). Use of hybrid chitosan membranes and MSC cells for promoting nerve regeneration in an axonotmesis rat model. *Neural Regeneration Research*, (in press).

[58] Gärtner, A., Pereira, T., Amorim, I., Ribeiro, J., & França, M. L. P. A-d-S. (2012). Use of poly(DL-lactide-ε-caprolactone) PLC membranes and MSC cells for promoting nerve regeneration in an axonotmesis rat model: in vitro and in vivo analysis. *Differentiation*, (submitted).

[59] Maurício, A. C., Gärtner, A., Armada-da-Silva, P., Amado, S., Pereira, T., Veloso, A. P., et al. (2011). Cellular Systems and Biomaterials for Nerve Regeneration in Neurotmesis Injuries. *Pignatello R, editor. Biomaterials Applications for Nanomedicine*, 978-9-53307-661-4, Available from: InTech.

[60] Luis, A. L., Rodrigues, J. M., Geuna, S., Amado, S., Shirosaki, Y., Lee, J. M., et al. (2008). Use of PLGA 90:10 scaffolds enriched with in vitro-differentiated neural cells for repairing rat sciatic nerve defects. *Tissue Eng Part A*, 14(6), 979-93, 2008/05/02.

[61] Luis, A. L., Rodrigues, J. M., Geuna, S., Amado, S., Simoes, M. J., Fregnan, F., et al. (2008). Neural cell transplantation effects on sciatic nerve regeneration after a standardized crush injury in the rat. *Microsurgery*, 28(6), 458-70, 2008/07/16.

[62] Amado, S., Rodrigues, J. M., Luis, A. L., Armada-da-Silva, P. A., Vieira, M., Gartner, A., et al. (2010). Effects of collagen membranes enriched with in vitro-differentiated N1E-115 cells on rat sciatic nerve regeneration after end-to-end repair. *J Neuroeng Rehabil*, 7, 7, 2010/02/13.

[63] Simoes, M. J., Amado, S., Gartner, A., Armada-Da-Silva, P. A., Raimondo, S., Vieira, M., et al. (2010). Use of chitosan scaffolds for repairing rat sciatic nerve defects. *Ital J Anat Embryol*, 115(3), 190-210, 2011/02/04.

[64] Maurício, A. C. Cellular Systems and Biomaterials for Nerve Regeneration in Neurotmesis Injuries.

[65] Brandl, F., Sommer, F., & Goepferich, A. (2007). Rational design of hydrogels for tissue engineering: impact of physical factors on cell behavior. *Biomaterials*, 28(2), 134-46, 2006/10/03.

[66] Fedorovich, N. E., Alblas, J., de Wijn, J. R., Hennink, W. E., Verbout, A. J., & Dhert, W. J. A. (2007). Hydrogels as Extracellular Matrices for Skeletal Tissue Engineering: State-of-the-Art and Novel Application in Organ Printing. *Tissue engineering*, 13(8), 1905-25.

[67] Coelho, J., Ferreira, P., Alves, P., Cordeiro, R., Fonseca, A., Góis, J., et al. (2010). Drug delivery systems: Advanced technologies potentially applicable in personalized treatments. *The EPMA Journal*, 1(1), 164-209.

[68] Rehfeldt, F., Engler, A. J., Eckhardt, A., Ahmed, F., & Discher, D. E. (2007). Cell responses to the mechanochemical microenvironment--implications for regenerative medicine and drug delivery. Adv Drug Deliv Rev '2007/09/29 , 59(13), 1329-39.

[69] Lee, M., Wu, B. M., & Dunn, J. C. (2008). Effect of scaffold architecture and pore size on smooth muscle cell growth. *Journal of biomedical materials research Part A*, 87(4), 1010-6, 2008/02/08.

[70] Seliktar, D. (2012). Designing cell-compatible hydrogels for biomedical applications. *Science*, 336(6085), 1124-8, 2012/06/02.

[71] Garg, T., Singh, O., Arora, S., & Murthy, R. (2012). Scaffold: a novel carrier for cell and drug delivery. *Critical reviews in therapeutic drug carrier systems*, 29(1), 1-63, 2012/02/24.

[72] Rihova, B. (2000). Immunocompatibility and biocompatibility of cell delivery systems. *Adv Drug Deliv Rev*, 42(1-2), 65-80, 2000/08/16.

[73] Lyons, F., Partap, S., & O'Brien, F. J. (2008). Part 1: scaffolds and surfaces. *Technology and health care : official journal of the European Society for Engineering and Medicine*, 16(4), 305-17, 2008/09/09.

[74] Martino, M. M., Mochizuki, M., Rothenfluh, D. A., Rempel, S. A., Hubbell, J. A., & Barker, T. H. (2009). Controlling integrin specificity and stem cell differentiation in 2D and 3D environments through regulation of fibronectin domain stability. *Biomaterials*, 30(6), 1089-97, 08/11/26.

[75] Schmidt, J. J., Rowley, J., & Kong, H. J. (2008). Hydrogels used for cell-based drug delivery. *Journal of Biomedical Materials Research Part A*, 87(4), 1113-22.

[76] Freyman, T. M., Yannas, I. V., & Gibson, L. J. (2001). Cellular materials as porous scaffolds for tissue engineering. *Progress in Materials Science*, 46(3-4), 273-82.

[77] Tejas, Shyam. K., & Mauli, A. (2008). Functions and Requirements of Synthetic Scaffolds in Tissue Engineering. *Nanotechnology and Tissue Engineering: CRC Press*, 53-86.

[78] Hoffman, A. S. (2002). Hydrogels for biomedical applications. *Advanced drug delivery reviews*, 54(1), 3-12.

[79] Tan, H., & Marra, K. G. (2010). Injectable, Biodegradable Hydrogels for Tissue Engineering Applications. *Materials*, 3(3), 1746-67.

[80] Yu, L., & Ding, J. (2008). Injectable hydrogels as unique biomedical materials. *Chemical Society reviews*, 37(8), 1473-81.

[81] Nguyen, M. K., & Lee, D. S. (2010). Injectable Biodegradable Hydrogels. *Macromolecular Bioscience*, 10(6), 563-79.

[82] Goessl, A., Tirelli, N., & Hubbell, J. A. (2004). A hydrogel system for stimulus-responsive, oxygen-sensitive in situ gelation. *Journal of biomaterials science*, Polymer edition, 15(7), 895-904, 2004/08/21.

[83] Nguyen, K. T., & West, J. L. (2002). Photopolymerizable hydrogels for tissue engineering applications. *Biomaterials*, 23(22), 4307-14.

[84] Shim, W. S., Yoo, J. S., Bae, Y. H., & Lee, D. S. (2005). Novel injectable pH and temperature sensitive block copolymer hydrogel. *Biomacromolecules*, 6(6), 2930-4, 2005/11/15.

[85] Borschel, G. H., Dennis, R. G., & Kuzon, W. M. Jr. (2004). Contractile skeletal muscle tissue-engineered on an acellular scaffold. *Plastic and reconstructive surgery*, 113(2), 595-602, discussion 3-4, 2004/02/06.

[86] Ahmed, T. A. E., Dare, E. V., & Hincke, M. (2008). Fibrin: a versatile scaffold for tissue engineering applications. *Tissue Engineering Part B: Reviews*, 14(2), 199-215.

[87] Huang, Y. C., Dennis, R. G., Larkin, L., & Baar, K. (2005). Rapid formation of functional muscle in vitro using fibrin gels. *J Appl Physiol*, 98(2), 706-13, 2004/10/12.

[88] Koning, M., Harmsen, M. C., van Luyn, M. J. A., & Werker, P. M. N. (2009). Current opportunities and challenges in skeletal muscle tissue engineering. *Journal of tissue engineering and regenerative medicine*, 3(6), 407-15.

[89] Lee, K. Y., & Mooney, D. J. (2012). Alginate: properties and biomedical applications. *Progress in polymer science*, 37(1), 106-26, 2011/11/30.

[90] Pawar, S. N., & Edgar, K. J. (2012). Alginate derivatization: a review of chemistry, properties and applications. *Biomaterials*, 33(11), 3279-305, 2012/01/28.

[91] Zorlutuna, P., Jeong, J. H., Kong, H., & Bashir, R. (2011). Stereolithography-Based Hydrogel Microenvironments to Examine Cellular Interactions. *Adv Funct Mater*, 21(19), 3642-51.

[92] Lei, Y., Gojgini, S., Lam, J., & Segura, T. (2011). The spreading, migration and proliferation of mouse mesenchymal stem cells cultured inside hyaluronic acid hydrogels. *Biomaterials*, 32(1), 39-47, 2010/10/12.

[93] Prestwich, G. D. (2011). Hyaluronic acid-based clinical biomaterials derived for cell and molecule delivery in regenerative medicine. *Journal of controlled release : official journal of the Controlled Release Society*, 155(2), 193-9, 2011/04/26.

[94] Gauvin, R., Parenteau-Bareil, R., Dokmeci, M. R., Merryman, W. D., & Khademhosseini, A. (2012). Hydrogels and microtechnologies for engineering the cellular microenvironment. *Wiley interdisciplinary reviews Nanomedicine and nanobiotechnology*, 4(3), 235-46, 2011/12/07.

[95] Fossett, E., & Khan, W. S. (2012). Optimising human mesenchymal stem cell numbers for clinical application: a literature review. *Stem cells international*, 2012, 465259, 2012/03/27.

[96] Le Blanc, K., & Ringden, O. (2005). Immunobiology of human mesenchymal stem cells and future use in hematopoietic stem cell transplantation. *Biol Blood Marrow Transplant*, 11(5), 321-34, 2005/04/23.

[97] Wakitani, S., Imoto, K., Yamamoto, T., Saito, M., Murata, N., & Yoneda, M. (2002). Human autologous culture expanded bone marrow mesenchymal cell transplanta-

tion for repair of cartilage defects in osteoarthritic knees. *Osteoarthritis and cartilage OARS, Osteoarthritis Research Society*, 10(3), 199-206, 2002/03/01.

[98]   Wang, L., Ott, L., Seshareddy, K., Weiss, M. L., & Detamore, MS. (2011). Musculoske-letal tissue engineering with human umbilical cord mesenchymal stromal cells. *Regen Med*, 6(1), 95-109, 2010/12/24.

[99]   Friedenstein, A. J., Petrakova, K. V., Kurolesova, A. I., & Frolova, G. P. (1968). Heter-otopic of bone marrow. Analysis of precursor cells for osteogenic and hematopoietic tissues. *Transplantation*, 6(2), 230-47, 1968/03/01.

[100] Togel, F., Weiss, K., Yang, Y., Hu, Z., Zhang, P., & Westenfelder, C. (2007). Vasculo-tropic, paracrine actions of infused mesenchymal stem cells are important to the re-covery from acute kidney injury. *American journal of physiology, Renal physiology*, 292(5), F1626-35, 2007/01/11.

[101] Zhang, M., Mal, N., Kiedrowski, M., Chacko, M., Askari, A. T., Popovic, Z. B., et al. (2007). SDF-1 expression by mesenchymal stem cells results in trophic support of car-diac myocytes after myocardial infarction. *FASEB journal : official publication of the Federation of American Societies for Experimental Biology*, 21(12), 3197-207, 2007/05/15.

[102] Mezey, E., & Chandross, K. J. (2000). Bone marrow: a possible alternative source of cells in the adult nervous system. *European journal of pharmacology*, 405(1-3), 297-302, 2000/10/18.

[103] Brazelton, T. R., Rossi, F. M., Keshet, G. I., & Blau, H. M. (2000). From marrow to brain: expression of neuronal phenotypes in adult mice. *Science*, 290(5497), 1775-9, 2000/12/02.

[104] Bongso, A., Fong-Y, C., & Gauthaman, K. (2008). Taking stem cells to the clinic: Ma-jor challenges. *Journal of Cellular Biochemistry*, 105(6), 1352-60.

[105] Conconi, M. T., Burra, P., Di Liddo, R., Calore, C., Turetta, M., Bellini, S., et al. (2006). CD105(+) cells from Wharton's jelly show in vitro and in vivo myogenic differentia-tive potential. *Int J Mol Med*, 18(6), 1089-96, 2006/11/08.

[106] Kadivar, M., Khatami, S., Mortazavi, Y., Shokrgozar, MA, Taghikhani, M., & Solei-mani, M. (2006). In vitro cardiomyogenic potential of human umbilical vein-derived mesenchymal stem cells. *Biochemical and Biophysical Research Communications*, 340(2), 639-47.

[107] Rantanen, J., Hurme, T., Lukka, R., Heino, J., & Kalimo, H. (1995). Satellite cell prolif-eration and the expression of myogenin and desmin in regenerating skeletal muscle: evidence for two different populations of satellite cells. *Laboratory investigation; a jour-nal of technical methods and pathology*, 72(3), 341-7, 1995/03/01.

Chapter 3

Biofabrication of Tissue Scaffolds

Ning Zhu and Xiongbiao Chen

Additional information is available at the end of the chapter

1. Introduction

Tissue engineering is an emerging interdisciplinary field that applies the principles of life science and engineering to produce engineered tissues for the repair and replacement of damaged tissues or organs [1]. In tissue engineering, tissue scaffolds play a crucial role. A tissue scaffold is a three-dimensional (3D) structure made from biological materials and biomaterials, which is used to facilitate cell/tissue growth and the transport of nutrients and wastes while degrading gradually itself. To fabricate such tissue scaffolds, a number of fabrication techniques have been developed and reported in the literature and these techniques can generally be classified into two categories: conventional and advanced. Conventional techniques [2], including solvent-casting, particulate-leaching, and freeze drying, can build scaffolds with interconnected porous structures. However, they offer little capacity to precisely control pore size, pore geometry, pore interconnectivity, and spatial distribution of pores or allow for the construction of internal channels within the scaffolds. Ideally, scaffolds should not only provide a supporting structure but also the chemical, mechanical, and biological signals required to respond to environmental stimuli. As an alternative to conventional scaffold fabrication methods, advanced fabrication techniques have recently been developed in tissue engineering, such as electrospinning [3], a nanotechnology-based fabrication technique, and rapid prototyping [4], a class of techniques by which a 3D scaffold is fabricated by laying down multiple, precisely formed layers in succession. With the development of such advanced tissue engineering fabrication techniques, the new concept of "biofabrication" has emerged. Biofabrication is defined as the production of complex living and non-living biological products from raw materials, such as living cells, molecules, extracellular matrices, and biomaterials. It has the potential to be the manufacturing paradigm of the 21st century and makes a significant contribution to the development of tissue engineering strategies [5].

2. Overview of scaffold-fabrication techniques

2.1. Conventional fabrication techniques

Many techniques are available to process synthetic and natural biomaterials into various scaffolds. These include conventional techniques, such as solvent-casting and particulate-leaching [6], gas foaming [7], phase separation [8], melt molding [9], and freeze drying [10], among others. An overview of these different techniques follows.

1.   Solvent-casting and particulate-leaching (Figure 1a):

Solvent-casting and particulate-leaching techniques involve using a polymer solution uniformly mixed with salt particles of a specific diameter. The solvent then evaporates leaving behind a polymer matrix with salt particles embedded throughout. The composite is immersed in water, where the salt leaches out to produce a porous structure [11]. Highly porous scaffolds with porosity values up to 93% and average pore diameters up to 500 µm can be formed using this technique. A disadvantage of this technique is that it can only be used to produce thin membranes up to 3 mm thick [12].

2.   Gas foaming (Figure 1b):

During the gas foaming process, molded biodegradable polymers are pressurized at high pressures with gas-foaming agents, such as CO_2 and nitrogen [13], water [14], or fluoroform [15], until the polymers are saturated. This results in nucleation and growth of gas bubbles with sizes ranging between 100 and 500 µm in the polymer. This technique has the advantage of being an organic solvent-free process; the major drawback is that the process may yield a structure with largely unconnected pores and a non-porous external surface [16].

3.   Phase separation (Figure 1c):

During the phase separation process, a polymer solution is quenched and undergoes a liquid-liquid phase separation to form two phases; a polymer-rich phase and a polymer-poor phase. The polymer-rich phase solidifies and the polymer poor phase is removed, leaving a highly porous polymer network [17]. The micro- and macro-structure of the resulting scaffolds are controlled by varying process parameters such as polymer concentration, quenching temperature, and quenching rate. The process is conducted at low temperatures, which is beneficial for the incorporation of bioactive molecules in the structure. Using phase separation techniques, nano-scale fibrous structure enables to be formed, which mimics natural extracellular matrix architecture and provides a better environment for cell attachment and function [18].

4.   Melt molding (Figure 1d):

Melt molding involves filling a mold with polymer powder and a porogen component and then heating to above the glass-transition temperature of the polymer while applying pressure to the mixture [19]. During the fabrication process, the raw materials will bind together to form a scaffold with designed specified external shape. Once the mold is removed, the porogen is leached out and the porous scaffold is then dried. Melt-molding with porogen-leaching is a non-solvent fabrication process that allows independent control of morphology and shape. Drawbacks include the possibility of residual porogen and high processing temperatures that preclude the ability to incorporate bioactive molecules.

5. Freeze drying (Figure 1e):

Polymeric porous scaffolds can be prepared by freeze drying. In the freezing stage, the polymer solution is cooled down to a certain temperature at which all materials are in a frozen state and the solvent forms ice crystals, forcing the polymer molecules to aggregate into the interstitial spaces. In the second phase, the solvent is removed by applying a pressure lower than the equilibrium vapor pressure of the frozen solvent. When the solvent is completely sublimated, a dry polymer scaffold with an interconnected porous microstructure remains [20, 21]. The porosity of the scaffolds depends on the concentration of the polymer solution; pore size distribution is affected by the freezing temperatures. Apart from fabricating porous scaffolds, this technique is also used to dry biological samples to protect their bioactivities [22].

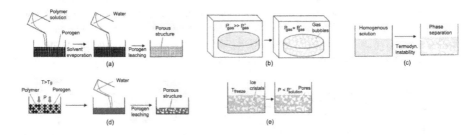

Figure 1. Schematic of conventional scaffold fabrication techniques: (a) solvent-casting and particulate-leaching process: A polymer solution is cast into a mold filled with porogen particles, then the solvent is allowed to evaporate and the porogen is leached out; (b) gas foaming process: Polymer samples are exposed to high pressure allowing saturation of the gas into the polymer; the subsequent gas pressure reduction causes the nucleation of bubbles; (c) phase separation process: A thermodynamical instability is established in a homogeneous polymer solution that separates into a polymer-rich and a polymer-poor phase; (d) melt molding process. A mold filled with polymer powder and porogen component is heated to above the polymer glass-transition temperature (T_g) and a pressure (P) is applied to the mixture. The porogen is then leached out, leaving a porous structure; (e) freeze drying process: A polymer solution is cooled down, leading to the formation of solvent ice crystals. Then the solvent is removed by using a pressure lower than the equilibrium vapor pressure of the solvent (P° solution), leaving a porous structure. (Modified from [23])

2.2. Advanced biofabrication techniques

1. Electrospinning

Electrospinning is a fabrication technique utilizing electrical charges to draw fine fibers up to the nanometer scale. The technique was invented by Cooley and Morton in 1902. The fiber electrospinning can also be traced back to the 1930s [24]. In the past decade, significant developments in electrospinning have allowed for creation of scaffolds with different materials and, hence, this technique has gained a high popularity in tissue engineering research.

Nanofibrous architectures are known to modulate effects on a wide variety of cell behaviors. Nanofibrous architectures can positively affect cell binding and spreading compared to micropore and microfibrous architectures (Figure 2). Nanofibrous scaffold architectures have larger surface areas to adsorb proteins than micro-architectures, presenting more binding sites to cell membrane receptors [25]. The exposure of additional cryptic binding sites may also be affected by adsorbed proteins. Furthermore, cells growing in a 3D nanofibrous structural environment are able to exchange nutrients and utilize receptors throughout their surface, while cells in flat culture conditions are limited to nutrient exchange on only one side. Electrospinning techniques have been widely employed to fabricate porous scaffolds with nanofibrous architectures that can mimic the structure and biological functions of the natural extracellular matrix [26]. This technique is able to generate fibers with diameters ranging from 2 nm to several micrometers using solutions of both natural and synthetic polymers, with small pore sizes and high surface area to volume ratios. A typical electrospinning setup includes three parts: a syringe pump containing the polymeric materials, a high voltage source to generate high electric field for spinning, and a collector to collect the fibers [27] (Figure 3). During scaffold fabrication, the following electrospinning parameters are very important with respect to the fiber morphology: polymer solution parameters (viscosity, molecular weight of polymer, polymer conductivity, surface tension), processing parameters (applied voltage, distance between tip and collector, flow rate), and environment parameters (humidity, temperature). Nanofibers with high surface area to volume ratios are most suitable for tissue engineering applications [28].

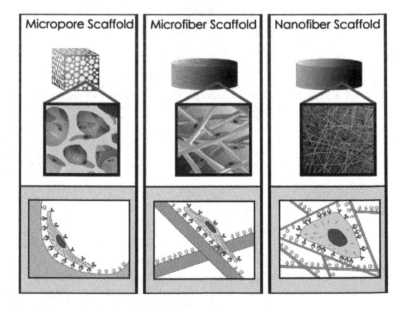

Figure 2. Scaffold architecture affects cell binding and spreading. (Modified from [25])

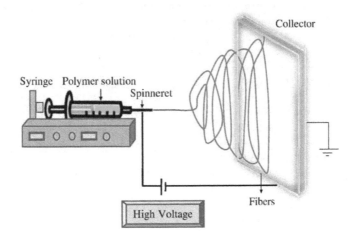

Figure 3. Schematic of electrospinning apparatus. (Modified from [29])

2. Rapid prototyping

As an alternative to conventional scaffold fabrication methods, a group of techniques based on rapid prototyping (RP) has recently been introduced within the tissue engineering field. RP techniques, based on computer assisted design (CAD) and manufacturing (CAM) techniques, allow for better control of scaffold internal microstructure and external macroshape compared to conventional fabrication techniques [4, 30]. Three basic RP system types: liquid-based, solid-based, and powder-based can be selected based on the properties of different scaffold biomaterials. The primary RP processes applied to tissue scaffold fabrication include stereolithography (SLA) [31], selective laser sintering (SLS) [32], fused deposition modeling (FDM) [33], three dimensional (3D) printing [34], and 3D plotting [35]. The choice of materials for the RP techniques includes various polymers, ceramics, and metals. Recently, RP techniques have also demonstrated their capacity for embedding living cells [36, 37] and growth factors [38] into scaffolds during the fabrication process and thus their utility for creating biomimetic tissue scaffolds.

Technology	Types	Materials	Advantages	Disadvantages	Tissue Engineering Applications
SLA	Liquid-based	Polymers, wax or wax compounds	Good mechanical strength; easy to remove support materials; easy to achieve small features	Limited to reactive resins (mostly toxic)	Bone [39], Heart valves [40].
SLS	Powder-based	Metals, ceramics, bulk polymers	Good mechanical strength; high accuracy; broad range of materials	Elevated temperatures; local high energy input; uncontrolled porosity	Bone [41, 42], Cartilage [43].
FDM	Solid-based	Some thermoplastic polymers/ ceramics	Low costs; good mechanical strength; versatile in lay-down pattern design	Elevated temperatures; small range of bulk materials	Bone [44], Adipose [45], Cartilage [46].
3D printing	Powder-based	powder of bulk polymers; ceramics	Fast processing; low costs; no toxic components; water used as binder	Material must be in powder form; weak bonding between powder particles; rough surface; trapped powder issue; might require post-processing	Bone [47],
3D plotting	Liquid-based or solid-based	Swollen polymers (hydrogels); thermoplastic polymers; reactive resins; ceramics	Broad range of materials and conditions; incorporation of cells and proteins	Slow processing; no standard condition; time consuming adjustment to new materials; low mechanical strength	Bone [48], Cartilage [49].

Table 1. RP techniques for tissue engineering

3. Applications of biofabrication to tissue engineering

3.1. Biofabrication and architectural design of scaffolds

The microstructure of scaffolds is increasingly believed to contribute significantly to the diffusion of nutrients and metabolic wastes, spatial organization of cell growth and the development of specific biological functions in tissues. A scaffold with high porosity is desirable for the easy diffusion of nutrients and metabolic wastes and is also beneficial for cell migration and neo-vascularization. A high surface area to volume ratio favors cell attachment and growth. The effect of scaffold pore size on tissue regeneration is also emphasized by experiments demonstrating that (1) an optimum pore size of 5 µm is good for neo-vascularization; (2) 5 - 15 µm pores are beneficial for fiberblast ingrowth; (3) 20 - 125 µm pores can affect the regeneration of adult mammalian skin; and (4) fibrovascular tissues require pores sizes greater than 500 µm [38, 50]. Advanced biofabrication techniques are able to design and precisely control the architecture of scaffolds. They can build scaffolds with reproducible morphology and microstructure that varies across the scaffold matrix to resemble natural tissues with complex hierarchical structures.

Conventional lyophilization can only form porous structures with random orientation. An improved technique for fabricating scaffolds with a linearly oriented architecture is called "freeze casting". Freeze casting facilitates directional solidification of solutions or slurries [51]. During freeze casting, the polymer solution is pipetted into a cylindrical mold fitted with a copper bottom plate and secured onto the temperature-controlled copper cold finger of the freeze casting system. The cold finger temperature is lowered at a constant cooling rate to a final temperature, resulting in the directional solidification of the material dispersion. When the ice is sublimated by freeze drying, the porous microstructure of the resulting scaffold is a negative template of the ice crystals. Freeze casting has been used to produce a wide range of porous, oriented scaffolds from organic and inorganic materials [51, 52]. This technique is also suitable for the fabrication of nerve conduit scaffolds with a featured porous structure that may guide axon growth.

Different scaffold fabrication techniques can be combined to capitalize on their respective positive features for varying applications. The combination of rapid prototyping with lyophilization, in which the polymer solution is dispensed on substrates with a controllable temperature and the strands formed are frozen and lyophilized to remove the solvent, is called "rapid freeze prototyping" technique [53]. This technique has the advantage of fabricating scaffolds with both sub-millimeter and micrometer sized pores [54] (Figure 4). The optimized porous scaffolds can accommodate tissue ingrowth at different scales, from cells to tissues. Scaffolds can also be cold processed so that the polymer can be bio-functionalized without compromising their function during manufacturing.

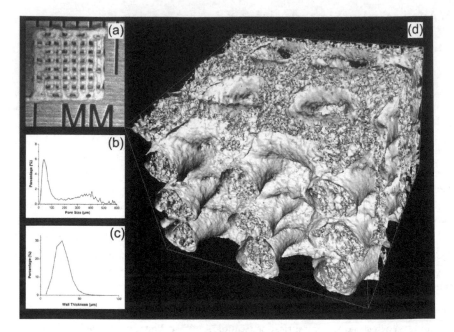

Figure 4. Scaffold fabricated by rapid freeze prototyping: (a) camera image of the scaffold, (b) pore size distribution of the scaffold, (c) wall thickness distribution of the scaffold, and (d) 3D reconstructed model of the scaffold using micro-tomography. (Modified from [54])

3.2. Biofabrication and scaffolds with living cells

Biofabrication of living structures with desired functionality has become a hot topic in tissue en-gineering in past few years. Conventional cell-seeding methods are inadequate for the develop-ment of *in vitro* tissue-test systems because they involve random placement of cells and, therefore, lack the precision necessary for spatial control. Conventional cell-seeding methods are also a type of 2D cell culture. In contrast, cell cultures in 3D structures allow for a more natu-ral cell attachment and focal adhesion in all directions. The most physiologically relevant cell morphology that can be attained on and in three-dimensional scaffolds will provide the best structural cues to regulate cell function [55, 56]. Different methods of fabricating 3D scaffolds with living cells have been developed. One of the methods is to spray living cells into the scaf-folds throughout the electrospinning process to produce nanofibrous 3D tissue scaffolds. In this method, cells are periodically sprayed from a pump-action spray bottle onto the developing scaffold during the electrospinning process [56]. The cells can be layered throughout the thick-ness of the scaffolds, but not incorporated into individual polymer nanofibers.

Living cells also can be directly electrospun, as fine composite threads encapsulating living cells, using a coaxial needle configuration and a biocompatible polymer [57, 58]. The poly-mer nanofibers accommodate the survival and proliferation of the cells. Advanced rapid prototyping techniques, such as bioprinting, are more capable of incorporating living cells into scaffolds than other techniques. Introducing cells at almost any arbitrary density and precisely into the desired location of a scaffold is possible by means of rapid prototyping. Hydrogel scaffolds, as delivery vehicles for cells, are suitable for bioprinting processes that seed living cells while constructing scaffolds with specific geometries [36]. A pneumatic dispenser system is used to bioprint the cell-associated scaffolds using polymer solution, such as alginate aqueous solutions. The fabrication parameters including pressure and nozzle velocity can be altered, thus affecting the viability of the cells [59]. Complete biological "scaffold free" tissue substitutes can also be engineered with specific compositions and shapes, by exploiting cell-cell adhesion and the ability of cultured cells to grow their own ECM; such approaches have the advantage of reducing and mediating inflammatory responses to biomaterials [60]. For this concept, extrusion-based bioprinting is an automated deposition method that can generate a fully biological construct which is structurally and functionally close to native tissues. Spherical or cylindrical multicellular units (the bio-ink) are delivered according to a computer-generated template with the hydrogel (the bio-paper) serving as the support material. The cells neither invade nor rearrange within the hydrogel, which keeps its integrity during post-printing fusion and can be easily removed to free the fused multicellular construct (Figure 5). The authentic tissues can be assembled through cell adhesion, cell sorting, and tissue fusion processes [37].

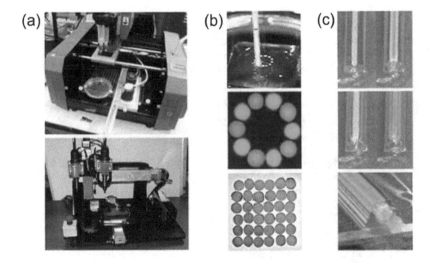

Figure 5. Scaffold-free bioprinting technology: (a) the bio-printer: 3D printing is achieved by means of a three-axis positioning system (stage in y and printing heads along x and z (top: Neatco, Carlisle, Canada; bottom: Organovo-Invetech, San Diego)); (b) spheroids with living cells are delivered one by one into the hydrogel bio-paper according to a computer script; (c) layer-by-layer deposition of cylindrical units of bio-paper (shown in blue) and multicellular cylindrical building blocks. The outcome of printing (spheroids in panel (b), multicellular cylinders in panel (c)) is a set of discrete units, which post-printing fuse to form a continuous structure. (Modified from [60])

4. Summary

Engineered scaffolds are playing an increasingly important role in tissue engineering. Scaffolds should not only have porous structures and provide mechanical support to new tissue regrowth but also have a complex mimetic hierarchical structure and biological features. Conventional scaffold fabrication techniques fail to meet these requirements for tissue regeneration. Biofabrication technologies have demonstrated potentials in this regard and can be used to create regenerative tissues or organs through the combination of state of the art fabrication techniques, materials science, and cell biology.

Author details

Ning Zhu and Xiongbiao Chen

Division of Biomedical Engineering, University of Saskatchewan, Saskatoon, SK, Canada

References

[1] Langer R, Vacanti JP. Tissue Engineering. Science 1993 May;260(5110):920-926.

[2] Liu C, Xia Z, Czernuszka JT. Design and development of three-dimensional scaffolds for tissue engineering. Chemical Engineering Research & Design 2007 Jul;85(A7): 1051-1064.

[3] Prabhakaran MP, Ghasemi-Mobarakeh L, Ramakrishna S. Electrospun composite nanofibers for tissue regeneration. Journal of Nanoscience and Nanotechnology 2011 Apr;11(4):3039-3057.

[4] Peltola SM, Melchels FPW, Grijpma DW, Kellomaki M. A review of rapid prototyping techniques for tissue engineering purposes. Annals of Medicine 2008;40(4): 268-280.

[5] Mironov V, Trusk T, Kasyanov V, Little S, Swaja R, Markwald R. Biofabrication: a 21st century manufacturing paradigm. Biofabrication 2009 Jun;1(2):022001.

[6] Hsu SH, Su CH, Chiu IM. A novel approach to align adult neural stem cells on micropatterned conduits for peripheral nerve regeneration: A feasibility study. Artificial Organs 2009 Jan;33(1):26-35.

[7] Yang Y, De Laporte L, Rives CB, Jang JH, Lin WC, Shull KR, et al. Neurotrophin releasing single and multiple lumen nerve conduits. Journal of Controlled Release 2005 Jun;104(3):433-446.

[8] Khorasani MT, Mirmohammadi SA, Irani S. Polyhydroxybutyrate (PHB) scaffolds as a model for nerve tissue engineering application: Fabrication and in vitro assay. International Journal of Polymeric Materials 2011;60(8):562-575.

[9] Pego AP, Poot AA, Grijpma DW, Feijen J. Biodegradable elastomeric scaffolds for soft tissue engineering. Journal of Controlled Release 2003 Feb;87(1-3):69-79.

[10] Huang YC, Huang YY, Huang CC, Liu HC. Manufacture of porous polymer nerve conduits through a lyophilizing and wire-heating process. Journal of Biomedical Materials Research Part B-Applied Biomaterials 2005 Jul;74B(1):659-664.

[11] Mikos AG, Thorsen AJ, Czerwonka LA, Bao Y, Langer R, Winslow DN, et al. Preparation and characterization of poly(L-lactic acid) foams. Polymer 1994 1994;35(5): 1068-1077.

[12] Mikos AG, Sarakinos G, Vacanti JP, Langer R, Cima LG, inventors. Biocompatible polymer membranes and methods of preparation of three dimensional membrane structures. United States Patent No. 5514378, 1996.

[13] Di Maio E, Mensitieri G, Iannace S, Nicolais L, Li W, Flumerfelt RW. Structure optimization of polycaprolactone foams by using mixtures of CO_2 and N_2 as blowing agents. Polymer Engineering and Science 2005 Mar;45(3):432-441.

[14] Haugen H, Ried V, Brunner M, Will J, Wintermantel E. Water as foaming agent for open cell polyurethane structures. Journal of Materials Science-Materials in Medicine 2004 Apr;15(4):343-346.

[15] Parks KL, Beckman EJ. Generation of microcellular polyurethane foams via polymerization in carbon dioxide .2. Foam formation and characterization. Polymer Engineering and Science 1996 Oct;36(19):2417-2431.

[16] Quirk RA, France RM, Shakesheff KM, Howdle SM. Supercritical fluid technologies and tissue engineering scaffolds. Current Opinion in Solid State & Materials Science 2004 Jun-Aug;8(3-4):313-321.

[17] Lee KWD, Chan PK, Feng XS. Morphology development and characterization of the phase-separated structure resulting from the thermal-induced phase separation phenomenon in polymer solutions under a temperature gradient. Chemical Engineering Science 2004 Apr;59(7):1491-1504.

[18] Ma PX, Zhang RY. Synthetic nano-scale fibrous extracellular matrix. Journal of Biomedical Materials Research 1999 Jul;46(1):60-72.

[19] Thomson RC, Wake MC, Yaszemski MJ, Mikos AG. Biodegradable polymer scaffolds to regenerate organs. Advances in Polymer Science 1995: 245-274.

[20] Pikal MJ, Shah S, Roy ML, Putman R. The secondary drying stage of freeze-dring kinetics as a function of temperature and chamber pressure. International Journal of Pharmaceutics 1990 May;60(3):203-217.

[21] Liapis AI, Bruttini R. A theory for the primary and secondary drying stages of the freeze-drying of pharmaceutical crystalline and amorphous solutes - comparison between experimental - data and theory. Separations Technology 1994 Jul;4(3):144-155.

[22] Bischof JC, He XM. Thermal stability of proteins. In: Lee RC, Despa F, Hamann KJ, editors. Cell Injury: Mechanisms, Responses, and Repair, 2005. p. 12-33.

[23] Puppi D, Chiellini F, Piras AM, Chiellini E. Polymeric materials for bone and cartilage repair. Progress in Polymer Science 2010 Apr;35(4):403-440.

[24] Subbiah T, Bhat GS, Tock RW, Pararneswaran S, Ramkumar SS. Electrospinning of nanofibers. Journal of Applied Polymer Science 2005 Apr 15;96(2):557-569.

[25] Stevens MM, George JH. Exploring and engineering the cell surface interface. Science 2005 Nov 18;310(5751):1135-1138.

[26] Huang ZM, Zhang YZ, Kotaki M, Ramakrishna S. A review on polymer nanofibers by electrospinning and their applications in nanocomposites. Composites Science and Technology 2003 Nov;63(15):2223-2253.

[27] Pham QP, Sharma U, Mikos AG. Electrospinning of polymeric nanofibers for tissue engineering applications: A review. Tissue Engineering 2006 May;12(5):1197-1211.

[28] Jain KK. Role of nanotechnology in developing new therapies for diseases of the nervous system. Nanomedicine 2006 Jun;1(1):9-12.

[29] Bhardwaj N, Kundu SC. Electrospinning: A fascinating fiber fabrication technique. Biotechnology Advances 2010 May-Jun;28(3):325-347.

[30] Yeong WY, Chua CK, Leong KF, Chandrasekaran M. Rapid prototyping in tissue engineering: challenges and potential. Trends in Biotechnology 2004 Dec;22(12):643-652.

[31] Karalekas DE. Study of the mechanical properties of nonwoven fibre mat reinforced photopolymers used in rapid prototyping. Materials & Design 2003 Dec;24(8):665-670.

[32] Wiria FE, Leong KF, Chua CK, Liu Y. Poly-epsilon-caprolactone/hydroxyapatite for tissue engineering scaffold fabrication via selective laser sintering. Acta Biomaterialia 2007 Jan;3(1):1-12.

[33] Hutmacher DW, Schantz T, Zein I, Ng KW, Teoh SH, Tan KC. Mechanical properties and cell cultural response of polycaprolactone scaffolds designed and fabricated via fused deposition modeling. Journal of Biomedical Materials Research 2001 May;55(2):203-216.

[34] Lam CXF, Mo XM, Teoh SH, Hutmacher DW. Scaffold development using 3D printing with a starch-based polymer. Materials Science & Engineering C-Biomimetic and Supramolecular Systems 2002 May 31;20(1-2):49-56.

[35] Landers R, Mulhaupt R. Desktop manufacturing of complex objects, prototypes and biomedical scaffolds by means of computer-assisted design combined with computer-guided 3D plotting of polymers and reactive oligomers. Macromolecular Materials and Engineering 2000 Oct;282(9):17-21.

[36] Khalil S, Sun W. Bioprinting endothelial cells with alginate for 3D tissue constructs. Journal of Biomechanical Engineering-Transactions of the ASME 2009 Nov;131(11).

[37] Mironov V, Kasyanov V, Drake C, Markwald RR. Organ printing: promises and challenges. Regenerative Medicine 2008 Jan;3(1):93-103.

[38] Yu D, Li Q, Mu X, Chang T, Xiong Z. Bone regeneration of critical calvarial defect in goat model by PLGA/TCP/rhBMP-2 scaffolds prepared by low-temperature rapid-prototyping technology. International Journal of Oral and Maxillofacial Surgery 2008 Oct;37(10):929-934.

[39] Chang PSH, Parker TH, Patrick CW, Miller MJ. The accuracy of stereolithography in planning craniofacial bone replacement. Journal of Craniofacial Surgery 2003 Mar; 14(2):164-170.

[40] Sodian R, Loebe M, Hein A, Martin DP, Hoerstrup SP, Potapov EV, et al. Application of stereolithography for scaffold fabrication for tissue engineered heart valves. ASAIO Journal 2002 Jan-Feb;48(1):12-16.

[41] Williams JM, Adewunmi A, Schek RM, Flanagan CL, Krebsbach PH, Feinberg SE, et al. Bone tissue engineering using polycaprolactone scaffolds fabricated via selective laser sintering. Biomaterials 2005 Aug;26(23):4817-4827.

[42] Cruz F, Simoes J, Coole T, Bocking C. Direct manufacture of hydroxyapatite based bone implants by Selective Laser Sintering, 2nd International Conference on Advanced Research and Rapid Prototyping (VRAP 2005), September 28 – October 1, 2005, Leiria, Portugal.

[43] Chen C-H, Chen J-P, Lee M-Y. Eeffects of gelatin modification on rapid prototyping PCL scaffolds for cartilage engineering. Journal of Mechanics in Medicine and Biology 2011 Dec;11(5):993-1002.

[44] Rohner D, Hutmacher DW, Cheng TK, Oberholzer M, Hammer B. In vivo efficacy of bone-marrow-coated polycaprolactone scaffolds for the reconstruction of orbital defects in the pig. Journal of Biomedical Materials Research Part B-Applied Biomaterials 2003 Aug 15;66B(2):574-580.

[45] Wiggenhauser PS, Mueller DF, Melchels FPW, Egana JT, Storck K, Mayer H, et al. Engineering of vascularized adipose constructs. Cell and Tissue Research 2012 Mar; 347(3):747-757.

[46] Koo S, Hargreaves BA, Gold GE, Dragoo JL. Fabrication of custom-shaped grafts for cartilage regeneration. The International Journal of Artificial Organs 2010 Oct;33(10): 731-737.

[47] Seitz H, Rieder W, Irsen S, Leukers B, Tille C. Three-dimensional printing of porous ceramic scaffolds for bone tissue engineering. Journal of Biomedical Materials Research Part B-Applied Biomaterials 2005 Aug;74B(2):782-788.

[48] Yilgor P, Sousa RA, Reis RL, Hasirci N, Hasirci V. 3D plotted PCL scaffolds for stem cell based bone tissue engineering. Macromolecular Symposia 2008 2008;269:92-99.

[49] El-Ayoubi R, Degrandpre C, DiRaddo R, Yousefi AM, Lavigne P. Design and dynamic culture of 3D-scaffolds for cartilage tissue engineering. Journal of Biomaterials Applications 2011 Jan;25(5):429-444.

[50] Whang K, Healy KE, Elenz DR, Nam EK, Tsai DC, Thomas CH, et al. Engineering bone regeneration with bioabsorbable scaffolds with novel microarchitecture. Tissue Engineering 1999 Spr;5(1):35-51.

[51] Wegst UGK, Schecter M, Donius AE, Hunger PM. Biomaterials by freeze casting. Philosophical Transactions of the Royal Society a-Mathematical Physical and Engineering Sciences 2010 Apr 28;368(1917):2099-2121.

[52] Zhang H, Cooper AI. Aligned porous structures by directional freezing. Advanced Materials 2007 Jun 4;19(11):1529-1533.

[53] Pham CB, Leong KF, Lim TC, Chian KS. Rapid freeze prototyping technique in bio-plotters for tissue scaffold fabrication. Rapid Prototyping Journal 2008;14(4):246-253.

[54] Zhu N, Li MG, Cooper D, Chen XB. Development of novel hybrid poly(l-lactide)/ chitosan scaffolds using the rapid freeze prototyping technique. Biofabrication 2011;3(3):034105.

[55] Albrecht DR, Underhill GH, Wassermann TB, Sah RL, Bhatia SN. Probing the role of multicellular organization in three-dimensional microenvironments. Nature Methods 2006 May;3(5):369-375.

[56] Seil JT, Webster TJ. Spray deposition of live cells throughout the electrospinning process produces nanofibrous three-dimensional tissue scaffolds. International Journal of Nanomedicine 2011 2011;6:1095-1099.

[57] Townsend-Nicholson A, Jayasinghe SN. Cell electrospinning: a unique biotechnique for encapsulating living organisms for generating active biological microthreads/ scaffolds. Biomacromolecules 2006 Dec 11;7(12):3364-3369.

[58] Hamid Q, Sun W, Asme. Coaxial electrospinning biopolymer with living cells, ASME 2010 First Global Congress on NanoEngineering for Medicine and Biology (NEMB2010), February 7-10, 2010, Houston, Texas, USA; Paper no. NEMB2010-13282, pp. 167-172.

[59] Khalil S, Sun W. Biopolyrner deposition for freefonn fabrication of hydrogel tissue constructs. Materials Science & Engineering C-Biomimetic and Supramolecular Systems 2007 Apr;27(3):469-478.

[60] Jakab K, Norotte C, Marga F, Murphy K, Vunjak-Novakovic G, Forgacs G. Tissue engineering by self-assembly and bio-printing of living cells. Biofabrication 2010 Jun; 2(2).

Chapter 4

Alignment of Cells and Extracellular Matrix Within Tissue-Engineered Substitutes

Jean-Michel Bourget, Maxime Guillemette,
Teodor Veres, François A. Auger and Lucie Germain

Additional information is available at the end of the chapter

1. Introduction

Most of the cells in our body are in direct contact with extracellular matrix (ECM) components which constitute a complex network of nano-scale proteins and glycosaminoglycans.
Those cells constantly remodel the ECM by different processes. They build it by secreting different proteins such as collagen, proteoglycans, laminins or degrade it by producing factors
such as matrix metalloproteinase (MMP). Cells interact with the ECM via specific receptors,
the integrins [1]. They also organize this matrix, guided by different stimuli, to generate patterns, essential for tissue and organ functions. Reciprocally, cells are guided by the ECM, they
modify their morphology and phenotype depending on the protein types and organization
via bidirectional integrin signaling [2-4]. In the growing field of tissue engineering [5], control
of these aspects are of the utmost importance to create constructs that closely mimic native tissues. To do so, we must take into account the composition of the scaffold (synthetic, natural,
biodegradable or not), its organization and the dimension of the structure.

The particular alignment patterns of ECM and cells observed in tissues and organs such as
the corneal stroma, vascular smooth muscle cells (SMCs), tendons, bones and skeletal muscles are crucial for organ function. SMCs express contraction proteins such as alpha-smooth-
muscle (SM)-actin, desmin and myosin [6] that are essential for cell contraction [6]. To result
in vessel contraction, the cells and ECM need to be organized in such a way that most cells
are elongated in the same axis. For tubular vascular constructs, it is suitable that SMCs align
in the circumferential direction, as they do in vivo [7, 8]. Another striking example of alignment is skeletal muscle cells that form long polynuclear cells, all elongated in the same axis.
Each cell generates a weak and short contraction pulse but collectively, it results in a strong,
long and sustained contraction of the muscle and, in term, a displacement of the member. In

the corneal stroma, the particular arrangement of the corneal fibroblasts (keratocytes) and ECM is essential to keep the transparency of this tissue [9-13]. Tendons also present a peculiar matrix alignment relative to the muscle axis. It gives a substantial resistance and exceptional mechanical properties to the tissue in that axis [14, 15]. Intervertebral discs [16], cartilage [17], dental enamel [18], and basement membrane of epithelium are other examples of tissues/organs that present peculiar cell and matrix organization. By reproducing and controlling those alignment patterns within tissue-engineered substitutes, a more physiological representation of human tissues could be achieved.

Taking into account the importance of cell microenvironment on the functionality of tissue-engineered organ substitutes, one can assume the importance of being able to customise the 3D structure of the biomaterial or scaffold supporting cell growth. To do so, some methods have been developed and most of them rely on topographic or contact guidance. This is the phenomenon by which cells elongate and migrate in the same axis as the ECM. Topographic guidance was so termed by Curtis and Clark [19] to include cell shape, orientation and movement in the concept of contact guidance described by Harrison [20] and implemented by Weiss [21, 22]. Therefore, if one can achieve ECM alignment, cells will follow the same pattern. Inversely, if cells are aligned on a patterned culture plate, the end result would be aligned ECM deposition [23].

The specific property of tissues or materials that present a variation in their mechanical and structural properties in different axis is called anisotropy. This property can be evaluated either by birefringence measurements [24, 25], mechanical testing in different axis [26], immunological staining of collagen or actin filaments [23] or direct visualisation of collagen fibrils using their self-fluorescence around 488 nm [27, 28].

Several techniques have been recently developed to mimic the specific alignment of cells within tissues to produce more physiologically relevant constructs. In this chapter, we will describe five different techniques, collagen gel compaction, electromagnetic field, electrospinning of nanofibers, mechanical stimulation and microstructured culture plates.

2. Methods to align cells and ECM in tissue-engineered constructs

2.1. Collagen gel

Collagen is the main constituent of the ECM [1], it is therefore logical to use it as a scaffold for tissue engineering [29, 30]. Collagen is produced by cells as a protocollagen strand that, upon enzymatic modification, will be able to assemble into procollagen triple helix and then into tropocollagen triple helix. Self-assembly of tropocollagen into collagen microfibrils is followed by lysyl oxidase crosslinking to finally form a collagen fiber [31]. For tissue engineering applications, collagen can be extracted from dermis of different species including bovine, porcine, avian and human [32, 33] and tissues such as human placenta [34]. Collagen monomer can be bought commercially from different providers. However, these solutions do not always contain the full-length collagen molecule, which can affect its properties.

Preparation of a collagen gel from these solutions is quite simple, the collagen solution, provided at pH 2, self-assemble at 37°C and at a neutral pH. Cells can be added to the solution after neutralisation and before casting of the gel, allowing for a uniform distribution of cells in the construct. As cells migrate and elongate into the gel, they will try to anchor themselves to the collagen fibers, but since the collagen gels are soft, cells will deform the fibril network causing the gel to compact [35]. If this contraction is controlled by applying a static constraint in one direction, the gel will contract differentially in the constrained and unconstrained axis. This will result in an anisotropic construct because collagen fibers and cells will become aligned in the constrained axis [34, 36, 37].

Thomopoulos et al. [28] used fibroblast populated collagen gels that were constrained either uniaxially or biaxially to evaluate the anisotropy generated in the gel. Uniaxial static strain resulted in gel contraction in the unconstrained axis and lead to a structural and mechanical anisotropy. They found no difference between tendon fibroblasts and cardiac fibroblasts in anisotropy generated in the construct. They also demonstrated that active remodeling of the gel by cells is not necessary for the development of anisotropy in collagen gel. Indeed, uniaxially constrained collagen gel without cells also become anisotropic. This surprising result could be explained by the force generated by collagen polymerisation [38]. They also developed a mathematical model to predict anisotropy in fibroblast-populated collagen gels [39]. They found that mechanical anisotropy could not be explained solely by collagen fibers alignment, but also take into account the redistribution of collagen fibers upon remodeling, nonaffine fiber kinematics [40, 41] and fiber lengths. Costa et al. [42] also investigated the mechanism of cell and matrix alignment in constrained collagen gels. They constrained fibroblast-containing collagen gels with different shapes (square, triangle and circle) and liberated one or more of the edges to create anisotropy into the gel. Contrasting with a previous report of Klebe et al. [43], they showed that fully constrained gels present random cell and matrix orientation. Nevertheless, on the basis of the results obtained in their study, Costa et al. proposed that rather than aligning along the local direction of greatest tension, cells orient parallel to the local free boundary. An interesting result was obtained with the round shape constrain. As expected, no alignment were present when gel was uniformly constrained, but when they cut a central hole in the construct, the gel contracted away from the central hole and cells aligned in the circumferential orientation. This result is consistent with previous results obtained in blood vessel reconstruction in which a collagen gel is contracting around a central mandrel causing circumferential cell alignment [34]. Grinnell and Lamke [44] cultured fibroblasts on hydrated collagen lattices. They found that cells reorganized the network and aligned the collagen fibrils in the plane of cell spreading, becoming more densely packed. They noted that the lattice has thinned to one-tenth of its original thickness.

Weinberg and bell [45] used collagen gel seeded with bovine cells to produce the first tissue-engineered blood vessel. This weak construct was supported by a Dacron mesh in order to sustain physiological pressure. This method was improved later by other groups to enhance mechanical properties of the collagen gel to get rid of the synthetic material, but those constructs were still too weak to be implanted. L'heureux et al. [34] produced such a tissue-engineered blood vessel using collagen gel. The gel was made of a mixture of human type I and III collagen at a final concentration of 3 mg/ml, it was seeded with human SMCs and finally casted around a cylindrical mandrel, forming the media layer. The anisotropic strain generated by the mandrel constraining gel compaction, combined to a manual detachment of the gel adhesion to the mandrel, caused a progressive circumferential alignment of the SMC. The same process was repeated to produce the adventitia, using human dermal fibroblast embedded in collagen gel and casted around the media layer. Contrasting with the result obtained with the SMC media layer, fibroblasts of the adventitial layer did not get self-oriented. This type of construct was still too weak to be implanted. This paper also showed that gel compaction speed is influenced by initial cell seeding concentration in the construct.

Collagen gel has also been used to engineered intervertebral disc. The highly organized annulus fibrosus which present a cell and matrix alignment, is contrasting with the nucleus pulposus showing random organization. Bowles et al. [16] isolated cells from both parts of the intervertebral disc and seeded them into collagen gels. Interestingly, cells kept their capacities to become organized or not when cultured in vitro and seeded into collagen gel constructs. Robert Tranquillo published several papers using collagen gel, mostly on engineered vascular constructs. Some of his work was done using magnetic alignment of fibers, it will be discussed in the following section. In 1992, they [46] described mathematical theories to understand the complex coupling of cell and matrix deformation in collagen gel populated with cells.

Thus, alignment of cells in collagen gel was one of the first cell alignment method applied to tissue engineering. It is easy to perform, relatively inexpensive and gives interesting results for specific applications. On the other hand, collagen gel do not show mechanical properties sufficient for load bearing application such as bone, cartilage, ligament and blood vessels, at least if it is used alone.

2.2. Electromagnetic field

Electromagnetic field (EMF) can affect multiple aspects of cell behavior and ECM remodeling. We are always in contact with EMF, either coming from the earth, high voltage lines or mobile phones [47, 48]. It is still unclear whether EMF are linked or not to health problems such as cancer, but this hypothesis seems unlikely in most cases [49]. Even if mobile phone usage is probably not linked with brain cancer, the capability of EMF to influence cells and extracellular matrix are clearly demonstrated [50-55]. It is therefore crucial to investigate this relation to first prevent potential deleterious exposure that might lead to health problem and second, to understand mechanisms and eventually develop novel medical therapies [56-58] as well as tissue engineering applications [59-63]. When exposed to a strong EMF, collagen, as well as other biomolecules such as fibrin, will align perpendicularly to the field. This phenomenon is caused by the negative diamagnetic anisotropy of the collagen molecules [64]. This property causes the polymerisation process to take place in a particular orientation. Tissue engineers have used this property to produce alignment of ECM scaffolds and cells in different reconstructed tissues. EMF was also shown to induce orientation of cells, including epithelial cells [65-67], fibroblasts [65, 68], erythrocytes [69] and osteoblasts [61, 70].

The tendency of biomolecules to align in an EMF has been demonstrated more than 30 years ago, but tissue engineering applications have arisen more recently. Strong EMF were proposed as a method to align fibrin polymer by Torbet et al. [71]. They reported that polymerisation of fibrin gels under a strong EMF resulted in oriented fibrin polymerisation. They also speculate right when proposing that this technique could be extended to other polymers and to living cells as it was done afterward. Twenty-six years later, the same researcher [72, 73] used EMF to align collagen fibers, in order to replicate the physiologic structure of the corneal stroma. This structure possesses a particular arrangement of aligned collagen fibers that cross each other orthogonally. This pattern was recreated by cycle of gelation-rotation-gelation of type I collagen under a 7 Tesla (T) EMF. When corneal fibroblasts, or keratocytes, are seeded in the construct, they align themselves by contact guidance in the local orientation of the scaffold. This technique was used to produce a hemi-cornea, composed of the stroma and the epithelial layer and showed promising results when grafted on an animal model [62]. Even if this represents a significant advance in corneal tissue engineering, the resulting corneal stroma substitute presents a slightly different geometry than native cornea. In a non-pathological cornea, the arrangement of orthogonal lamellas within the stroma consist of a mesh of orthogonal collagen lamellas that are woven together in multilayer. This arrangement provides the cornea with a strong mechanical resistance while remaining a transparent structure [74-77]. Reproducing this geometry over the normal thickness of the stroma seems quite difficult using this layer-by-layer technique. Kotani et al [70] studied the effect of EMF on bone formation and orientation. They have shown that, when exposed to a strong EMF of 8 T, osteoblasts oriented parallel to the field. In contrast, when osteoblasts and collagen are mix together, the alignment of both constituents is perpendicular to the field, as for collagen alone. This supposed that contact guidance is a stronger inducer of cell alignment than EMF. Two years later, [61] they showed that exposure of mouse osteoblasts to a strong EMF improved differentiation and matrix synthesis in vitro. They also demonstrated that ectopic bone formation in vivo is stimulated by EMF. When pellets of collagen (1.2 mg/pellet, bovine) containing bone morphogenic protein 2 (5 μg/pellet, human recombinant) are implanted subcutaneously and exposed to an 8 T EMF, bone formation was exacerbated and aligned parallel to the EMF.

Robert Tranquillo used EMF as a method to align cells and ECM in tissue-engineered constructs [59, 63, 78, 79], with a particular focus on media substitutes. In 1993, Guido et al. [24] developed a quantitative method to study cells and fibrils orientation when submitted to an EMF. This method used time-lapse image analysis and live automated birefringence measurements to quantify this phenomenon. Tranquillo et al. [59] showed that a 4.7 T EMF could orient collagen fibrillogenesis resulting in a circonferential orientation, in order to create a media equivalent. Barocas et al. [80] compared four different fabrication conditions for a media equivalent composed of SMC embedded in a collagen gel that were either submitted to EMF and/or mandrel compaction. Compaction of the gel around a central mandrel by SMCs induced a circumferential alignment of cells and collagen fibers, as demonstrated previously [34]. Magnetic circumferential alignment was performed prior gel compaction to produce prealigned gels. When those gels were allowed to contract freely, the circumferential alignment was lost, but when a mandrel was present, the alignment was better than with EMF alone. This method can also be used to guide neurite outgrowth of neural cells. Dubey et al. used collagen [81] and fibrin [82] aligned gel to control outgrowth of neurite. When fibers were aligned, neurite outgrowths were stimulated and could therefore grow longer than random aligned controls.

Retrospectively, this method is effective for biological scaffold such as collagen and fibrin, but to our knowledge, alignment of synthetic materials such as poly(glycolic acid) (PGA) or poly(D,L-lactide-co-glycolide) (PLGA) has not been performed yet. This technique requires a special apparatus capable of generating a strong EMF. Cell viability does not seem to be affected by EMF, allowing for a uniform cell distribution in the construct.

2.3. Electrospun nanofiber

Electrospinning of nanofibers is an interesting approach to produce scaffold for tissue engineering [83-89]. This technique can be used to produce aligned scaffold that will dictate cell elongation by contact guidance [90]. The process of producing polymer microfiber using electrostatic forces was patented in 1934 by Formhals [91] but tissue engineering applications such as musculoskeletal [92] and vascular [93] has been developed recently. Electrospinning can be performed with simple setup consisting of a syringe pump, a high voltage source, and a rotating collector [85]. Precise description of the different possible setups and techniques have been reviewed in details previously [94]. Briefly, a polymer solution is hanging at the tip of a syringe needle by surface tension. When an electric current is applied, EMF results in charge repulsion within the polymer solution, causing the initiation of a jet. Solvent evaporate while jet is traveling, resulting in polymerisation into fibers, which are captured by a collector [94]. Depending on settings and polymers used, those fibers can range from 3 nm to greater than 5 μm in diameter [95]. This technique has been used to engineer many types of scaffolds for tissue engineering [90] including synthetic polymer such as poly(D,L-lactide-co-glycolide) (PLGA) [96], poly-(ε-caprolactone) (PCL) [97], 50:50 poly(L-lactic acid-co-ε-caprolactone) (PLCL) fibers [98], or natural polymer such as collagen [99] or fibrin [100] for various tissue applications. It is also possible to create composite scaffolds by spinning different polymer solution either together or consecutively on the same target. Due to the great plasticity of the technique, it is simple to engineer different patterns to guide cell fate in the desired direction. In order to do so, a rotating mandrel can be used to collect the fiber, resulting in aligned nanofibers [101].

Jose et al. [102] developed an aligned nanofibrous scaffold for bone tissue engineering. This scaffold is a nanocomposite copolymer of PLGA and nano-hydroxyapatite (HA). Fiber diameters, glass transition temperature, storage modulus and degradation rate were characterized for different concentration of nano-HA from 0 to 20%. Briefly, average fiber diameters were augmented from 300 nm for PLGA to 700 nm for 20% nano-HA but formed aggregate at those high concentration. Fiber alignment capability was not influenced by nano-HA concentration. Mechanical properties of the composite material were modulated by nano-HA concentration, it acted as a reinforcement agent at lower concentration (1% and 5 %) but induced defects in the structure at higher concentrations (10 % and 20 %). Influences were also seen in degradation rate and storage modulus. In order to show cell compati-

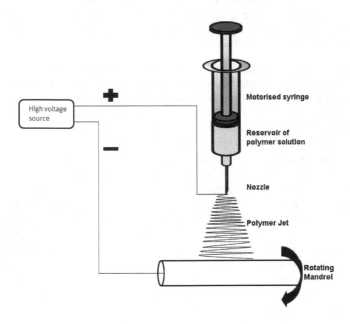

Figure 1. Schematization of an electrospinning setup. The polymer solution is positively charged while the rotating mandrel is negative. The solution is pushed through the nozzle at constant speed. The solvent evaporates while the jet is travelling, resulting in fibers formation.

bility, a collagen component was added to the PLGA (20:80) [103], and human mesenchymal stem cells (MSCs) were used for the demonstration. Thomas et al. [104] investigated the effect of rotation speed on scaffold alignment, mechanical properties and morphologies. They used a nanofibrous mesh of PCL collected at zero, 3,000 and 6,000 rpm for bone tissue engineering. When the collector rotation speed is increased, more aligned fibers were produced. This resulted in a modification of the morphology and mechanical properties of individual fibers and of the resulting scaffold. Interestingly, the hardness and Young's modulus of individual fibers were diminished while increasing rotation speed, but opposite results were obtained when the whole resulting scaffold was analysed. Ultimate tensile strength of the scaffold in the axis of alignment rises from 2.2 to 9.6 MPa when rotation speed was increased from 0 to 6,000 rpm. This result could be explained by increasing fiber alignment and packing as well as a decrease in inter-fiber pore size when rotation speed is increased. Li et al. [92] performed a similar study on rotation speed. They used electrospun aligned nanofibrous scaffold to control anisotropy into tissue-engineered musculoskeletal constructs. Their scaffolds were also made of a biodegradable PCL polymer, casted on a rotating target to align fibers. Increasing the rotation speed of the shaft from 0 to 9.3 m/s (0 to 7,000 rpm) produced more aligned fibers, to a maximum of 94 % of fibers aligned within a 20° angle range, at maximum speed. Alignment of the ECM leads to an increase in the isotropic tensile modulus ranging from 2.1 MPa for unaligned controls to 11.6 MPa for the aligned substrate at 9.3 m/s. Human MSCs and meniscus fibrochondrocytes, seeded on these aligned scaffolds, attached and elongated in the fibers direction. It is also possible with this technique to produce successive layers at different angles by changing the rotation vector.

Teh et al. [105] produced a silk fibroin (SF) hybrid scaffold for ligament regeneration. Silk is an interesting material for tissue engineering, but the hyper-allergenic sericin component must be removed. It has an interesting degradation rate and show remarkable mechanical properties. Silk was previously used to culture fibroblasts and keratinocytes [106]. The new design proposed by Teh et al. is composed of a bilayered SF, contained a knitted SF fibrous mesh layer and an aligned SF electrospun fibers cast on rotating rods. This construct was seeded with MSCs before rolling it into a cylindrical ligament analog. They found that MSCs differentiation into ligament fibroblast was enhanced by the alignment of the fibers. This resulted in an improvement of tensile properties from 125 to 158 N after 14 days and in an increase of ligament-related protein levels such as collagen I and III as well as Tenascin-c. Xu et al. [93] produced an aligned polymer nanofibrous scaffold for blood vessel reconstruction. They used a biodegradable copolymer of poly(L-lactid-co-ε-caprolactone) [P(LLA-CL)] (75:25), aligned using a rotating disc. They demonstrated that human coronary SMCs elongated and migrated in the direction of the fibers and express a spindle-like contractile phenotype with better adherence and proliferation than on control polymer. Yang et al. [107] used a fibrous scaffold to guide neural cells. They used mouse neural stem cells seeded in a poly(L-Lactic acid) (PLLA) nano/micro fibrous scaffolds made by electrospinning. By using two different concentrations of the PLLA solution, 2% and 5%, they were able to cast nanofibers of 150 to 500 nm and microfibers of 800 to 3000 nm, respectively. They have shown that cell elongation and neurite outgrowth is parallel to fiber's direction. They found that the differentiation of neural precursor cells was higher on nanofibers than on microfibers but independent of cell alignment.

Collagen scaffold produced by electrospinning was done by Matthews et al. [108]. In this paper, they set the basis for electrospinning of collagen fibers for tissue engineering application by varying different parameters (collagen source and concentration, solvent, input voltage). With optimal conditions found in this study, they obtained a matrix containing collagen fibers of 100 nm of diameter that exhibited a 67 nm banding pattern, characteristic of native collagen fibers. They cultured aortic SMCs into this collagen scaffold and obtained uniform distribution of cells into the construct. Zhong et al. [109] went further with collagen nanofibrous scaffolds for fibroblast culture. They used calf skin type I collagen, at 80 mg/ml, electrospunned over a wheel rotating at 15 m/s and formed fibrils of 180 nm, which is smaller than the unaligned ones that have an average diameter of 250 nm. They treated their collagen construct with glutaraldehyde vapor (30%) to enhance the biostability of the scaffold. After seeding the construct with rabbit conjunctiva fibroblasts, they measured cell adhesion, proliferation, morphology and interaction with the scaffold. In addition to cell alignment, they noted a lower cell adhesion but higher cell proliferation on aligned constructs.

Given that electrospinning is a versatile technique to produce aligned ECM for tissue engineering, by modifying the casting parameters (rotation speed, input voltage, distance from target, dimension of the tip) or the composition of the solution (type of polymer, solvent, concentration) it is possible to produce different structures in terms of fiber diameters and composition. It is also possible to cast successive layers with different orientations to obtain a complex scaffold. This technique will certainly be perfected in the future using computerized and robotized set-up to produce reproducible and complex scaffolds for various tissue engineering applications.

2.4. Microstructured culture plates

As explained above, topographic guidance is the process by which cells respond to the particular arrangement of their environment by modifying their shape and migration vectors [110]. In vivo, cell environment is composed mostly of native collagen molecules and proteoglycans, in vitro, researchers tried to mimic the cues given by proteins to influence cell fate. Those cues can come from different structures resembling or not collagen molecules and have been discuss in previous pages. In the following section, it is the very structure of the culture plate that dictates the organization of cells. To do so, gratings of various dimensions and shapes are created by various methods into a cell-compatible plastic and cells are seeded over it.

Among the different methods to create and control the type and the shape of the guiding structures, there are very interesting and versatile approaches using microfabrication processes analog to the ones developed by the microelectronic industry [111, 112].

Structures with features ranging from nano- to tens of microns scale matching both the ECM proteins or cells dimension can now be created. These techniques can be adapted to different polymers for various applications and use either polymer casting, micromachining or thermoforming. This section will focus on the most common process that uses photolithography and hot embossing as an example. Briefly, a pattern is printed in chromium on a quartz plate to form the mask for photolithography. A photoresist is poured over a silicon plate and exposed to UV light under the mask. The resist is then developed in organic solvent to reveal the pattern and obtain the first wafer (master). This master wafer is then replicated in a polydimethylsiloxan (PDMS) mold that is cured into the silicon wafer. PDMS can be used for cell culture or be replicated on another substrate. In order to replicate it, hot embossing with an intermediate epoxy wafer is used to finally obtain the desired pattern in the chosen polymer.

Numerous types of materials could be used for the final cell culture step. Polystyrene is an interesting material due to its great biocompatibility, being used regularly for cell culture flask [113]. Teixeira et al. [114] have shown that corneal epithelial cells take an elongated shape and aligned themselves along with grooves and ridges as small as 70 nm. They tested various lengths of grooves and ridges to show that cell alignment is similar from 70 nm to 850 nm ridges but is reduced with 1900 nm ridges. Those lengths were chosen to match the approximate dimension of the basement membrane features. In another paper [115], they showed similar results using corneal stromal fibroblasts (keratocytes). They obtain 70% of aligned fibroblasts with pitch (sum of groove and ridge) larger than 800 nm where as few as 35% of epithelial cells were aligned in the features direction. This is a logical result considering how fibroblastic cells elongate and migrate more than epithelial cells, they are therefore more prone or easy to align.

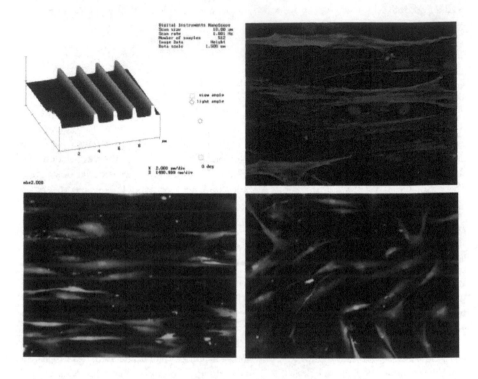

Figure 2. A) Atomic force microscopy of a sample used for replica molding. The master wafer represents the inverse (the negative) of the final results in polystyrene. B) Smooth muscle cells on a microstructured substrate of grooves (1 um) and ridges (4 um) after 1 day of culture. Cells are elongated in the direction of the microstructured pattern. C-D) Human dermal fibroblasts (GFP+) cultured on the same microstructured substrate (C) or on flat plastic (D) after 1 day.

Isenberg et al. [116] cultured SMCs on 50 μm wide and 5 μm deep gratings. They used a combination of photolithography and hot embossing [117] to reproduce patterns of ridges and grooves on polystyrene substrate coated with a thermoresponsive polymer, poly(N-iso-propylacrylamide) (PIPAAm) compatible with cell culture [118]. They seeded human aortic SMC on these microtextured culture substrates and allow them to form cell sheets. At room temperature, the cell sheet spontaneously detach from the culture substrate and can be manipulated. In this paper, they have shown that cells elongated and migrated in the direction of the grooves but did not evaluate mechanical or structural anisotropy. In 2012, [119] they tested those parameters and showed mechanical anisotropy in the resulting media layer that mimic the organization of the native vessel.

Guillemette et al. [23] used photolithography and hot embossing to create a pattern of ridges and grooves (4 μm wide, 500 nm deep) in a thermoplastic elastomer, the styrene-(ethylene/ butylene)-styrene block co-polymer (SEBS) [120]. Aligned sheets of SMCs, dermal fibroblasts and corneal fibroblasts were produced using the self-assembly or cell sheet engineering approach [121, 122]. All three cell types aligned in the direction of the long axis of the ridges and grooves, for the cells in direct contact with the substrate. Cells grown with ascorbic acid produced ECM and formed tissues comprising many cell layers [119]. Interestingly, suprabasal cell layer that is in contact with the first cell layer aligned themselves with a shift angle from the previous layer characteristic of the cell type. Guillemette et al. [123] used a combination of micromolding and laser microablation to culture cardiac muscle cells. A pattern of grooves and ridges was designed so that wide grooves could be ablated using a laser to create a porous mesh for cardiac cells to grow. Two different pore shapes were studied, square pores and rectangle pores to increase anisotropy. It was shown that square holes are less effective than rectangle holes in aligning cells within the long axis, and that the combination of rectangle holes and grooves gives better alignment than rectangle holes alone. This demonstration pertains to the classic action of cell alignment on an ECM, and improvement of cell functionality as an end result.

2.5. Mechanical strain

Many cells in the human body are subjected to mechanical stress that dictates their phenotype and orientation. This adaptive process starts within the embryo, but is driven by stress and controlled by morphogen gradients or other cues still to be identified. Mechanical stress is probably an inducer for some cell alignment, such as in vasculogenesis [124].

Cell alignment, induced following compaction of collagen gel around a mandrel [34], is driven by mechanical strain anisotropy. For blood vessel reconstruction, a circumferential constraint causes cell and ECM to align circumferentially, as long as the scaffolding gel could move freely in the longitudinal direction. Nevertheless, there is a particular interest in applying mechanical stimulation to different tissue-engineered constructs including vessel, bone, cartilage and ligament, for the induction of alignment and maturation.

Mechanical strain, as a method to align cells and matrix in order to improve functionality, was extensively used in vascular tissue engineering. Mostly via transluminal pressurisation or via a circulating medium in a specifically designed bioreactor. It has been shown by Kanda et al.[125] that a dynamic deformation of 5% at 60 Hertz of a ring of collagen gel containing SMCs will cause cells and ECM to align in the circumferential direction. Niklason et al. [126] has shown that vascular substitutes, made using a PGA scaffold, submitted to pulsed flow for weeks improved mechanical properties, resulting in a burst pressure of more than 2000 mmHg. In this study, cell and matrix alignment was not investigated. Nerem's team has shown that collagen gels present improved mechanical properties and circumferential alignment of the ECM when submitted to a cyclic deformation of 10% at 1 Hz frequency [127] and this process was driven by the ECM remodeling by matrix metalloproteinase 2 [128-130]

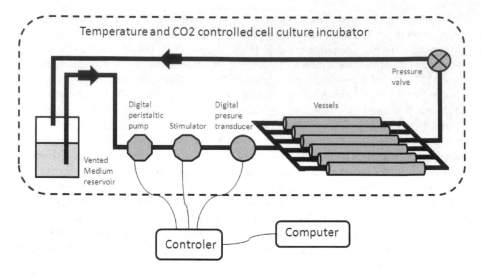

Figure 3. Design of a bioreactor for mechanical strain stimulation of tissue-engineered cylindrical constructs. The culture medium is pumped from the medium reservoir, which is vented through a 0.22 μm sterile air filter, with a computer controlled peristaltic pump. The stimulator is composed of a computer-controlled piston that can generate a cyclic strain in the vessels. The pressure transducer monitors the variation in pressure. The pressure valve ensures an adequate pressure to be built in the vessels. Such devices are commercially available.

Grenier et al. [131, 132] demonstrated that SMCs sheets produced by self-assembly [26, 121, 133] can undergo collagen reorganization following an uniaxial static stretch. More recently, Gauvin et al. [134] extended this experiment using human dermal fibroblast sheets with dynamic stimulation. Constructs were subjected for 3 days to either a static strain of 10%, or a dynamic mechanical stimulation of 10% at 1 Hz. As expected, cells and ECM aligned in the strain axis when submitted to either static or dynamic mechanical stimulation. Ultimate tensile strength and tensile modulus were increased in dynamic mechanical stimulation as compared to unstrained controls and to static strain. Therefore, it demonstrated that mechanical stimulation contributed to establishment of anisotropy in the structure and improves mechanical properties of cell sheet based constructs.

Isenberg et al. [135] evaluated the effects of mechanical strain on media equivalent with an experimental design that isolate its effect from other confounding factors such as gel compaction, creep fatigue and fiber alignment. Therefore, they waited 2 weeks for gel compaction to stabilize, used ribose cross links to fix fiber orientation and to prevent creep deformation. Finally, they placed the construct on distensible latex tubing in a custom designed chamber to produce a pure circumferential strain. They found that modulus and ultimate tensile strength were augmented when the constructs were stimulated for 5 weeks (no change at 2 weeks), at 5% strain, 0,5 Hz and 12.5% duty cycle. Therefore, they demonstrated that independently of the effect on cell and ECM alignment, mechanical strain increased the mechanical properties of collagen based media substitutes.

2.6. Other techniques

There are other techniques that have been developed to align cells and ECM that were not discussed yet. Some of these techniques were too specific or not enough common to give them a complete section, however a quick overview of some of these methods will be given below.

The first method that will be discussed in this section is shear stress. This force is of great importance for blood vessels where it dictates the longitudinal alignment of endothelial cells. This longitudinal configuration is really important for cell function and disturbance in blood flow cause the alignment to be lost. In vessel branching for example, it is associated with endothelial dysfunction, atherosclerosis development and thrombus formation [136]. This capability of endothelial cells to sense the shear stress and align themselves in response to the stimuli rely on specialized cell component called primary cilia [137-139]. This capability can be reproduced in vitro using either a laminar flow chamber [140, 141] or a bioreactor for transluminal flow, either on reconstructed [121] or native [142] endothelium. To induce an alignment response of endothelial cells in vitro, it is important to take into account the parameters that influence the resulting shear stress on endothelium. Those parameters are: vessel section surface, fluid flow and fluid viscosity. Alignment of endothelial cells is influenced by wall shear stress intensity, exposure time and turbidity [110].

A second method, also dependant on shear, was recently developed by McClendon et al. [143] and takes advantage of the biocompatibility of the peptide amphiphile (PA) [144, 145] to produce circumferentially aligned tubes acting as scaffold for arterial tissue engineering. The PA is contained in a liquid crystalline solution that form aligned domains that can be trapped in a gel showing macroscopic alignment by applying low shear rates and ionic crosslink. The interesting point about this technique is the possibility of incorporating cells while forming the scaffold, allowing for full cell penetration into the culture substrate. Therefore, they encapsulated SMCs into their construct and showed that cells proliferated and aligned themselves in the direction of the scaffold, without depending on external stimuli or gel compaction.

Another method for cell alignment is by printing a protein pattern on a culture surface. Cells seeded on these surfaces will adhere and migrate preferentially on the printed pattern resulting in an aligned culture. Thakar et al. [146] used this technique to align vascular SMCs on collagen strip of various width, in order to investigate the relationship between morphology and function of these cells. This interesting technique is difficult to use in a tissue engineering perspective because cells will gradually invade the unprinted region of the surface and therefore alignment of cells will be gradually lost over time.

3. Discussion

The field of tissue engineering has moved forward at great speed in the last two decades, as shown by the rapid augmentation of the number of publication with the terms "tissue engineering" on Pubmed. Researchers have built models for in vitro testing and substitutes that work well within different animal models. On the other hand, there are only a few tissue engineering products that have been tested in humans and even fewer that have moved on as FDA approved product for the market. The words "tissue engineering" allowed retrieval of 46 records on clinicaltrials.gov at the end of august 2012. Beside complications regarding regulatory affairs to get a product accepted, falling in a category between medical device and pharmaceutical drugs [147, 148], some substitutes failed to show adequate mechanical properties to do the job right. Creating more physiological substitutes by recreating the geometry of native ECM and cells is a quite interesting way to improve resistance without introducing a new material or create a thicker construct.

In this chapter, some of the existing techniques that have been published to produce tissue-engineered constructs showing a customised geometry were reviewed. Most of these techniques have been developed for other applications, and adapted later for tissue engineering. Alignment of collagen fibers in collagen gel constrained uniaxially is probably the oldest one, it is a quite simple technique where cell align themselves in the axis of the constraint. This model has been combined with EMF alignment of biomolecules, a more complex technique that direct ECM assembly in a desired orientation. Electrospun nanofibers are becoming more popular in the field and the simple modification of adding a rotating target make it an interesting technique for ECM alignment. The recent advances in microfabrication have made it easy to produce the custom culture substrates that present nanoscale structures at the ECM level. While contact or topographic guidance has been studied quite a while ago, this capability of cells to align themselves in the direction of grooves and ridges of certain dimension is interesting for tissue engineering applications, especially with cell sheet engineering. Finally, mechanical strain is a strong inducer of cell alignment that dictates the geometry of cells in our body. This technique is of great interest for load bearing applications such as cartilage, bone or vascular tissue engineering. Each of the technique mentioned above have advantages and drawbacks, and some of them are dependent on the type of tissue desired.

Constrained collagen gel compaction is a simple technique that is compatible with cell seeding prior gelation, allowing for a uniform cell distribution throughout the construct. On the other hand, collagen gel presents poor mechanical properties, making them unsuitable for load bearing applications such as vascular tissue engineering. The development of hydrogels has helped to partially overcome this problem [29]. Alignment of ECM and cells in EMF is an effective technique but it necessitate state-of-the-art apparatus, not commonly available in a lab, in order to generate an EMF between 4 T and 8 T. As for collagen gels, cells can be added into the solution to have a uniform cell distribution. This technique seems to be restricted at this time to biomolecules, therefore limiting its application field. It can be combined with controlled collagen gel compaction to produce a more potent alignment. Electrospinning of polymer fibers is a very interesting technique that can be applied to a lot of different kinds of polymers by simply modifying the parameters of casting. This technique is particularly effective for tubular constructs since using a cylindrical mandrel as the target will directly create the desired construct. However, it is not possible to seed cells while casting the construct. Therefore, cells will need to penetrate the construct on their own, causing cell distribution to be potentially non homogenous if the construct is too thick or not enough porous to allow for cell migration. Microstructured culture plate is an effective technique, especially for cell sheet engineering or self-assembly. This approach relies on the capacity of cells to secrete and organize ECM. When grown on structured substrate, cells will align the extracellular matrix in the direction of the grooves. With this technique, it is possible to create complex design of cell alignment by modifying the surface topography. This is the only method described here that does not rely on a pre-existing scaffolding material. On the other hand, producing those cell culture substrates is long and costly, needing access to a microfabrication clean room containing expensive apparatus. Mechanical strain can be applied by a number of different setups depending on the construct type. This technique is effective to align the whole construct in a preferred direction, but complex patterns cannot be created. The cost of this technique depends on the setting that could be computer-controlled or not. Mechanical stress must be precisely controlled since a strain that would be too strong could lead to creeping of the construct or affect cell viability or ECM integrity.

4. Conclusion

The future of tissue engineering relies on the production of more complex structures, composed of many cell types that will interact together. In order to do so, cells must be assembled together in a structure that mimics their native microenvironment. Techniques to align and organize scaffolds will continue to go forward and new technologies will arise, pushed by the constant need for tissue-engineered constructs for organ transplantation.

Author details

Jean-Michel Bourget[1,2,3], Maxime Guillemette[4], Teodor Veres[5], François A. Auger[1,2] and Lucie Germain[1,2]

1 Laval University LOEX center, Tissue Engineering And Regenerative Medecine : LOEX – FRQS Research Center of the "Centre Hospitalier Affilié Universitaire de Québec", Canada

2 Department of Surgery, Faculty of Medicine, Laval University, Quebec, Canada

3 National Research Council Canada, Boucherville, PQ, Canada

4 Physics Department, Faculty of Science and Engineering, Laval University, and Medical Physics Unit, "Centre Hospitalier Universitaire de Québec", Québec, QC, Canada

5 Life Sciences Division, National Research Council Canada, Biomedical Engineering, McGill University, National Research Council Canada, Boucherville, PQ, Canada

References

[1] Alberts B. Molecular biology of the cell. 5th ed. New York: Garland Science; 2008.

[2] Delon I, Brown NH. Integrins and the actin cytoskeleton. Curr Opin Cell Biol. 2007;19:43-50.

[3] Arnaout MA, Mahalingam B, Xiong JP. Integrin structure, allostery, and bidirectional signaling. Annu Rev Cell Dev Biol. 2005;21:381-410.

[4] Wiesner S, Legate KR, Fassler R. Integrin-actin interactions. Cell Mol Life Sci. 2005;62:1081-99.

[5] Langer R, Vacanti JP. Tissue engineering. Science. 1993;260:920-6.

[6] Koubassova NA, Tsaturyan AK. Molecular mechanism of actin-myosin motor in muscle. Biochemistry (Mosc). 2011;76:1484-506.

[7] Holzapfel GA, Sommer G, Gasser CT, Regitnig P. Determination of layer-specific mechanical properties of human coronary arteries with nonatherosclerotic intimal thickening and related constitutive modeling. Am J Physiol Heart Circ Physiol. 2005;289:H2048-58.

[8] Wolinsky H, Glagov S. Structural Basis for the Static Mechanical Properties of the Aortic Media. Circ Res. 1964;14:400-13.

[9] Robert L, Legeais JM, Robert AM, Renard G. Corneal collagens. Pathol Biol (Paris). 2001;49:353-63.

[10] Pinsky PM, van der Heide D, Chernyak D. Computational modeling of mechanical anisotropy in the cornea and sclera. J Cataract Refract Surg. 2005;31:136-45.

[11] Kamma-Lorger CS, Hayes S, Boote C, Burghammer M, Boulton ME, Meek KM. Effects on collagen orientation in the cornea after trephine injury. Mol Vis. 2009;15:378-85.

[12] Boote C, Elsheikh A, Kassem W, Kamma-Lorger CS, Hocking PM, White N, et al. The influence of lamellar orientation on corneal material behavior: biomechanical and structural changes in an avian corneal disorder. Invest Ophthalmol Vis Sci. 2011;52:1243-51.

[13] Boote C, Kamma-Lorger CS, Hayes S, Harris J, Burghammer M, Hiller J, et al. Quantification of collagen organization in the peripheral human cornea at micron-scale resolution. Biophys J. 2011;101:33-42.

[14] Lewis G, Shaw KM. Modeling the tensile behavior of human Achilles tendon. Biomed Mater Eng. 1997;7:231-44.

[15] Lynch HA, Johannessen W, Wu JP, Jawa A, Elliott DM. Effect of fiber orientation and strain rate on the nonlinear uniaxial tensile material properties of tendon. J Biomech Eng. 2003;125:726-31.

[16] Bowles RD, Williams RM, Zipfel WR, Bonassar LJ. Self-assembly of aligned tissue-engineered annulus fibrosus and intervertebral disc composite via collagen gel contraction. Tissue Eng Part A. 2010;16:1339-48.

[17] Jeffery AK, Blunn GW, Archer CW, Bentley G. Three-dimensional collagen architecture in bovine articular cartilage. J Bone Joint Surg Br. 1991;73:795-801.

[18] Paine ML, Snead ML. Protein interactions during assembly of the enamel organic extracellular matrix. J Bone Miner Res. 1997;12:221-7.

[19] Curtis ASG, Clark P. The Effects of Topographic and Mechanical-Properties of Materials on Cell Behavior. Critical Reviews in Biocompatibility. 1990;5:343-62.

[20] Harrison RG. The reaction of embryonic cells to solid structures. Journal of Experimental Zoology. 1914;17:521-44.

[21] Weiss P. In vitro experiments on the factors determining the course of the outgrowing nerve fiber. Journal of Experimental Zoology. 1934;68:393-448.

[22] Weiss P. Experiments on Cell and Axon Orientation Invitro - the Role of Colloidal Exudates in Tissue Organization. Journal of Experimental Zoology. 1945;100:353-86.

[23] Guillemette MD, Cui B, Roy E, Gauvin R, Giasson CJ, Esch MB, et al. Surface topography induces 3D self-orientation of cells and extracellular matrix resulting in improved tissue function. Integr Biol (Camb). 2009;1:196-204.

[24] Guido S, Tranquillo RT. A methodology for the systematic and quantitative study of cell contact guidance in oriented collagen gels. Correlation of fibroblast orientation and gel birefringence. J Cell Sci. 1993;105 (Pt 2):317-31.

[25] Vidal BC. Form birefringence as applied to biopolymer and inorganic material supraorganization. Biotech Histochem. 2010;85:365-78.

[26] Gauvin R, Guillemette M, Galbraith T, Bourget JM, Larouche D, Marcoux H, et al. Mechanical properties of tissue-engineered vascular constructs produced using arterial or venous cells. Tissue Eng Part A. 2011;17:2049-59.

[27] Brightman AO, Rajwa BP, Sturgis JE, McCallister ME, Robinson JP, Voytik-Harbin SL. Time-lapse confocal reflection microscopy of collagen fibrillogenesis and extracellular matrix assembly in vitro. Biopolymers. 2000;54:222-34.

[28] Thomopoulos S, Fomovsky GM, Holmes JW. The development of structural and mechanical anisotropy in fibroblast populated collagen gels. J Biomech Eng. 2005;127:742-50.

[29] Parenteau-Bareil R, Gauvin R, Berthod F. Collagen-Based Biomaterials for Tissue Engineering Applications. Materials. 2010;3:1863-87.

[30] Yarlagadda PK, Chandrasekharan M, Shyan JY. Recent advances and current developments in tissue scaffolding. Biomed Mater Eng. 2005;15:159-77.

[31] Shoulders MD, Raines RT. Collagen structure and stability. Annu Rev Biochem. 2009;78:929-58.

[32] Cliche S, Amiot J, Avezard C, Gariepy C. Extraction and characterization of collagen with or without telopeptides from chicken skin. Poultry Science. 2003;82:503-9.

[33] Parenteau-Bareil R, Gauvin R, Cliche S, Gariepy C, Germain L, Berthod F. Comparative study of bovine, porcine and avian collagens for the production of a tissue engineered dermis. Acta Biomater. 2011;7:3757-65.

[34] L'Heureux N, Germain L, Labbe R, Auger FA. In vitro construction of a human blood vessel from cultured vascular cells: a morphologic study. J Vasc Surg. 1993;17:499-509.

[35] Tranquillo RT, Durrani MA, Moon AG. Tissue engineering science: consequences of cell traction force. Cytotechnology. 1992;10:225-50.

[36] Lopez Valle CA, Auger FA, Rompre P, Bouvard V, Germain L. Peripheral anchorage of dermal equivalents. Br J Dermatol. 1992;127:365-71.

[37] Barocas VH, Tranquillo RT. An anisotropic biphasic theory of tissue-equivalent mechanics: the interplay among cell traction, fibrillar network deformation, fibril alignment, and cell contact guidance. J Biomech Eng. 1997;119:137-45.

[38] Eastwood M, Porter R, Khan U, McGrouther G, Brown R. Quantitative analysis of collagen gel contractile forces generated by dermal fibroblasts and the relationship to cell morphology. J Cell Physiol. 1996;166:33-42.

[39] Thomopoulos S, Fomovsky GM, Chandran PL, Holmes JW. Collagen fiber alignment does not explain mechanical anisotropy in fibroblast populated collagen gels. J Biomech Eng. 2007;129:642-50.

[40] Chandran PL, Barocas VH. Affine versus non-affine fibril kinematics in collagen networks: theoretical studies of network behavior. J Biomech Eng. 2006;128:259-70.

[41] Chandran PL, Barocas VH. Deterministic material-based averaging theory model of collagen gel micromechanics. J Biomech Eng. 2007;129:137-47.

[42] Costa KD, Lee EJ, Holmes JW. Creating alignment and anisotropy in engineered heart tissue: role of boundary conditions in a model three-dimensional culture system. Tissue Eng. 2003;9:567-77.

[43] Klebe RJ, Caldwell H, Milam S. Cells transmit spatial information by orienting collagen fibers. Matrix. 1989;9:451-8.

[44] Grinnell F, Lamke CR. Reorganization of hydrated collagen lattices by human skin fibroblasts. J Cell Sci. 1984;66:51-63.

[45] Weinberg CB, Bell E. A blood vessel model constructed from collagen and cultured vascular cells. Science. 1986;231:397-400.

[46] Tranquillo RT, Murray JD. Continuum model of fibroblast-driven wound contraction: inflammation-mediation. J Theor Biol. 1992;158:135-72.

[47] Takebayashi T, Varsier N, Kikuchi Y, Wake K, Taki M, Watanabe S, et al. Mobile phone use, exposure to radiofrequency electromagnetic field, and brain tumour: a case-control study. Br J Cancer. 2008;98:652-9.

[48] Swerdlow AJ, Feychting M, Green AC, Leeka Kheifets LK, Savitz DA. Mobile phones, brain tumors, and the interphone study: where are we now? Environ Health Perspect. 2011;119:1534-8.

[49] Miyakoshi J. Effects of static magnetic fields at the cellular level. Prog Biophys Mol Biol. 2005;87:213-23.

[50] Zhong C, Zhao TF, Xu ZJ, He RX. Effects of electromagnetic fields on bone regeneration in experimental and clinical studies: a review of the literature. Chin Med J (Engl). 2012;125:367-72.

[51] Costin GE, Birlea SA, Norris DA. Trends in wound repair: cellular and molecular basis of regenerative therapy using electromagnetic fields. Curr Mol Med. 2012;12:14-26.

[52] Liu YX, Tai JL, Li GQ, Zhang ZW, Xue JH, Liu HS, et al. Exposure to 1950-MHz TD-SCDMA Electromagnetic Fields Affects the Apoptosis of Astrocytes via Caspase-3-Dependent Pathway. PLoS One. 2012;7:e42332.

[53] Ongaro A, Varani K, Masieri FF, Pellati A, Massari L, Cadossi R, et al. Electromagnetic fields (EMFs) and adenosine receptors modulate prostaglandin E(2) and cytokine release in human osteoarthritic synovial fibroblasts. J Cell Physiol. 2012;227:2461-9.

[54] Vincenzi F, Targa M, Corciulo C, Gessi S, Merighi S, Setti S, et al. The anti-tumor effect of a(3) adenosine receptors is potentiated by pulsed electromagnetic fields in cultured neural cancer cells. PLoS One. 2012;7:e39317.

[55] Lu YS, Huang BT, Huang YX. Reactive Oxygen Species Formation and Apoptosis in Human Peripheral Blood Mononuclear Cell Induced by 900 MHz Mobile Phone Radiation. Oxid Med Cell Longev. 2012;2012:740280.

[56] Dube J, Rochette-Drouin O, Levesque P, Gauvin R, Roberge CJ, Auger FA, et al. Restoration of the transepithelial potential within tissue-engineered human skin in vitro and during the wound healing process in vivo. Tissue Eng Part A. 2010;16:3055-63.

[57] Dube J, Rochette-Drouin O, Levesque P, Gauvin R, Roberge CJ, Auger FA, et al. Human keratinocytes respond to direct current stimulation by increasing intracellular

calcium: preferential response of poorly differentiated cells. J Cell Physiol. 2012;227:2660-7.

[58] Sun LY, Hsieh DK, Yu TC, Chiu HT, Lu SF, Luo GH, et al. Effect of pulsed electromagnetic field on the proliferation and differentiation potential of human bone marrow mesenchymal stem cells. Bioelectromagnetics. 2009;30:251-60.

[59] Tranquillo RT, Girton TS, Bromberek BA, Triebes TG, Mooradian DL. Magnetically orientated tissue-equivalent tubes: application to a circumferentially orientated media-equivalent. Biomaterials. 1996;17:349-57.

[60] Tsai MT, Chang WH, Chang K, Hou RJ, Wu TW. Pulsed electromagnetic fields affect osteoblast proliferation and differentiation in bone tissue engineering. Bioelectromagnetics. 2007;28:519-28.

[61] Kotani H, Kawaguchi H, Shimoaka T, Iwasaka M, Ueno S, Ozawa H, et al. Strong static magnetic field stimulates bone formation to a definite orientation in vitro and in vivo. J Bone Miner Res. 2002;17:1814-21.

[62] Builles N, Janin-Manificat H, Malbouyres M, Justin V, Rovere MR, Pellegrini G, et al. Use of magnetically oriented orthogonal collagen scaffolds for hemi-corneal reconstruction and regeneration. Biomaterials. 2010;31:8313-22.

[63] Morin KT, Tranquillo RT. Guided sprouting from endothelial spheroids in fibrin gels aligned by magnetic fields and cell-induced gel compaction. Biomaterials. 2011;32:6111-8.

[64] Worcester DL. Structural origins of diamagnetic anisotropy in proteins. Proc Natl Acad Sci U S A. 1978;75:5475-7.

[65] Méthot S, Moulin V, Rancourt D, Bourdages MG, D., Plante M, Auger FA, et al. Morphological changes of human skin cells exposed to a DC electric field in vitro using a new exposure system. Can J Chem Eng. 2001;79:668-77.

[66] Messerli MA, Graham DM. Extracellular electrical fields direct wound healing and regeneration. Biol Bull. 2011;221:79-92.

[67] Zhao M, McCaig CD, Agius-Fernandez A, Forrester JV, Araki-Sasaki K. Human corneal epithelial cells reorient and migrate cathodally in a small applied electric field. Curr Eye Res. 1997;16:973-84.

[68] Sunkari VG, Aranovitch B, Portwood N, Nikoshkov A. Effects of a low-intensity electromagnetic field on fibroblast migration and proliferation. Electromagn Biol Med. 2011;30:80-5.

[69] Higashi T, Yamagishi A, Takeuchi T, Kawaguchi N, Sagawa S, Onishi S, et al. Orientation of erythrocytes in a strong static magnetic field. Blood. 1993;82:1328-34.

[70] Kotani H, Iwasaka M, Ueno S, Curtis A. Magnetic orientation of collagen and bone mixture. Journal of Applied Physics. 2000;87:6191-3.

[71] Torbet J, Freyssinet JM, Hudry-Clergeon G. Oriented fibrin gels formed by polymerization in strong magnetic fields. Nature. 1981;289:91-3.

[72] Torbet J, Malbouyres M, Builles N, Justin V, Roulet M, Damour O, et al. Orthogonal scaffold of magnetically aligned collagen lamellae for corneal stroma reconstruction. Biomaterials. 2007;28:4268-76.

[73] Torbet J, Dickens MJ. Orientation of skeletal muscle actin in strong magnetic fields. FEBS Lett. 1984;173:403-6.

[74] Meek KM, Fullwood NJ. Corneal and scleral collagens--a microscopist's perspective. Micron. 2001;32:261-72.

[75] Meek KM, Boote C. The organization of collagen in the corneal stroma. Exp Eye Res. 2004;78:503-12.

[76] Hayes S, Boote C, Lewis J, Sheppard J, Abahussin M, Quantock AJ, et al. Comparative study of fibrillar collagen arrangement in the corneas of primates and other mammals. Anat Rec (Hoboken). 2007;290:1542-50.

[77] Meek KM, Boote C. The use of X-ray scattering techniques to quantify the orientation and distribution of collagen in the corneal stroma. Prog Retin Eye Res. 2009;28:369-92.

[78] Dickinson RB, Guido S, Tranquillo RT. Biased cell migration of fibroblasts exhibiting contact guidance in oriented collagen gels. Ann Biomed Eng. 1994;22:342-56.

[79] Girton TS, Dubey N, Tranquillo RT. Magnetic-induced alignment of collagen fibrils in tissue equivalents. Methods Mol Med. 1999;18:67-73.

[80] Barocas VH, Girton TS, Tranquillo RT. Engineered alignment in media equivalents: magnetic prealignment and mandrel compaction. J Biomech Eng. 1998;120:660-6.

[81] Dubey N, Letourneau PC, Tranquillo RT. Guided neurite elongation and schwann cell invasion into magnetically aligned collagen in simulated peripheral nerve regeneration. Exp Neurol. 1999;158:338-50.

[82] Dubey N, Letourneau PC, Tranquillo RT. Neuronal contact guidance in magnetically aligned fibrin gels: effect of variation in gel mechano-structural properties. Biomaterials. 2001;22:1065-75.

[83] Kumar PR, Khan N, Vivekanandhan S, Satyanarayana N, Mohanty AK, Misra M. Nanofibers: effective generation by electrospinning and their applications. J Nanosci Nanotechnol. 2012;12:1-25.

[84] Jin L, Wang T, Zhu ML, Leach MK, Naim YI, Corey JM, et al. Electrospun fibers and tissue engineering. J Biomed Nanotechnol. 2012;8:1-9.

[85] Castano O, Eltohamy M, Kim HW. Electrospinning technology in tissue regeneration. Methods Mol Biol. 2012;811:127-40.

[86] Nisbet DR, Forsythe JS, Shen W, Finkelstein DI, Horne MK. Review paper: a review of the cellular response on electrospun nanofibers for tissue engineering. J Biomater Appl. 2009;24:7-29.

[87] Sill TJ, von Recum HA. Electrospinning: applications in drug delivery and tissue engineering. Biomaterials. 2008;29:1989-2006.

[88] Murugan R, Ramakrishna S. Design strategies of tissue engineering scaffolds with controlled fiber orientation. Tissue Eng. 2007;13:1845-66.

[89] Teo WE, Ramakrishna S. A review on electrospinning design and nanofibre assemblies. Nanotechnology. 2006;17:R89-R106.

[90] Liao S, Li B, Ma Z, Wei H, Chan C, Ramakrishna S. Biomimetic electrospun nanofibers for tissue regeneration. Biomed Mater. 2006;1:R45-53.

[91] Formhals A. Process and apparatus for preparing artificial threads. In: Patent U, editor. USA1934.

[92] Li WJ, Mauck RL, Cooper JA, Yuan X, Tuan RS. Engineering controllable anisotropy in electrospun biodegradable nanofibrous scaffolds for musculoskeletal tissue engineering. J Biomech. 2007;40:1686-93.

[93] Xu CY, Inai R, Kotaki M, Ramakrishna S. Aligned biodegradable nanofibrous structure: a potential scaffold for blood vessel engineering. Biomaterials. 2004;25:877-86.

[94] Pham QP, Sharma U, Mikos AG. Electrospinning of polymeric nanofibers for tissue engineering applications: a review. Tissue Eng. 2006;12:1197-211.

[95] Subbiah T, Bhat GS, Tock RW, Pararneswaran S, Ramkumar SS. Electrospinning of nanofibers. Journal of Applied Polymer Science. 2005;96:557-69.

[96] Li WJ, Laurencin CT, Caterson EJ, Tuan RS, Ko FK. Electrospun nanofibrous structure: a novel scaffold for tissue engineering. J Biomed Mater Res. 2002;60:613-21.

[97] Li WJ, Danielson KG, Alexander PG, Tuan RS. Biological response of chondrocytes cultured in three-dimensional nanofibrous poly(epsilon-caprolactone) scaffolds. J Biomed Mater Res A. 2003;67:1105-14.

[98] Geng X, Kwon OH, Jang J. Electrospinning of chitosan dissolved in concentrated acetic acid solution. Biomaterials. 2005;26:5427-32.

[99] Venugopal J, Ramakrishna S. Biocompatible nanofiber matrices for the engineering of a dermal substitute for skin regeneration. Tissue Eng. 2005;11:847-54.

[100] Peretti GM, Randolph MA, Zaporojan V, Bonassar LJ, Xu JW, Fellers JC, et al. A biomechanical analysis of an engineered cell-scaffold implant for cartilage repair. Annals of Plastic Surgery. 2001;46:533-7.

[101] Boland ED, Bowlin GL, Simpson DG, Wnek GE. Electrospinning of tissue engineering scaffolds. Abstracts of Papers of the American Chemical Society. 2001;222:U344-U.

[102] Jose MV, Thomas V, Johnson KT, Dean DR, Nyairo E. Aligned PLGA/HA nanofibrous nanocomposite scaffolds for bone tissue engineering. Acta Biomater. 2009;5:305-15.

[103] Jose MV, Thomas V, Xu Y, Bellis S, Nyairo E, Dean D. Aligned bioactive multi-component nanofibrous nanocomposite scaffolds for bone tissue engineering. Macromol Biosci. 2010;10:433-44.

[104] Thomas V, Jose MV, Chowdhury S, Sullivan JF, Dean DR, Vohra YK. Mechano-morphological studies of aligned nanofibrous scaffolds of polycaprolactone fabricated by electrospinning. J Biomater Sci Polym Ed. 2006;17:969-84.

[105] Teh TK, Toh SL, Goh JC. Aligned hybrid silk scaffold for enhanced differentiation of mesenchymal stem cells into ligament fibroblasts. Tissue Eng Part C Methods. 2011;17:687-703.

[106] Min BM, Lee G, Kim SH, Nam YS, Lee TS, Park WH. Electrospinning of silk fibroin nanofibers and its effect on the adhesion and spreading of normal human keratinocytes and fibroblasts in vitro. Biomaterials. 2004;25:1289-97.

[107] Yang F, Murugan R, Wang S, Ramakrishna S. Electrospinning of nano/micro scale poly(L-lactic acid) aligned fibers and their potential in neural tissue engineering. Biomaterials. 2005;26:2603-10.

[108] Matthews JA, Wnek GE, Simpson DG, Bowlin GL. Electrospinning of collagen nanofibers. Biomacromolecules. 2002;3:232-8.

[109] Zhong S, Teo WE, Zhu X, Beuerman RW, Ramakrishna S, Yung LY. An aligned nanofibrous collagen scaffold by electrospinning and its effects on in vitro fibroblast culture. J Biomed Mater Res A. 2006;79:456-63.

[110] Nelson CM, Tien J. Microstructured extracellular matrices in tissue engineering and development. Curr Opin Biotechnol. 2006;17:518-23.

[111] Clark P, Connolly P, Curtis AS, Dow JA, Wilkinson CD. Topographical control of cell behaviour. I. Simple step cues. Development. 1987;99:439-48.

[112] Kumar A, Whitesides GM. Features of Gold Having Micrometer to Centimeter Dimensions Can Be Formed through a Combination of Stamping with an Elastomeric Stamp and an Alkanethiol Ink Followed by Chemical Etching. Applied Physics Letters. 1993;63:2002-4.

[113] Walboomers XF, Ginsel LA, Jansen JA. Early spreading events of fibroblasts on microgrooved substrates. J Biomed Mater Res. 2000;51:529-34.

[114] Teixeira AI, Abrams GA, Bertics PJ, Murphy CJ, Nealey PF. Epithelial contact guidance on well-defined micro- and nanostructured substrates. J Cell Sci. 2003;116:1881-92.

[115] Teixeira AI, Nealey PF, Murphy CJ. Responses of human keratocytes to micro- and nanostructured substrates. J Biomed Mater Res A. 2004;71:369-76.

[116] Isenberg BC, Tsuda Y, Williams C, Shimizu T, Yamato M, Okano T, et al. A thermoresponsive, microtextured substrate for cell sheet engineering with defined structural organization. Biomaterials. 2008;29:2565-72.

[117] Sarkar S, Dadhania M, Rourke P, Desai TA, Wong JY. Vascular tissue engineering: microtextured scaffold templates to control organization of vascular smooth muscle cells and extracellular matrix. Acta Biomater. 2005;1:93-100.

[118] Okano T, Yamada N, Okuhara M, Sakai H, Sakurai Y. Mechanism of cell detachment from temperature-modulated, hydrophilic-hydrophobic polymer surfaces. Biomaterials. 1995;16:297-303.

[119] Isenberg BC, Backman DE, Kinahan ME, Jesudason R, Suki B, Stone PJ, et al. Micropatterned cell sheets with defined cell and extracellular matrix orientation exhibit anisotropic mechanical properties. J Biomech. 2012;45:756-61.

[120] Guillemette MD, Roy E, Auger FA, Veres T. Rapid isothermal substrate microfabrication of a biocompatible thermoplastic elastomer for cellular contact guidance. Acta Biomater. 2011;7:2492-8.

[121] L'Heureux N, Paquet S, Labbe R, Germain L, Auger FA. A completely biological tissue-engineered human blood vessel. Faseb J. 1998;12:47-56.

[122] Auger FA, Rémy-Zolghadri M, Grenier G, Germain L. The Self-Assembly Approach for Organ Reconstruction by Tissue Engineering. e-biomed: The Journal of Regenerative Medicine. 2000;1:75-86.

[123] Guillemette MD, Park H, Hsiao JC, Jain SR, Larson BL, Langer R, et al. Combined technologies for microfabricating elastomeric cardiac tissue engineering scaffolds. Macromol Biosci. 2010;10:1330-7.

[124] Risau W, Flamme I. Vasculogenesis. Annu Rev Cell Dev Biol. 1995;11:73-91.

[125] Kanda K, Matsuda T. Mechanical stress-induced orientation and ultrastructural change of smooth muscle cells cultured in three-dimensional collagen lattices. Cell Transplant. 1994;3:481-92.

[126] Niklason LE, Gao J, Abbott WM, Hirschi KK, Houser S, Marini R, et al. Functional arteries grown in vitro. Science. 1999;284:489-93.

[127] Seliktar D, Black RA, Vito RP, Nerem RM. Dynamic mechanical conditioning of collagen-gel blood vessel constructs induces remodeling in vitro. Ann Biomed Eng. 2000;28:351-62.

[128] Seliktar D, Nerem RM, Galis ZS. The role of matrix metalloproteinase-2 in the remodeling of cell-seeded vascular constructs subjected to cyclic strain. Ann Biomed Eng. 2001;29:923-34.

[129] Seliktar D, Nerem RM, Galis ZS. Mechanical strain-stimulated remodeling of tissue-engineered blood vessel constructs. Tissue Eng. 2003;9:657-66.

[130] Seliktar D, Zisch AH, Lutolf MP, Wrana JL, Hubbell JA. MMP-2 sensitive, VEGF-bearing bioactive hydrogels for promotion of vascular healing. J Biomed Mater Res A. 2004;68:704-16.

[131] Grenier G, Remy-Zolghadri M, Bergeron F, Guignard R, Baker K, Labbe R, et al. Mechanical loading modulates the differentiation state of vascular smooth muscle cells. Tissue Eng. 2006;12:3159-70.

[132] Grenier G, Remy-Zolghadri M, Larouche D, Gauvin R, Baker K, Bergeron F, et al. Tissue reorganization in response to mechanical load increases functionality. Tissue Eng. 2005;11:90-100.

[133] Pricci M, Bourget JM, Robitaille H, Porro C, Soleti R, Mostefai HA, et al. Applications of human tissue-engineered blood vessel models to study the effects of shed membrane microparticles from T-lymphocytes on vascular function. Tissue Eng Part A. 2009;15:137-45.

[134] Gauvin R, Parenteau-Bareil R, Larouche D, Marcoux H, Bisson F, Bonnet A, et al. Dynamic mechanical stimulations induce anisotropy and improve the tensile properties of engineered tissues produced without exogenous scaffolding. Acta Biomater. 2011;7:3294-301.

[135] Isenberg BC, Tranquillo RT. Long-term cyclic distention enhances the mechanical properties of collagen-based media-equivalents. Ann Biomed Eng. 2003;31:937-49.

[136] Resnick N, Yahav H, Shay-Salit A, Shushy M, Schubert S, Zilberman LC, et al. Fluid shear stress and the vascular endothelium: for better and for worse. Prog Biophys Mol Biol. 2003;81:177-99.

[137] Van der Heiden K, Egorova AD, Poelmann RE, Wentzel JJ, Hierck BP. Role for primary cilia as flow detectors in the cardiovascular system. Int Rev Cell Mol Biol. 2011;290:87-119.

[138] Lu D, Kassab GS. Role of shear stress and stretch in vascular mechanobiology. J R Soc Interface. 2011;8:1379-85.

[139] Egorova AD, van der Heiden K, Poelmann RE, Hierck BP. Primary cilia as biomechanical sensors in regulating endothelial function. Differentiation. 2012;83:S56-61.

[140] Tremblay PL, Huot J, Auger FA. Mechanisms by which E-selectin regulates diapedesis of colon cancer cells under flow conditions. Cancer Res. 2008;68:5167-76.

[141] Ishida T, Peterson TE, Kovach NL, Berk BC. MAP kinase activation by flow in endo-
       thelial cells. Role of beta 1 integrins and tyrosine kinases. Circ Res. 1996;79:310-6.

[142] Muller JM, Chilian WM, Davis MJ. Integrin signaling transduces shear stress--de-
       pendent vasodilation of coronary arterioles. Circ Res. 1997;80:320-6.

[143] McClendon MT, Stupp SI. Tubular hydrogels of circumferentially aligned nanofibers
       to encapsulate and orient vascular cells. Biomaterials. 2012;33:5713-22.

[144] Hartgerink JD, Beniash E, Stupp SI. Self-assembly and mineralization of peptide-am-
       phiphile nanofibers. Science. 2001;294:1684-8.

[145] Webber MJ, Kessler JA, Stupp SI. Emerging peptide nanomedicine to regenerate tis-
       sues and organs. J Intern Med. 2010;267:71-88.

[146] Thakar RG, Ho F, Huang NF, Liepmann D, Li S. Regulation of vascular smooth mus-
       cle cells by micropatterning. Biochem Biophys Res Commun. 2003;307:883-90.

[147] Hellman KB, Johnson PC, Bertram TA, Tawil B. Challenges in tissue engineering and
       regenerative medicine product commercialization: building an industry. Tissue Eng
       Part A. 2011;17:1-3.

[148] Johnson PC, Bertram TA, Tawil B, Hellman KB. Hurdles in tissue engineering/regen-
       erative medicine product commercialization: a survey of North American academia
       and industry. Tissue Eng Part A. 2011;17:5-15.

Chapter 5

Autograft of Dentin Materials for Bone Regeneration

Masaru Murata, Toshiyuki Akazawa,
Masaharu Mitsugi, Md Arafat Kabir, In-Woong Um,
Yasuhito Minamida, Kyung-Wook Kim,
Young-Kyun Kim, Yao Sun and Chunlin Qin

Additional information is available at the end of the chapter

1. Introduction

Regenerative medicine is based on advanced and applied biomaterials science. Biomaterials have a major impact on the patient cure for improving the quality of life. We have been challenging to develop bioabsorbable dentin materials (Murata et al, 2011; Murata et al, 2012), harmonized with bone remodelling, by using the supersonic and acid-etching technology (Akazawa et al, 2012).

While human bone autograft was done in 19th century, human dentin autograft for bone augmentation was reported in IADR 2003. The first clinical case was a sinus lifting using auto-dentin for bone augmentation (Murata, 2003). Dentin is acellular matrix, while bone include osteocytes. Very interestingly, biochemical components in dentin and bone are almost similar. They consist of body fluid (10%), collagen (18%), non-collagenous proteins (NCPs: 2%) and hydroxyapatite (HAp: 70%) in weight volume (Fig. 1). Demineralized dentin matrix (DDM) and demineralized bone matrix (DBM) are mainly type I collagen with growth factors such as bone morphogenetic proteins (BMPs) (Urist, 1965) and fibroblast growth factors (FGFs) (Fig. 2) (Butler et al.,1977; Murata et al, 2010a,b).

Korea Tooth Bank (KTB) was established in Seoul 2009 for an unique service of tooth-derived graft materials. The medical service system is the preparation and delivery of the tooth-derived materials on demand (Kim et al,2010; Kim et al, 2012). The tooth-derived materials were named as auto-tooth graft materials, which divided into the block-type and powder-type (Park et al., 2010). The block-type material, which is hydrated in 0.9% NaCl solution for 15-30 min before use, can be cut by operators with surgical knife or scissors. Recently, the enamel-dentin grafting has been becoming a realistic alternative to the bone grafting in Korea. We have thought the non-functional teeth as native resources of various graft materials and have achieved the medical recycle of patient-own teeth as novel materials for bone regeneration in Japan and Korea. This matrix-based bone therapy is *Dental Innovation* early in 21st century. Our innovative technique will expand from East Asia to the world.

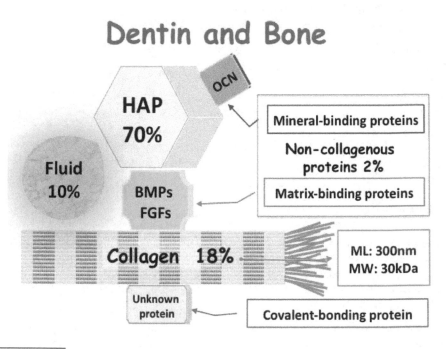

BMPs, FGFs: matrix-binding proteins in NCPs. OCN: mineral-binding proteins in NCPs; Collagen: mainly type I collagen

Figure 1. Chemical components (w/v%) of human dentin and bone;

2. Biochemistry of human dentin

Dentin and bone are mineralized tissues and almost similar in chemical components. They consist of body fluid, collagen, non-collagenous proteins (NCPs) and hydroxyapatite (HAp) in weight volume (Fig. 1). The NCPs in dentin and bone are secreted into the ECM in the process of biomineralization. The category is termed the SIBLING (Small Integrin-Binding Ligand, N-linked Glycoprotein) family that includes dentin sialophosphoprotein (DSPP), dentin matrix protein 1 (DMP1), bone sialoprotein (BSP) and osteopontin (OPN) (Fisher et al, 2001; Qin et al, 2007; Sun et al, 2010; Qin et al, 2011).

Both DDM and DBM are composed of predominantly type I collagen (95%) and matrix-binding proteins such as BMPs (Murata et al., 2000; Akazawa et al., 2006; Murata et al., 2007). BMPs, transforming growth factor-beta (TGF-β), insulin growth factor-I (IGF-I) and IGF-II were detected in human dentin (Finkelman et al., 1990). In the rabbit study, completely demineralized dentin matrix induced bone in the muscle at 4 weeks, while calcified dentin induced bone at 8-12 weeks after implantation (Yeoman & Urist, 1967; Bang & Urist, 1967). Many researchers made effort to discover dentin-derived BMPs. (Butler et al., 1977; Urist et al., 1982; Kawai & Urist., 1989; Bessho et al., 1990). In our study, human DDM and human DBM induced bone and cartilage independently in the subcutaneous tissues at 4 weeks (Murata et al, 2010b). These results indicated that highly calcified tissues such as cortical bone and calcified dentin are not earlier in osteoinduction and osteoconduction than spongy bone, DBM, and DDM. The delayed inductive properties of the calcified dentin and bone may be related to the inhibition of BMPs-release by HAp crystals (Huggins et al., 1970).

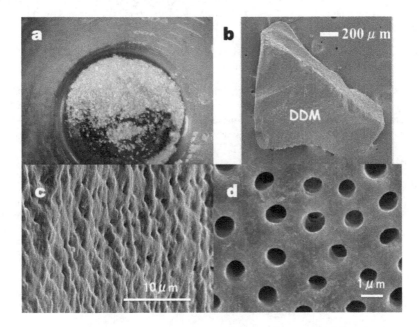

a: wet granules, b,c,d: SEM of DDM granule. Note: dentinal tubes

Figure 2. Crushed tooth granules and SEM photos of demineralized dentin matrix (DDM)

DDM is defined as an acid-insoluble dentin collagen that is absorbable, but hard to digest in human body (Fig. 2). DDM is acellular biomatrix with the micro-tube structure. DDM and DBM possess the ability to coagulate blood plasmas (Huggins & Reddi., 1973). The coagulation action of blood plasma by DDM should become advantageous for surgical operations.

Dentin formation is a dynamic and complicated process, involving interplays among a number of molecules including type I collagen, NCPs and prtoteoglycans, which work collectively to precisely control the site and rate of apatite formation. Type I collagen secreted by odontoblasts forms the scaffold, upon which HAp crystals are deposited. In addition to type I collagen, the extracelluar matrix contains a number of NCPs which play critical roles in the initiation and regulation of HAp crystals (Qin et al., 2011).

3. Clinical study of human dentin

3.1. Case 1: Bone augmentation, 17 year-old female

Patient: A 17-year-old female presented with missing teeth (#11). Clinical and radiological examinations revealed atrophied bone and fractured root residue in the region (Fig. 3a,b). Her medical history was unremarkable.

Surgical procedure 1: Four wisdom teeth were extracted for the preparation of tooth-derived materials (block-type, powder-type).

Preparations of dentin materials: The extracted molar was divided into the crown portion and the root portion. The crown portion was crushed under the cooling. The crushed granules were decalcified in 0.6N HCl solution, rinsed in cold distilled water and freeze-dried. On the other hand, the root portion was perforated by using a round bar to create a porous structure. The root with many holes was decalcified in 0.6N HCl solution, rinsed and freeze-dried. These biomaterials are named as auto-tooth bone (ATB) by KTB.

Surgical procedure 2: This patient-own blood sample was centrifuged and the middle layer was collected as fibrin glue (so called concentrated growth factors: CGF) (Fig. 4a,b). The different ATB materials were immersed in 0.9% NaCl solution before use (Fig. 4c). Additionally, ATB granules were mixed with the fibrin glue (CGF) prepared from autologous blood (Fig. 4d,e). The root-dentin material was divied into 2 parts by using a knife. A titanium fixture (Nobel Replace Tapered NP: 16mm) was implanted into the atrophied bone under local anesthesia (Fig. 3c,d). The root-dentin wall was grafted into the bone defect (fixture-exposed region) as veneer graft (Fig. 4f). The composite of ATB and fibrin contributed to the attachment between the grafted root-dentin and the muco-periosteal flap (Fig. 5a,b,c).

Results and discussion: This patient was successfully restored with the dental implant and the autograft of 2 types of ATB (root-on, powders) with autologous fibrin glue (Fig. 5d). Properly hydrated ATB should facilitate its adaption to the bone defect due to its elasticity and flexibility. The results demonstrated that autogenous tooth could be recycled as the innovative biomaterials.

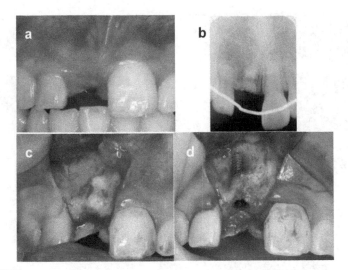

a: intraoral initial view (before operation), Note: a missing tooth (#11) b: X-ray photo, Note: radio-opacity of residual root c: exposed bone, Note: concave shape d: view just after Ti. fixture implantation, Note: labial bone defect

Figure 3. Case 1: Auto-tooth bone graft for implant placement, 17 year-old girl;

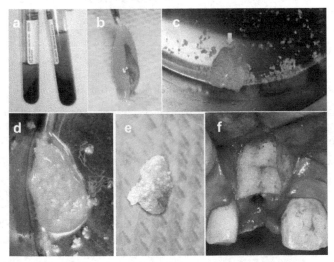

a: blood after centrifugation, Note: 3 layers b: fibrin glue; middle layer in 4a c: wettable ATB materials (block-type ⇩, powder-type) d,e: composite of powder and fibrin glue f: covering with block-type of dentin

Figure 4. Case 1: Auto-tooth bone (ATB) graft for implant placement, 17 year-old girl

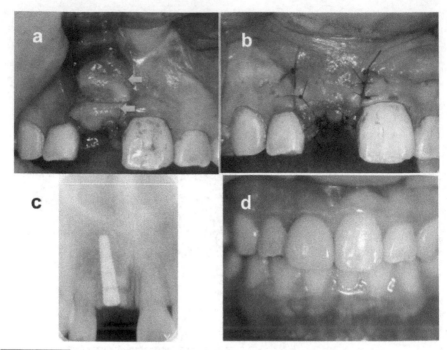

a: fibrin glue including ATB powders (⇔) b: repositioned flap. Note: suture with nylon c: X-ray photo just after operation d: final view after prosthetic restoration

Figure 5. Case 1: Auto-tooth bone graft for implant placement, 17 year-old girl

3.2. Case 2: DDM onlay graft and tooth autograft, 25 year-old female

Patient: A 25-year-old female presented with missing teeth (#46). She lost the first molar about 12 years ago. A clinical examination revealed an atrophied bone in the region. Her medical history was unremarkable.

Surgical procedure 1: A non-functional vital tooth (#28) was extracted and immediately crushed with saline ice by our newly developed tooth- mill (Osteo-Mill®, Tokyo Iken Co., Ltd) at 12000rpm for 30 sec (Fig. 6) (Patent: 4953276). Briefly, vessel and blade were made in ZrO_2. The crushed tooth-granules were decalcified in 2% HNO_3 solution for 20 min (Murata et al., 2009). The DDM granules including cementum were rinsed in cold distilled water. Cortical perforations were performed in the atrophied bone, and DDM were immediately autotransplanted on the perforated bone under local anesthesia.

Surgical procedure 2: At 4 months after the first operation, a non-functional vital tooth (#18) was extracted and received the immediate root canal filling (RCF), using a new fixation device (Fig. 7). The device was developed for tooth transplantation and replantation (Patent: 4866994).

After the bone biopsy for the tissue observation and the preparation of transplated cavity, tooth autograft was carried out into the host bone (Fig. 8a,b,d).

Results and discussion: The biopsy tissue showed that DDM granules were received to host, and partially replaced by new bone (Fig. 8e). This case was onlay graft of DDM on perforated cortical bone (Murata et al, 1999; Murata et al, 2000). Though RCF is generally carried out at more than 4 weeks after tooth transplantation, we did immediate RCF, using the medical device. This patient was successfully restored with her own 2 teeth. This case was the immediate tooth autotransplantition with the immediate root canal filling at 4 months after DDM autograft in 2009.

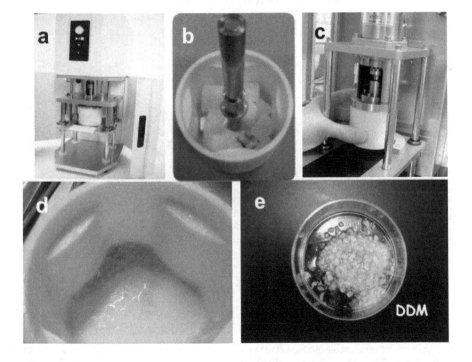

a: mill, b: tooth with ice blocks, c: ZrO$_2$ vessel, d: crushed tooth, e: DDM granules before clinical use.

Figure 6. Preparation of DDM using automatic tooth mill (Osteo-Mill®, Tokyo Iken)

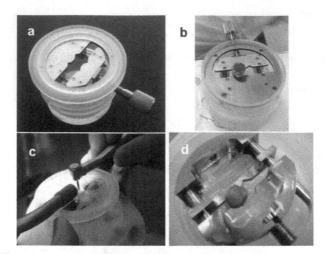

a: whole view, Note: the device developed for tooth transplantation and replantation b: fixed tooth, Note: correspondence to all teeth c: crown treatment, Note: periodontal ligament tissue protected from infected fine particles d: root view, Note: keeping blood even after cutting and root canal filling

Figure 7. New device for protecting periodontal ligament cells (Mr.FIX®, Tokyo Iken)

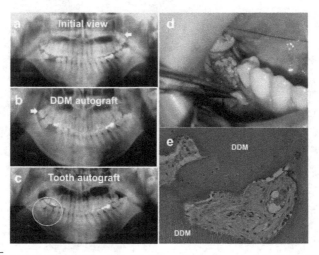

a: initial X-ray photo: missing tooth (#46) and atrophied bone. Non-functional tooth (⇐) for DDM b: just after DDM graft. Non-functional tooth (⇒) for next tooth autograft c: tooth auto-transplantation at 4 months after DDM graft d: DDM autograft on perforated cortical bone before suture e: biopsy: mature bone connected with DDM residue (HE section)

Figure 8. Case 2: 24 year-old woman

4. Supersonic and acid-etching method for Dentin geometry

Compact structure inhibits the body fluid permeation and the cell invasion into the inside of the materials. Generally, this situation is called a material wall. Dentin and cortical bone have compact structure. We have been challenging to develop new dentin materials, using a supersonic and acid-etching technology (Akazawa et al., 2009; Akazawa et al., 2010; Akazawa et al., 2012). The surface structure design of dentin by the supersonic treatment might easily produce new functional scaffolds, which control the bio-absorption rate and the adsorption ability for protein and cells. Figure 9 shows the dissolution efficiencies of human dentin granules, which were demineralized for 5-45 min in 2.0%-HNO$_3$ solutions by the supersonic treatment at 600W. A photograph inside Fig.9 is Digital microscopic view of DDM, dissolution for 30 min in 2.0%- HNO$_3$ by the supersonic treatment at 600W and 28 kHz.

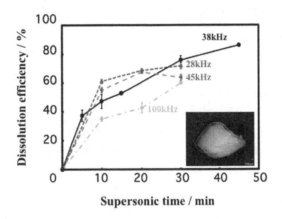

Figure 9. Dissolution efficiencies of human dentin granules, demineralized for 5-45 min in 2.0%-HNO$_3$ by supersonic treatment at 600W. Inside photo: Digital microscopic DDM view, dissolution for 30 min in 2.0%- HNO$_3$ by supersonic treatment at 600W and 28 kHz.

The innovative technology can create the adequate geometry and the surface structure of commercially available materials (Akazawa et al., 2012). Geometrical factors will improve the performance of biomaterials for bone regeneration (Reddi, 1974: Kuboki et al, 1995; Murata et al, 1998). Biomaterials science should support and develop the advanced regenerative therapy using tooth-derived materials for patients in the near future.

Acknowledgment

This project was greatly supported by the grant (consortium: 2004-5) of Japan Ministry of Economy, Trade and Industry, and Korea Tooth Bank Co. Ltd. The authors would like to thank WISM Mutoh Co. Ltd., and Tokyo Iken Co. Ltd., for developing the devices (Patents: 4866994, 4953276).

Author details

Masaru Murata[1], Toshiyuki Akazawa[2], Masaharu Mitsugi[3], Md Arafat Kabir[1], In-Woong Um[4], Yasuhito Minamida[1], Kyung-Wook Kim[5], Young-Kyun Kim[6], Yao Sun[7,8] and Chunlin Qin[8]

1 Health Sciences University of Hokkaido, Japan

2 Hokkaido Organization, Japan

3 Takamatsu Oral and Maxillofacial Surgery, Japan

4 Korea Tooth Bank Co. Ltd, Korea

5 Dankok University, Korea

6 Seoul National University, Korea

7 Harbin Medical University, China

8 Texas A&M Health Science Center Baylor College of Dentistry, USA

References

[1] Akazawa, T., Murata, M., Sasaki, T., Tazaki, J., Kobayashi, M., Kanno, T., Matsushima, K., & Arisue, M. (2006). Biodegradation and bioabsorption innovation of the functionally graded cattle-bone-originated apatite with blood compatibility. J Biomed Mater Res, 76A., 1., 44-51.

[2] Akazawa, T., Murata, M., Hino, J., Nakamura, K., Tazaki, J., Kikuchi, M., & Arisue, M. (2007). Materials design and application of demineralized dentin/apatite composite granules derived from human teeth. Archives of Bioceramics Research, 7., 25-28.

[3] Akazawa, T., Murata, M., Tazaki, J., Nakamura, K., Hino, J., Ito, I., Yamamoto, M., Tabata, Y., Takahata, M., & Ito, M.(2009). Biomimetic microstructure and biocompatibility of functionally graded hydroxyapatite derived from animal bone by a supersonic dissolution - Precipitation method- . Bioceramics 22, 22., 155-158.

[4] Akazawa, T., Murata, M., Takahata, M., Xianjun, D., Abe, Y., Nakamura, K., Hino, J., Tazaki, J., Ito, K., Ito, M., Iwasaki, N., Minami, A., Nakajima, T., & Sakamoto, M. (2010). Characterization of microstructure and bio-absorption of the hydroxyapatite

ceramics modified by a partial dissolution-precipitation technique using supersonic treatment. Journal of the Ceramic Society of Japan, 118., 6., 535-540.

[5] Akazawa, T., Murata, M., Tabata, Y., & Ito, M.(2012). Bone regeneration (ISBN) Chapter: biomimetic microstructure and biocompatibility of hydroxyapatite porous ceramics designed by a partial dissolution-precipitation technique with supersonic treatment. INTECK Publisher, Croatia, pp275-292

[6] Akazawa, T., Murata, M., Hino, J., Nagano, F., Shigyo, T, Nomura, T, Inano, H., Ita-bashi, K., Yamagishi, T, Nakamura, K., Takahashi, T., Iida, S., Kashiwazaki, H. (2012). Surface structure and biocompatibility of demineralized dentin matrix granules soaked in a simulated body fluid. Applied Surface Science, in press.

[7] Bang, G. & Urist, MR. (1967). Bone induction in excavation chambers in matrix of de-calcified dentin. Arch Surg, 94., 6., 781-789.

[8] Bessho, K., Tagawa, T., & Murata, M. (1990). Purification of rabbit bone morphoge-netic protein derived from bone, dentin, and wound tissue after tooth extraction. J Oral Maxillofac Surg, 48., 162-169.

[9] Butler, WT., Mikulski, A., Urist, MR., Bridges, G., & Uyeno, S. (1977). Noncollage-nous proteins of a rat dentin matrix possessing bone morphogenetic activity. J Dent Res, 56., 228-232.

[10] Finkelman, RD., Mohan, S., Jennings, JC., Taylor, AK., Jepsen, S., & Baylink, DJ. (1990). Quantitation of growth factors IGF-I, SGF/IGF-II, and TGF-beta in human dentin. J Bone Miner Res., 5., 7., 717-23.

[11] Fisher L.W., Torchia D.A., Fohr B., Young M.F., & Fedarko N.S. (2001). Flexible struc-tures of SIBLING proteins, bone sialoprotein, and osteopontin. Biochem Biophys Res Commun., 280: 460-465.

[12] Huggins, CB., Wiseman, S., & Reddi, AH. (1970). Transformation of fibroblasts by al-logeneic and xenogeneic transplants of demineralized tooth and bone. J Exp Med, 132., 1250-1258.

[13] Huggins, CB., & Reddi, AH. (1973). Coagulation of blood plasma of guinea pig by the bone matrix. Proc Natl Acad Sci U S A., 70., 3., 929-33.

[14] Inoue, T., Deporter, DA., & Melcher, AH. (1986). Induction of chondrogenesis in muscle, skin, bone marrow, and periodontal ligament by demineralized dentin and bone matrix in vivo and in vitro. J Dent Res, 65., 12-22.

[15] Ito, K., Arakawa, T., Murata, M., Tazaki, J., Takuma, T., & Arisue, M. (2008). Analysis of bone morphogenetic protein in human dental pulp tissues. Archives of Bioceram-ics Research, 8., 166-169.

[16] Kawai, T., & Urist, MD. (1989). Bovine tooth-derived bone morphogenetic protein. J Dent Res, 68., 1069-1074.

[17] Kawakami, T., Kuboki, Y., Tanaka, J., Hijikata, S., Akazawa, T., Murata, M., Fujisawa, R., Takita, H., & Arisue, M. (2007). Regenerative Medicine of Bone and Teeth. Journal of Hard Tissue Biology, 16(3),95-113.

[18] Kim, YK., Kim, SG., Byeon, JH., Lee, HJ., Um, IU., Lim, SC., & Kim, SY. (2010). Development of a novel bone grafting material using autogenous teeth. Oral Surg Oral Med Oral Pathol Oral Radiol Endod., 109., 4., 496-503.

[19] Kim, YK.(2012). Bone graft material using teeth. Journal of the Korean Association of Oral and Maxillofacial Surgens, 38., 3, 134-138.

[20] Kuboki, Y., Saito, T., Murata, M., Takita, H., Mizuno, M., Inoue, M., Nagai, N. & Poole, R. (1995). Two distinctive BMP-carriers induce zonal chondrogenesis and membranous ossification, respectively; geometrical factors of matrices for cell-differentiation. Connective Tissue Research, 31., 1-8.

[21] Murata, M., Inoue, M., Arisue, M., Kuboki, Y., & Nagai, N. (1998). Carrier-dependency of cellular differentiation induced by bone morphogenetic protein (BMP) in ectopic sites. Int J Oral Maxillofac Surg, 27., 391-396.

[22] Murata, M., Huang, BZ., Shibata, T., Imai, S., Nagai, N., & Arisue, M. (1999). Bone augmentation by recombinant human BMP-2 and collagen on adult rat parietal bone. Int J Oral Maxillofac Surg, 28., 232-237.

[23] Murata, M., Maki, F., Sato, D., Shibata, T., & Arisue, M. (2000). Bone augmentation by onlay implant using recombinant human BMP-2 and collagen on adult rat skull without periosteum. Clin Oral Impl Res, 11., 289-295.

[24] Murata, M. (2003). Autogenous demineralized dentin matrix for maxillary sinus augmentation in human. The first clinical report. 81th International Association for Dental Research, Geteburg, Sweden, 2003, June.

[25] Murata, M., Akazawa, T., Tazaki, J., Ito, K., Sasaki, T., Yamamoto, M., Tabata, Y., & Arisue, M. (2007). Blood permeability of a novel ceramic scaffold for bone morphogenetic protein-2. J Biomed Mater Res, 81B., 2., 469-475.

[26] Murata, M., Akazawa, T., Tazaki, J., Ito, K., Hino, J., Kamiura, Y., Kumazawa, R., & Arisue, M. (2009). Human Dentin autograft for bone regeneration - Automatic pulverizing machine and biopsy –. Bioceramics 22, 22., 745-748.

[27] Murata, M., Kawai, T., Kawakami, T., Akazawa, T., Tazaki, J., Ito, K., Kusano, K., & Arisue, M. (2010a). Human acid-insoluble dentin with BMP-2 accelerates bone induction in subcutaneous and intramuscular tissues. Journal of the Ceramic Society of Japan, 118., 6., 438-441.

[28] Murata, M., Akazawa, T., Takahata, M., Ito, M., Tazaki, J., Hino, J., Nakamura, K., Iwasaki, N., Shibata,T., & Arisue, M. (2010b). Bone induction of human tooth and bone crushed by newly developed automatic mill. Journal of the Ceramic Society of Japan, 118., 6., 434-437.

[29] Murata, M., Akazawa, T., Mitsugi, M., Um, IW., Kim, KW., & Kim, YK. (2011). Human Dentin as Novel Biomaterial for Bone Regeneration, Biomaterials - Physics and Chemistry, Rosario Pignatello (Ed.), ISBN: 978-953-307-418-4, INTECK publisher, Croatia, pp127-140.

[30] Murata, M., Sato, D., Hino, J., Akazawa, T., Tazaki, J., Ito, K., & Arisue, M. (2012). Acid-insoluble human dentin as carrier material for recombinant human BMP-2. J Biomed Mater Res, 100A., 571-577.

[31] Park, SM., Um, IW., Kim, YK., & Kim, KW. (2012). Clinical application of auto-tooth bone garaft material. Journal of the Korean Association of Oral and Maxillofacial Surgens, 38.,1., 2-8.

[32] Qin C., D'Souza R., & Feng J.Q. (2007). Dentin matrix protein 1 (DMP1): new and important roles for biomineralization and phosphate homeostasis. J Dent Res 86:1134-1141

[33] Qin C., Brunn J.C., Jones J., George A., Ramachandran A., Gorski J.P., & Butler W.T. (2011). A comparative study of sialic acid-rich proteins in rat bone and dentin. Eur J Oral Sci 109: 133-141.

[34] Reddi, AH. (1974). Bone matrix in the solid state:geometric influence on differentiation of fibroblasts. Adv Biol Med Phys, 15., 1-18.

[35] Sun, Y., Lu, Y., Chen, S., Prasad, M., Wang, X., Zhu, Q., Zhang, J., Ball, H., Feng, J., Butler, WT., & Qin, C. (2010). Key proteolytic cleavage site and full-length form of DSPP. J Dent Res 89: 498-503.

[36] Togari, K., Mitazawa, K., Yagihashi, K., Tabuchi, M., Maeda, H., Kawai, Y., & Goto, S. (2011). Bone regeneration by demineralized dentin matrix in skull defects of rats. Journal of Hard Tissue Biology, 21(1),25-33.

[37] Urist, MR. (1965). Bone: Formation by autoinduction. Science, 150., 893-899.

[38] Urist, MR., Mizutani, H., Conover, MA., Lietze, A., & Finerman, GA. (1982) Dentin, bone, and osteosarcoma tissue bone morphogenetic proteins. Prog Clin Biol Res, 101., 61-81.

[39] Yeomans, JD. & Urist, MR. (1967). Bone induction by decalcified dentine implanted into oral, osseous and muscle tissues. Arch Oral Biol, 12., 999-1008.

Chapter 6

The Integrations of Biomaterials and Rapid Prototyping Techniques for Intelligent Manufacturing of Complex Organs

Xiaohong Wang, Jukka Tuomi, Antti A. Mäkitie,
Kaija-Stiina Paloheimo, Jouni Partanen and
Marjo Yliperttula

Additional information is available at the end of the chapter

1. Introduction

In the human body, an organ is a composite of different tissues in an ordered structural unit to serve a common function [1]. Ordinarily, cells self-assemble into tissues before forming an organ. There are at least three different tissues in a complex organ, such as the liver, heart, and kidney. Currently, complex organ failures are the first cause of mortality in developed countries despite advances in pharmacological, interventional, and surgical therapies [2]. Orthotopic organ transplantation is severely limited by the problems of donor shortage and immune rejections [3]. Extracorporeal support systems perform some specific functions within a limited time period [4]. Cell encapsulation techniques face the problems of capsule loss, low stability, and poor efficiency [5]. Cell sheet technique cannot rescue tissues with increased thicknesses above 80 μm [6]. Decellularized matrices are hard to be repopulated by multiple cell types [7]. On the other hand, stem cell research has emerged as one of the most high-profile and promising areas of 21st century science [8-10]. Typically, autologous adipose-derived stem cells (ADSCs) represent one of the most abundant, easily cultured, rapidly expanded, and multipotent cell source [11]. It has been a long-term goal in this field to manufacture complex organs from biocompatible materials (including non-immune patient derived cells) and computer-aided design (CAD) models in a fast, easy, cheap and automatic manner.

To manufacture a complex organ, cells act like building blocks and have special functions. A comprehensive multidisciplinary effort from biology, implantable biomaterials, and rapid prototyping (RP) technology is extraordinarily needed. A biomaterial is defined as any matter, surface, or construct that interacts with biological systems [12]. It may be an autograft, allograft or xenograft transplant material, or a nature derived or laboratory synthesized chemical component. Biomaterials are often used and/or adapted for a medical application, and thus comprise whole or part of a living structure or biomedical device which performs, augments, or replaces a natural function [13]. RP, also referred to as additive manufacturing (AM) or solid freeform fabrication (SFF), is a set of manufacturing processes which can deposit materials layer-by-layer until a CAD model with freeform geometry has been built. RP technology, which has been widely used in the automatic fabrication of complex geometric structure areas, carries the promise to become the most convenient and reliable technique for manufacturing of complex organs in the coming years [14-18].

Over the last two decades, tissue-engineering researchers have devoted themselves to seeding cells onto a porous biodegradable scaffold material to direct cell differentiation and functional assembly into three-dimensional (3D) tissues [19]. This strategy has achieved a great success in simple tissue/organ regeneration [20]. However, it is extremely difficult for this strategy to be used in creating a branched vascular system or a complex organ regenerative template mimicking the native ones with similar mechanical and biological properties. Similar to building a nuclear power plant for complex organ manufacturing, there is a significant gap between simple tissue/organ engineering and complex organ manufacturing approaches both in fabrication technique employed and ultimate goal achieved (Table 1) [14-18].

Complex organ manufacturing	Nuclear power plant building
Cells	Bricks, nuclear reactors
Synthetic, natural polymers	Steel
Crosslinking agents	Cements
Vascular systems	Water and light pipes
Nerve system	Electric control system
Multi-nozzle rapid prototyping machines	Cranes
CAD models	Blueprints
Construction	Architecture

Table 1. Analogues between complex organ manufacturing and nuclear power plant building.

The ultimate goal of complex organ manufacturing is to fabricate hybrid biomaterial (including living cells, even gene/protein) structures over a range of size scales (i.e. from a few micrometers to a few millimeters). We herein provide insights into some special integrations of biomaterials and RP techniques towards the purpose of intelligent freeform manufacturing of complex organs. The most successful and promising integrations have been highlighted; meanwhile the future development directions have been highlighted.

2. Biomaterials and RP techniques in thousands of postures

As stated above, biomaterials, usually acting as synthetic frameworks (referred as scaffolds, matrices, or constructs), can be categorized into different groups according to their supply sources, existence states, chemical properties as well as biomedical applications. Typically, patient specific blood, cells (especially stem cells), acellular matrices, tissues and organs are a kind of biomaterials with no immune reactions. More than 100 implantable biomaterials have been reported in different forms, such as bulks, blocks, membranes, sheets, beads, hydrogels, fibers, sutures, plates, nets, meshs, tubes, non-woven fabrics, porous scaffolds (or sponges), heart valves, intraocular lenses, dental implants, pacemakers, biosensors, etc [21-23]. However, very few of them are suitable for complex organ manufacturing purposes. For biomedical applications, biocompatibility, biodegradability and processing ability are among the most crucial issues one should consider. In most cases the implantable biomaterial has to be nontoxic, biocompatible, and biodegradable. Therefore, stringent criteria must be met before proceeding to clinical applications.

Especially, hydrogels are a family of natural or synthetic polymers with high water contents. During the last twenty years, hydrogels have been an important class of soft tissue repair materials or cell delivering vehicles that can be fabricated in the form of 3D micro-periodic structures by colloidal templating [24], interference lithography [25], direct-writing [26], ink-jet printing [27], and two-photon polymerization (2PP) [28].

In the last four decades, significant advances have been made in the progress of scaffold fabrication techniques for biomedical applications. For example, synthetic and natural biodegradable polymers, such as polylactic acid (PLA) [29], poly(lactic/glycolic) acid (PLGA) [30], collagen [31], hyaluronic acid [32] and chitosan [33], are often used as pure implantable biomaterials or tissue engineering scaffolds.

In parallel with the development of biomaterials, the number of commercial RP techniques has expanded rapidly during the last decade. More than 30 different RP techniques have been applied in the most diverse industries. Several companies are now using RP technologies for plastic, wood and metal product manufacturing. For example, Siemens, Phonak Widex, and other hearing aid manufactures use selective laser sintering (SLS) techniques to produce hearing aid shells. Align technology uses SLS techniques to fabricate molds for producing clear braces ("aligners"). And Boeing and its suppliers use SLS techniques to produce ducts and similar parts for F-18 fighter jets [34]. Around 20 of the RP techniques have been adapted in the field of regenerative medicine [35]. Basically, these adaptations can be classified into three major groups hinged on the RP working principles (Figure 1): (i) nozzle-based extruding/assembling/deposition systems, e.g. fused deposition modeling (FDM) (Figure 1A) [36], pressure assisted manufacturing (PAM), low-temperature deposition manufacturing (LDM), and bio-plotters (3DB) (Figure 1B) [37,38], which deposit materials either thermally or chemically through pens/syringes/nozzles; (ii) laser/photolithography-based writing systems, e.g. laser-guided direct writing, which arrange meterials/cells by laser beams [39,40] or photopolymerize a liquid (resin, powder, or wax) in stereolithography (SLA or STL) (Figure 1C) [36,41], or sinter powdered material in SLS systems (Figure 1D)

[42]; (iii) printing-based inkjeting systems, e.g. 3D printing (3DP) systems and wax-based
systems, which print a chemical binder onto a powder bed and print two types of wax materials in sequence (Figure 1 E) [36].

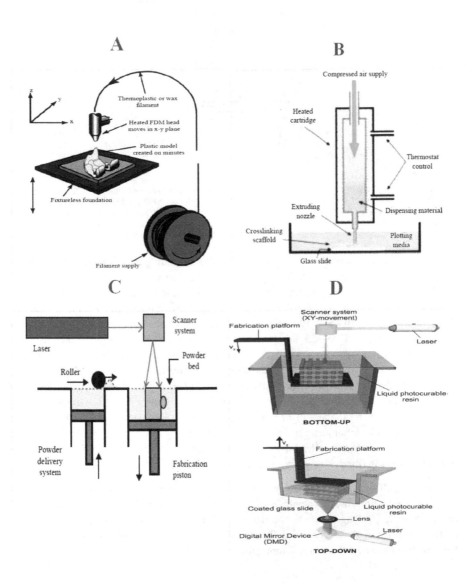

E

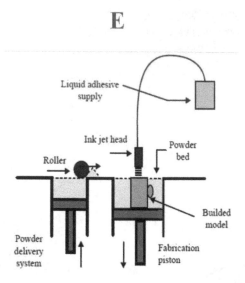

Figure 1. Working principles of various rapid prototyping systems: A) Schematic illustration of the nozzle-based FDM process [36]. B) Scheme of a nozzle-based 3D-Bioplotter heated cartridge setup [37,38]. C) Schematic of the laser-based SLS techniques [36]. D) Schemes of two laser-based of stereolithography (SLA or STL) setups [39]. Upper: a bottom-up system whereby the laser scans the surface for the curing of the photosensitive materials. Bottom: a top-down setup with dynamic digital light projection to cure a complete 2D layer at once. E) Schematic of the 3DP systems [36].

Although most of the adapted techniques can be used in building complex geometrical shapes with CAD modelling, every technique group is subjected to a limited biomaterial incorporation ability and has its own drawbacks in creating 3D living organs. For example, Chu and coworkers have developed design-for-manufacturing rules for their lattice mesostructure fabrication technique with a STL system. Lattice structures tend to have geometry variations in three dimensions [43]. However, this system is not fully capable of creating a branched vascular system, which is vitally important in the context of organ manufacturing to direct spatially heterogeneous tissue development. On the other hand, Arcaute and coworkers have encapsulated human dermal fibroblasts in a synthetic poly(ethylene glycol)-dimethacrylate hydrogel by a SLA technique. Without porous structures and biodegradable properties of the synthetic polymers, it is hard for the cells to form tissues inside the hydrogel [44]. The integrations of biomaterials and RP techniques can form a huge "family tree" with many different combinations. Figure 2 summarizes the integrations of biomaterials with RP techniques and their potential usages in complex organ manufacturing.

Currently, as the concepts of "factory in a box" and "desktop manufacturing" are expanding, new applications of RP techniques in architectural design and 3D construct building increase speedily. Among the most popular RP techniques, the Fab@Home equipments with an average price of about 3000 US dollars are among the most convenient and cost effective RP instruments used in biomaterial fabrication field [45].

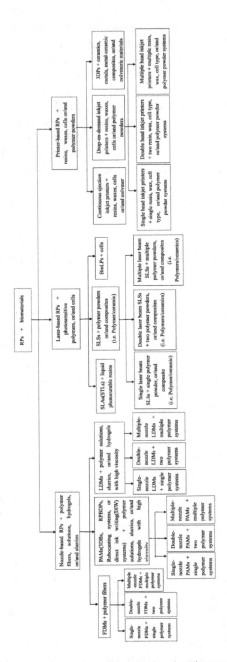

Figure 2. A "family tree" indicates various integrations of biomaterials and rapid prototyping techniques.

At present, the concepts of "scaffolds", "tissues", and "organs" are rather confused both in scientific and industrial areas. Most researchers and manufacturers in the area of tissue engineering like to label their RP products as "scaffolds", "tissues", or "organs". It is reasonable to describe an accellular porous 3D structure with a micro-scale internal architecture but without cells as a "scaffold". However, those with living cells incorporated should be defined as "constructs". Especially, those with cells have already connected to each other to perform special functions should be called "tissues". As described in the beginning of the introduction section, those with more than three different tissue types inside a construct should be called "organs". Simple organs, such as the bladder and blood vessels, should have less than or equal to three tissue types, while complex organs, such as the liver, heart, and kidney, should posses more than three tissue types. With these definitions, it is easier to distinguish which RP technique will be useful in complex organ manufacturing.

3. The integrations of biomaterials with RP techniques for complex organ manufacturing

The ability to put material only into a specific location where it is desired could have a profound impact on how parts are designed and manufactured [46]. Similarly, the ability to put different biomaterials (including different cell types) to exact sites where they are desired could have a profound impact on how complex organs are designed and manufactured. For example, in a complex organ, such as the liver, at least three different cell types (hepatocytes, stellate cells, and Kupffer cells) are required that function in a construct along with the three common cell types of a vascular system. The fundamental unit of the liver, the acinus, has a typical radius of 500 μm. Within this structure at least six cell types interact with one another to coordinate the diversity of liver functions [46]. The spatially heterogeneous arrangements of multi-tissues make all the traditional, or existing techniques incapable of completing this ambitious task.

Over the last ten years, the integration of biomaterials with RP techniques in creating special 3D constructs for various biomedical applications has emerged. The ability to use data from clinical imaging techniques like magnetic resonance imaging (MRI), computerized tomography (CT) or patient-specific data makes RP techniques particularly useful for biomedical applications. Several research groups have adapted different RP techniques to assemble (or print) cell-laden constructs directly from computer-programmed design models with high resolution (Table 2) [47-64]. Six unique intelligent RP devices as well as their primary products are shown in Figure 3[47-52, 65-67]. These processes have demonstrated some possibilities in the area of complex organ manufacturing. The pros and cons of these techniques in complex organ manufacturing are outlined in Table 2. Those with only porous 3D scaffolds are not included here because these integrations have been reported extensively in the former reviews [36,37,44,68-79].

Technique	Pros	Cons	Refs
3D inkjet bioprinting (3DP) in and Pittsburgh Clemson University, USA	Several thermosensitive hydrogels can be used as biopaper; low viscosity cell suspensions or aggregates can be used as bioink; Cell viability greater than 85%.	Complex 3D constructs are difficult to realize; limited feature height (< 5 μm); lack of structural support for cell layer or cell aggregates; tissue formation into lines depends on cell or cell aggregate fusion or assembling; poor mechanical properties.	[47, 48]
3D direct-write bioprinting in University of Cornell and Arizona, USA.	Low and high viscosity hydrogels, including type 1 collagen and alginate can be used; high cell viability (up to 98%); flexible geometric shapes.	Cell viability depends largely on the inner diameter of the gauge tip, collagen concentration and extraction environments; difficult to control the collage gel state.	[49, 50]
3D fiber deposition (3DF) in University Medical Center Utrecht, The Netherlands.	High viscosity hydrogels, such as Pluronic F127, Matrigel, alginate and agarose, can be used; multiple cell types can be incorporated; homogeneous and heterogeneous structures can be created.	Limited materials can be used; limited height of 3D construct (< 10 μm); difficult cell-cell interactions; poor mechanical properties.	[51, 52]
3D single/double syringe cell assembling (or pressure assisted manufacturing (PAM)) in Tsinghua University, China.	Gelatin-based hydrogels can be used; a wide range of biological components can be incorporated; variable and hybrid geometric shapes; high cell viability (more than 98%); easy for long-term storage and transportation.	Limited materials can be used; weaker mechanical properties.	[53 - 60]
Double-nozzle low-temperature deposition manufacturing (DLDM) in Tsinghua University, China.	A wide range of biomaterials including both synthetic and natural polymers can be used; a wide range of biological components can be incorporated; arbitrarily hybrid geometric shapes; high mechanical properties; easy for long-term storage and transportation.	Material viscosity and temperature dependent.	[61 - 64]

Table 2. Comparison of different cell-laden rapid prototyping techniques in complex organ manufacturing

Due to the heterogeneous properties of complex organs both in geometrical structures and material components, emphases should be given to those RP techniques with further development possibilities in the further integrations of biomaterials and equipments. In the following part of this section, some special two or multiple syringe/nozzle techniques are highlighted. In Harvard Medical School, Lee and coworkers have printed a collagen hydrogel precursor, fibroblasts and keratinocytes into a quasi 3D structure for skin repair using a robotic platform (Figure 3D) [65]. The procedure involves printing a layer of liquid collagen to act as a hydrogel precursor. The liquid collagen is crosslinked with a nebulized aqueous crosslinking agent (sodium bicarbonate) to form a hydrogel that provides structural integrity for the subsequent cell suspensions. In fact, this technique is an extension of the above mentioned 3DP or 3DB robotic system with additional syringes as "cartridges" to load two cell suspensions and hydrogel precursors. Highly viable proliferation of each cell layer (85% for keratinocytes and 95% for fibroblasts) was observed on both planar and non-planar surfaces. For thin tissue/organ (such as skin/bladder) manufacturing, this technique is a right choice. However, for complex organ manufacturing, some intrinsic shortcomings, such as limited printing height, and difficult to control the collagen gelation process, made this technique almost incapable.

In University Medical Center Utrecht, The Netherlands, Prof. J Alblas's group, a special bio-scaffolder pneumatic dispensing system (SYS + ENG) was adapted for printing cell-laden bone tissue repair hydrogels. High viscosity alginate (10% w/v) and BD Matrigel™ (10% w/v) hydrogels were employed. A limited ten-layer rectangular 3D construct of 10 ×10 mm with spacing between fibers of 0.8-2.5 mm and a thickness of 100 μm was fabricated and subsequently crosslinked in a $CaCl_2$ solution [51]. In spite of the limited height, the interconnected channels are still necessary for oxygen and nutrient delivery, as well as for tissue formation and vascular ingrowth. There are two critical drawbacks of this technique in complex organ manufacturing. The first is the poor mechanical properties of the cell-laden alginate or matrigel hydrogel for use as vascular systems. The second is that low viscosity hydrogels (including alginate and matrigel) are hard to be assembled into 3D constructs.

In university of Missouri, Norotte and coworkers used agarose rods as a molding template to print multicellular spheroids with their special bioprinter to form a tubular cell-laden structure (Figure 3E) [66]. After the fabrication stage, they manually pulled the agarose rods out of the tube, and concluded that it is a time consuming and labor-/spheroid- intensive procedure.

4. Some outstanding achievements made in Tsinghua University

In parallel with the above mentioned RP approaches, a series of RP technologies have been explored extensively by Professor XH Wang's group at the Center of Organ Manufacturing, Department of Mechanical Engineering, Tsinghua University, China. State-of-the-art of the layer-by-layer modeling, material incorporation, and manufacturing principles of these techniques can be found in some of the pertaining references. The advantages and disadvantages of these approaches to be used in complex organ manufacturing have also been listed in Table 2. Previous studies have demonstrated their abilities to engineer complex 3D tissues using various single/double nozzle/syringe RP systems. In the following section some technical specifications are highlighted.

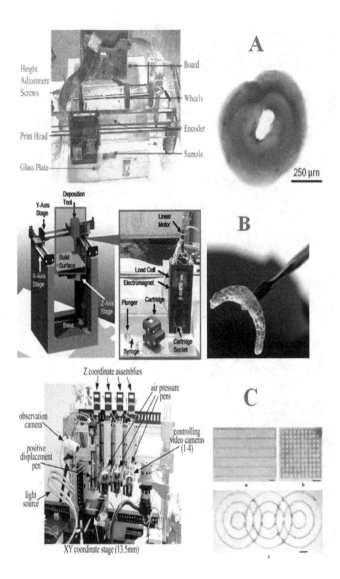

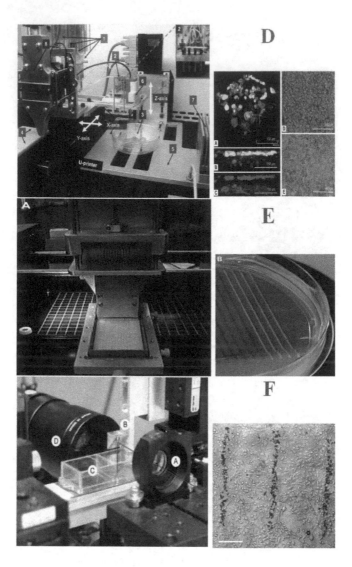

Figure 3. Several unique intelligent rapid prototyping devices and their functional cell-laden products: A) The inkjet cell printer and its bagel-like quasi-3D structure developed in Clemson University, prof. T Boland's group [47]. B) The robotic printing platform and its crescent construct made in Cornell University, prof. LJ Bonassar's group [49]. C) The direct-write system and its preliminary 3D figures developed in University of Arizona, prof. SK Williams' group [50]. D) A modular tissue printing platform with 4 'cartridges' to load cell suspensions and hydrogel precursors developed in Brigham and Women's Hospital, Harvard Medical School, Prof. S.-S. Yoo's group [65]. E) A bioprinting tubular structure with cellular cylinders developed in University of Missouri, Columbia, USA, Prof. G Forgacs' group [66]. F) A laser-guided direct writing (LGDW) system and its patterned factor-linked beads on a stem cell monolayer with micrometer accuracy (Bar = 200 μm) developed in University of Minnesota, prof. D.J. Odde's group [67].

4.1. The single syringe cell assembling technique

Figure 4 shows some of the cell assembling results using our first generation cell assembling system. A gelatin based hydrogel system, such as gelatin, gelatin/chitosan, gelatin/hyaluronan, gelatin/alginate, gelatin/fibrinogen or gelatin/alginate/fibrinogen, was integrated with a single syringe cell-assembling machine to obtain the necessary space and stabilizing factors for cell survival and tissue formation [53-58]. A single cell type was deposited at an ambient temperature (1~10°C) layer by layer in a chamber as the sol state material was transferred into a hydrogel. Grid hepatic tissues, endodermis, and adipose tissues have been regenerated by using this single syringe cell-assembly machine at about 8°C. The gelatin based hydrogel network provided stabilization support for the 3D constructs during the fabrication and post culture stages. This mild deposition temperature is favorable for biological property preservation as increased Joule heating can result in loss of cell viabilities and bioactivities. During the culture period, the gelatin based hydrogel served as both a mass transportation template for tissue development and an extracellular matrix accommodation mimicking the microenvironment in native organs. The use of the natural gelatin based hydrogels was clearly highlighted the distinct advantage of this cell assembly technique for fabricating living tissue analogs. A shortage of the single nozzle/syringe systems was that, these systems lack the ability to easily create parts with spatial heterogeneous materials. Consequently, two double nozzle/syringe RP systems have been explored to deposit different materials at different temperatures.

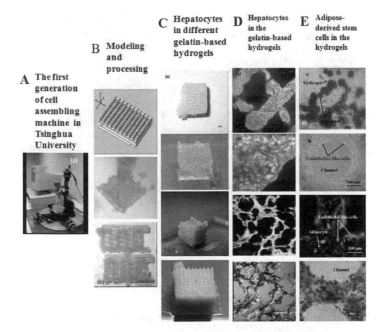

Figure 4. Hepatocyte and adipose-derived stem cell (ADSC) assembling based on the first generation of cell assembling technique developed in Tsinghua University, prof. XH Wang' group [53-58]

4.2. The double syringe cell assembling technique

Different from the above single syringe cell assembling technique, a double syringe cell assembling technique was developed in Tsinghua Unversity with a updated software and hardware. Gradient and cylindrical architectures consist of two different cell-laden hydrogels have been fabricated at a temperature range of 8 – 10℃ [59,60]. Two cell lines encapsulated in the similar gelatin-based hydrogels were put into different regions or compartment in a construct (Figure 5). The embedded branched networks enable culture medium to flow through the entire construct with unparalleled geometric complexity. However, there is a fatal shortcoming of this system to be used in complex organ manufacturing. The mechanical weak properties of the gelatin-based hydrogel made it impossible to connect the branched construct to an *in vivo* vascular system to endure anti-suture anastomosis and blood pressure even after a long-term *in vitro* culture period.

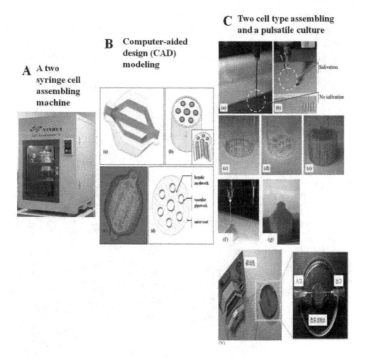

Figure 5. Cell assembling based on a two syringe RP technique developed in Tsinghua University, prof. XH Wang' group. Two different cell types in the gelatin-based hydrogels can be assembled simultaneously into a construct [59-60].

4.3. The combination of cell assembly and cryopreservation techniques

With the advantages of the gelatin-based hydrogel, cryoprotectants (e.g. dimethyl sulfoxide (DMSO), glycerol, and dextran-40) can be incorporated into the cell/hydrogel system and the constructs can be stored at low temperature (below -80℃) directly after the fabrication stage (Figure 6). This incorporation technique represents a significant advancement towards the cell-laden product storage and transport, potentially resulting in labor and resource saving, clinical availability and medical convenience [80-82]. With the gelatin-based hydrogel various bio-factors including macromolecular cell growth factors, small chemical regulators, and even genes/drugs can be easily incorporated to the deposition or assembling systems. This approach is suitable for some special natural thermosetting polymers' (e.g. gelatin and agarose) deposition and opens a new avenue for complex organ manufacturing.

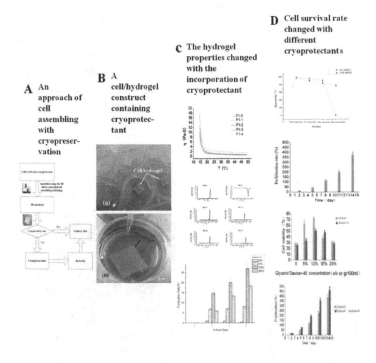

Figure 6. The combination of cell assembly and cryopreservation techniques, developed in prof. XH Wang' group [80-82].

4.4. The double-nozzle low-temperature deposition manufacturing (DLDM) system

The creation of a geometrically complex branched vascular system is a subject of broad fundamental and technological interest in complex organ manufacturing. With the DLDM system it is easy to deposit two different material systems, especially both synthetic and natural polymer systems simultaneously in a construct (Figure 7). Grid, tubular and elliptic structures with both synthetic and natural polymers, such as PU/gelatin and PU/collagen, have been produced at a low-temperature range of -20 - -30 ℃ [61-64]. As shown in Figure 7C, PU and collagen were successfully assembled into a tubular double layer construct. In Figure 7D, an elliptic hybrid hierarchical PU-cell/hydrogel construct with branched and grid internal channels was realized. Cells can survival the heterogeneous fabrication, polymerization/ crosslinking, and even storage stages with a high recovery proliferation ability. Figure 7D demonstrates that the external out coat was made of a PU/tetraglycol solution to provide mechanical support for the whole construct. The internal branched and grid channels were made of a cell/dimethyl sulfoxide (DMSO) containing gelatin/alginate/fibrinogen hydrogel to encapsulate ADSCs. Both the out coat PU and compartment cell/hydrogel layers possess microporous, which permit water, oxygen and other small molecules to pass. During the fabrication stage, a low temperature in the range of -20 - -30 ℃ around the nozzles is an important factor to control the sol-gel transformation of the material systems. If the temperature is set too high, the deposited fiber (strand) cannot solidify to form a stable 3D structure. On the other hand, if the temperature is set too low, the fiber is frozen too quickly to fuse with the previous deposited layer. An optimum deposition temperature has played a central role in putting the heterogeneous material systems at the desired locations in the construct.

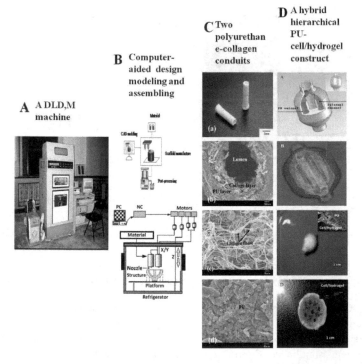

Figure 7. A DLDM technique developed in Tsinghua University, prof. XH Wang' group. An elliptical hybrid hierarchical polyurethane and cell/hydrogel construct was fabricated using the DLDM system [61-64].

This DLDM technique has demonstrated some outstanding merits in complex organ manufacturing with two different material systems that are technologically and biologically incapable to produce using the other existing or traditional RP techniques. The potential applications of the assembled elliptic hybrid hierarchical constructs are diverse, such as cell-cell interaction analyses, stem cell differentiation tracing (pursuing), chemical drug screening, and pathogenic mechanism studies. The synthetic PU system can provide elaborate compartments for cell/hydrogel accommodation. In these compartments, the composition of the cell/hydrogel mixture becomes the key factor in ensuring spatially uniform cell distribution, survival, proliferation and differentiation. By encapsulating the cell/hydrogel mixture in the PU compartments, the composition and proportion of hydrogel components can be easily adjusted to meet the necessary requirements for mimicking the natural cellular arrangements. A maximal cell density (hydrogel-poor and cell-rich) can be easily achieved in the compartment. The use of gelatin-based hydrogel can even be avoided completely in this system, irrespective of stabilization of the construct. Compared with the pure cell/gelatin/alginate/fibrin construct made by the single/double RP systems, the hybrid hierarchical network can provide much higher mechanical stability and pressure resistance abilities when it is applied to *in vitro* pulsatile cultures and *in vivo* blood vessel anastomoses. Some experiments have proved that the 3D constructs with intrinsic interconnected branched and grid channels were easily adapted to an *in vitro* pulsatile culture and *in vivo* implantation system [83-86].

5. A four-nozzle low-temperature deposition manufacturing (FLDM) system

At present, a FLDM system is under development in professor XH Wang's group [18]. Figure 8 demonstrates the outlook of the machine and a primary try on a liver lobe like structure construction. Compared with the DLDM RP system, two more nozzles have been equipped. Thus, two more cell types can be incorporated simultaneously into a construct. This amplified integration possesses some outstanding advantages towards complex organ manufacturing: (i) hierarchically organization of multiple population of cells and growth factors in a more intricate physiologically mimicking geometry; (ii) simultaneously deposition of one scaffold material, a vascular system with two main cell types, and one parenchymal cell type in a more elegant native tissue-specific phenotype; (iii) computer definition of the fluid paths and macro/microstructures in a more patient specific manner; and (iv) spatial distribution of multi-tissue boundaries and fluorescent biomarkers in a more controllable pattern. This FLDM RP system makes it possible to partially control over the design, modeling and fabrication of a highly hierarchical liver lobe like construct in a rapid, convenient, and cost effective manner.

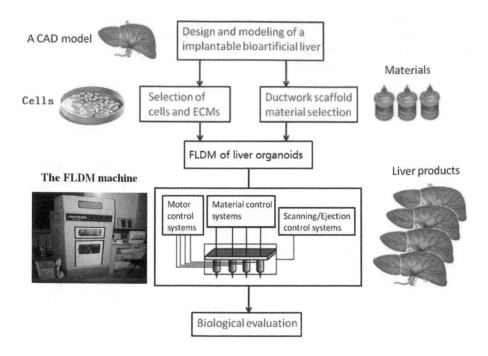

Figure 8. A schematic description of the modeling and manufacturing processes of four liver lobe-like constructs with a FLDM RP system developed in Tsinghua University, prof. XH Wang' group [18].

6. Emphases to some technical specifications

Theoretically, RP technology is able to produce any required complex shape. The standard modeling and deposition technologies enable the hybrid hierarchically ordered patterns to be generated in an automatic, convenient, and inexpensive manner. Again, we use the liver as an example. In a liver lobe at least 6 different cell types are structured as repeated units. These units can achieve high oxygen exchange and nutrient supply for a mass of cells where the cell sizes are in the range of ~20 μm. This geometry enables a high degree of processing optimization, which provides the opportunity for RP designers and manufacturers to control readily the distribution of different cells in a construct. Stimulated by this motivation, many groups have tried different RP systems with only thin or quasi-3D cell containing structures so far. Someone even claims to use scaffold free cell aggregates to print organs. This has been proven to be a time-consuming process and cells can not find their respective places in a complex organ without the support of scaffold materials.

Different from all the existing techniques, the gelatine-based hydrogel has been explored extensively as an internal scaffold material with the single/double syringe/nozzle RP techniques in the author's own group Tsinghua University. Aqueous gelatin solution is an amorphous natural hydrogel in which cells can be encapsulated, extruded and deposited at desired positions [87-90]. This solution is flexible with a gelation temperature of 20℃ and allow the diffusion of hydrophilic substrates. The sol-gel transform property makes it possible to deposit the gelatin-based cell-laden hydrogel at a large range of temperature (from 20℃ to -30℃). However, this hydrogel is not stable at 37℃. The mechanical properties of the gelatin-based hydrogels are notoriously inadequate and prohibit the use in stress-loaded implants. To improve the stability of the gelatin-based hydrogels, alginate and fibrinogen were incorporated. Sodium alginate (composed of mannuronic and guluronic (G) dimmers) is a biocompatible and biodegradable polymer, and has been widely used in cell encapsulation technology, although the biocompatibility of the alginates in relation to their composition is a matter of debate. Sodium alginate can be reversibly cross-linked by divalent cations, such as Ca^{+2} and Mg^{+2}, to form a relatively stable hydrogel. Fibrin, derived from blood fibrinogen, is another natural biocompatible and biodegradable polymer, which has been widely used as sealant and adhesive during surgery. With the catalyzing of thrombin smaller fibrinogen molecules can polymerize to form a stable fibrin hydrogel.

In addition to being able to build complex structures with precision and accuracy, it is equally important that the mechanical properties of the supporting materials are suitable for the intended applications. A novel linear elastomeric polyurethane from soft polycaprolactone (PCL) and polyethylene glycol (PEG) segments, and hexamethylene diisocyanate (HDI) chain extender has been synthesized in the authors' own group and used as an external scaffold material. This PU possesses tunable biodegradability, excellent biocompatibility and compatible mechanical properties with animal veins [91,92]. Long-term *in vivo* biocompatibility and biodegradability of the PU have been proven with a rabbit model. It has successfully repaired nerve and vein defects without any detected side effects, such as thrombosis, inflammation, intimal hyperplasia, and calcification. The excellent mechanical properties, biocompatibilities, adjust abilities and processing abilities have made this kind of polymer to be outstanding from the other existing synthetic scaffold biomaterials, such as polyhydroxybutyrate (PHB) [93], poly(D,L-lactic-co-glycolic acid) (PLGA) [94], and poly(tetrafluoroethylene) (PTFE) [95].

To date, the most widely recognized advantage of the RP technology (i.e. layered manufacturing methodology) is the relative ease of automatically manufacture of complex geometric shapes with heterogeneous structures composed of multi-material regions. Complex organ manufacturing aims to automatically produce complex organs directly from CAD models with high sophisticated RP techniques. Since the earlier concept of complex organ manufacturing using both synthetic and natural scaffold biomaterials and multi-nozzle RP techniques was first introduced in 2007, the present technique was developed gradually [13-18]. As displayed in Figure 7D, the virtual elliptic construct with branched fluidic network has been designed and fabricated according to a pre-defined CAD software. The integration of the DLDM RP technique with the cell cryopreservation technique together with the mechanically strong enough synthetic PU scaffold enables us to efficiently produce spatially hetero-geneous cell-laden tissue/organ substitutes that would otherwise be challenging to achieve [61-64]. This integrated technique therefore has the potential to lead a big revolution in the fields of tissue engineering and regenerative medicine.

It is expected that in the following several years these integrated RP technologies will see their major break-through development stage and play a key role in complex organ manu-facturing area. With the proper integrations of biomaterials and enabling RP techniques, it is possible for us to address all the challenges involved in complex organ manufacturing and to make the realization of complex organ manufacturing both feasible and practical. These proper integrations also benefit some of other related areas, such as high throughput drug screening, stem cell differentiation induction, fluorescent dye discovering, energy metabolite model establishing and cancer/stem cell behavior controlling.

7. Concluding remarks

The goal of complex organ manufacturing is to directly fabricate multiple cell types into an organ substitute using a multiple nozzle RP system. Analogous to the process of building a nuclear power plant, complex organ manufacturing requires the ability to control the posi-tions of many cell types, internal/external scaffold materials, and even cell growth factors on the nano-, micro-, and macro-scales with respect to each others. The integrations of biomate-rials and RP techniques have significantly improved the ability to manufacture cell-laden constructions with predefined geometries under the instructions of CAD models or medical data (for example, patient-specific images). Especially, recent advances in DLDM and FLDM RP techniques in Tsinghua University have leveraged these progresses. Although still at its infant stages and associated with numerous problems, ever-increasing evidence supports the intriguing hypothesis that the integrations of multiple biomaterials (including multiple cell types) and multiple nozzle RP techniques will eventually change the traditional practi-ces and make the dreams of complex organ manufacturing come true. It is expected that in the future, most of the reconstructive disciplines of complex organ manufacturing will be fully revised by the development of new multiple nozzle RP systems with optimal safety, easy manipulation ability and maximum reliability. Multiple nozzle RP techniques will un-doubtedly play an important role in the future complex organ manufacturing area. Cells in the engineered construct will potentially behave as comfortably as in their natural *in vivo* environment. Further studies are therefore needed to elucidate and determine the funda-mental structure-function relationships of diverse tissues in a complex organ, the nutrition supply systems and the heterogeneous structural cues to promote full functional realization in a complex organ. Ever increasing evidences have indicated that with the right integra-tions of biomaterials and RP techniques, a brand-new era of complex organ manufacturing like the rising sun, is on the horizon.

Acknowledgment

The Project was Supported by the State Key Laboratory of Materials Processing and Die & Mould Technology, Huazhong University of Science and Technology (No. 2012 - P03), the National Natural Science Foundation of China / the Research Grants Council of Hong Kong (NSFC/RGC, No. 50731160625), the National Natural Science Foundation of China (No. 81271665), the National Natural Science Foundation of China (No. 30970748), the Cross-Strait Tsinghua Cooperation Basic Research (No.2012THZ02-3), the National High Tech 863 Grant (No. 2009AA043801), the Finland Distinguished Professor program (FiDiPro) of Tekes (No. 40041/10).

Author details

Xiaohong Wang[1,2,3*], Jukka Tuomi[1], Antti A. Mäkitie[1,4], Kaija-Stiina Paloheimo[1], Jouni Partanen[1] and Marjo Yliperttula[5]

*Address all correspondence to: wangxiaohong@tsinghua.edu.cn

1 Business Innovation Technology (BIT) Research Centre, School of Science and Technology, Aalto University, Aalto, Finland

2 Key Laboratory for Advanced Materials Processing Technology, Ministry of Education & Center of Organ Manufacturing, Department of Mechanical Engineering, Tsinghua University, Beijing, P.R. China

3 State Key Laboratory of Materials Processing and Die & Mould Technology, Huazhong University of Science and Technology, Wuhan, P.R. China

4 Department of Otolaryngology - Head & Neck Surgery, Helsinki University Hospital and University of Helsinki, Helsinki, Finland

5 Division of Biopharmaceutics and Pharmacokinetics, Faculty of Pharmacy, University of Helsinki, Helsinki, Finland

References

[1] Widmaier EP, Raff H, Strang KT. Vander's Human Physiology. 2003 11th Ed. McGraw-Hill. ISBN 9870073049625.

[2] Walther G, Gekas J, Bertrand DF. Amniotic stem cells for cellular cardiomyoplasty: promises and premises. Catheterization and Cardiovascular Inter Ventions 2009;73:917-924.

[3] Aikawa E, Nahrendorf M, Sosnovik D, Lok VM, Jaffer FA, Aikawa M, Weissleder R. Multimodality molecular imaging identifies proteolytic and osteogenic activities in early aortic valve disease. Circulation 2007;115L:377-386.

[4] Demetriou AA, Brown RS Jr, Busuttil RW, Fair J, McGuire BM, Rosenthal P, Am Esch JS II, Lerut J, Nyberg SL, Salizzoni M, Fagan EA, de Hemptinne B, Broelsch CE, Muraca M, Salmeron JM, Rabbin JM, Metselaar HJ, Pratt D, De La Mata M, McChesney LP, Everson GT, Lavin PT, Sterens AC, Pitkin Z, Solomon BA. Prospective, randomized multicenter, controlled trial of a bioartificial liver in treating acute liver failure. Ann Surg 2004;239(5):660-670.

[5] Orive G, Hernández RM, Gascón AR, Calafore R, Chang TMS, de Vos P. Hortelano G, Hunkeler D, Lacík I, Pedraz JL. History, challenges and perspectives of cell microencapsulation. Trends Biotechnol 2004;22:87-92.

[6] Sekine H, Shimizu T, Yang J, Kobayashi E, Okano T. Pulsatile myocardial tubes fabricated with cell sheet engineering. Circulation 2006;114[suppl I]:I-87- I-93.

[7] Moniaux N, Faivre J. A reengineered liver for transplantation. Journal of Hepatology 2011;54:386-387.

[8] Planat-Benard V, Silvestre J-S, Cousin B, André M, Nibbelink M, Tamarat R, Clergue M, Manneville C, Saillan-Barreau C, Duriez M, Tedgui A, Levy B, Pénicaud L, Casteilla L. Plasticity of human adipose lineage cells toward endothelial cellls. Circulation 2004;109:656-663.

[9] Simper D, Stalboerger PG, Panetta CJ, Wang S, Caplice NM. Smooth muscle progenitor cells in human blood. Circulation 2002;106:1199-1204.

[10] Rowley JA, Sun Z, Goldman D, Mooney DJ. Biomaterials to spatially regulate cell fate. Adv Mater 2002;14(12):886-889.

[11] Caplan AI. Mesenchymal stem cell. J Orthop Res 1991; 9(5): 641-650.

[12] en.wikipedia.org/wiki

[13] Wang XH, Ma JB, Wang YN, He BL. Bone repair in radii and tibias of rabbits with phosphorylated chitosan reinforced calcium phosphate cements. Biomaterials. 2002;23(21):4167-4176

[14] Wang XH, Yan YN, Zhang RJ. Gelatin-based hydrogels for controlled cell assembly. In: Ottenbrite RM, ed. Biomedical Applications of Hydrogels Handbook. New York: Springer, 2010;269-284.

[15] Wang XH, Yan YN, Zhang RJ Rapid prototyping as a tool for manufacturing bioartificial livers. Trends Biotechnol 2007;25:505-513.

[16] Wang XH, Yan YN, Zhang RJ. Recent trends and challenges in complex organ manufacturing. Tissue Eng Part B 2010;16:189-197.

[17] Wang XH, Zhang QQ. Overview on "Chinese–Finnish workshop on biomanufacturing and evaluation techniques. Artificial Organs 2011;35(10):E191- E193.

[18] Wang XH. Intelligent freeform manufacturing of complex organs. Artificial Organs.
2012; doi:10.1111/j.1525-1594.2012.01499.x

[19] Langer R, Vacanti JP. Tissue Engineering. Science 1993;260:920-926.

[20] Oberpenning F, Meng J, Yoo J J, Atala A. De novo reconstitution of a functional
mammalian urinary bladder by tissue engineering. Nature Biotechnol
1999;17:149-155.

[21] Ramakrishna S, Mayer J, Wintermantel E, Leong KW. Biomedical applications of pol-
ymer-composite materials: a review. Comp Sci Technol 2001;61(9):1189-1224.

[22] Vert M. Aliphatic polyesters: great degradable polymers that cannot do everything.
Biomacromolecules 2005;6(2):538-546.

[23] Piskin E. Biodegrdable polymers as biomaterials. J Biomater Sci Polym Edi
1994;6:775-795.

[24] Lee Y-J, Braun PV. Tunable inverse opal hydrogel PH sensors. Adv Mater 2003;
5(7-8): 563-566.

[25] Kang JH, Moon JH, Lee SK, Park SG, Jang SG, Yang S. Thermoresponsive hydrogel
photonic crystals by three-dimensional holographic lithography. Adv Mater
2008;20(16):3061-3065.

[26] Barry 111 RA, Shepherd RF, Hanson JN, Nuzzo RG, Wiltzius P, Lewis JA. Direct-
write assembly of 3D hydrogel scaffolds for guided cell growth. Adv. Mater. 2009;
21(23): 2407-2410.

[27] Calvert P. Inkjet printing for materials and devices. Chem Mater 2001;13(10):
3299-3305.

[28] Liska R, Schuster M, Infuhr R, Turecek C, Fritscher C, Seidl B, Schmidt V, Kuna L,
Haase A, Varga F. Photopolymers for rapid prototyping. 2007;4(4):505-510.

[29] Mikos AG, Thorsen AJ, Czerwonka LA, Bao Y, Langer R, Winslow DN, Vacanti JP.
Preparation and characterization of poly(l-lactic acid) foams. Polymer 1994;35(5):
1068-1077.

[30] Karp JM, Shoichet MS, Davies JE. Bone formation on two-dimensional poly(DL-lac-
tide-co-glycolide) (PLGA) films and three-dimensional PLGA tissue engineering
scaffolds in vitro. J Biomed Mater Res A 2003;64A(2):388-396.

[31] Sai P, Babu M. Collagen based dressings - a review. Burn 2000;26(1):54-62.

[32] Khademhosseini A, Eng G, Yeh J, Fukuda J, Blumling 111 J, Langer R, Burdick JA. J
Biomed Mater Res A 2006; 79(3):522-532.

[33] Wang XH, Ma JB, Wang YN, He BL. Structural characterization of phosphorylated chitosan and their applications as effective additives of calcium phosphate cements. Biomaterials 2001;22(16): 2247-2255.

[34] Chu C, Graf G, Posen DW. Design for additive manufacturing of cellular structures. Compter-aided design and applications 2008;5(5):680-696.

[35] Chua LK, Leong KF, Lim CS. Rapid prototyping: principles and applications. Singapore: World Scientific Publishing 2004.

[36] Azari A, Nikzad S. The evolution of rapid prototyping in dentistry: a review. Rapid Prototyping J 2009;15(3): 216-225.

[37] Pfister A, Landers R. Laib A, Hübner U, Schmelzeisen R. Biofunctional rapid prototyping for tissue engineering applications: 3D bioplotting versus 3D printing. J Polymer Science Part A Polymer Chem 2004;42(3):624-638.

[38] Maher PS, Keatch RP, Donnelly K, Mackay RE, Paxton JZ. Construction of 3D biological matrices using rapid prototyping technology. Rapid Prototyping J 2009;15(3): 204-210.

[39] Yeong WY, Chua CK, Leong KF, Chandrasekaran M, Lee MW. Indirect fabrication of collagen scaffold based on inkjet printing technique. Rapid Prototyping J 2006;12(4): 229-237.

[40] Odde DJ, Renn MJ. Laser-guided direct writing of living cells. Biotechnol Bioeng 2000;67:312-318.

[41] Tan KH, Chua CK, Leong KF, Cheah CM, Gui WS, Tan WS, Wiria FE. Selective laser sintering of biocompatible polymers for applications in tissue engineering. Bio-Medical Materials and Engineering 2005;15(1-2):113-124.

[42] Billiet T, Vandenhaute M, Schelfhout J, Vlierberghe SV, Dubruel P. A review of trends and limitations in hydrogel-rapid prototyping for tissue engineering. Biomaerials 2012;33(26): 6020-6041.

[43] Chu J, Engelbrecht S, Graf G, Rosen DW. A comparison of synthesis methods for cellular structures with application to additive manufacturing. Rapid Prototyping J 2010;16:275-283.

[44] Arcaute K, Mann BK, Wicker RB. Stereolithography of three-dimensional bioactive poly(ethylene glycol) constructs with encapsulated cells. Ann Biomed Eng 2006;34(9): 1429-1441.

[45] Malone E, Lipson H. Fab@Home: the personal desktop fabricator kit. Rapid Prototyping J 2007;13(4):245-255.

[46] Bhatia SN, Chen CS. Tissue engineering at the micro-scale. Biomedical Microdevices 1999;2:131-144.

[47] Boland T, Xu T, Damon B, Cui X. Application of inkjet printing to tissue engineering. Biotechnol J 2006;1(9):910-917.

[48] Cooper GM, Miller ED, DeCesare GE, Usas A, Lensie EL, Bykowski MR, Huard J, Weiss LE, Losee JE, Campbell PG. Inkjet-based biopatterning of bone orphogenetic protein-2 to spatially control calvarial bone formation. Tissue Eng Part A 2010;16:1749-1759.

[49] Cohen DL, Malone E, Lipson H, Bonassar LJ. Direct freeform fabrication of seeded hydrogels in arbitrary geometries. Tissue Eng 2006;12:1325-1335.

[50] Smith CM, Stone AL, Parkhill RL, Stewart RL, Simpkins MW, Kachurin AM, Warren WL, Williams SK. Three-dimensional bioassembly tool for generating viable tissue-engineered constructs. Tissue Eng 2004;10:1566-1576.

[51] Fedorovich NE, Schuurman W, Wijnberg HM, Prins H-J, van Weeren PR, Malda J, Alblas J, Dhert WJA. Biofabrication of osteochondral tissue equivalents by printing topologically defined, cell-laden hydrogel scaffolds. Tissue Eng Part C 2012;18:33-44.

[52] Fedorovich NE, Alblas J, Hennink WE, Öner FC, Dhert WJA. Organ printing: the future of bone regeneration? Trends Biotechnol 2011;29:601-606.

[53] Yan YN, Wang XH, Xiong Z, Liu HX, Liu F, Lin F, Wu RD, Zhang RJ, Lu QP. Direct construction of a three-dimensional structure with cells and hydrogel. J Bioact Compat Polym 2005;20:259-69.

[54] Yan YN, Wang XH, Pan YQ, Liu HX, Cheng J, Xiong Z, Lin F, Wu RD, Zhang RJ, Lu QP. Fabrication of viable tissue-engineered constructs with 3D cell-assembly technique. Biomaterials 2005;26:5864-5871.

[55] Wang XH, Yan YN, Pan YQ, Wang, Xiong Z, Liu HX, Cheng J, Liu F, Lin F, Wu RD, Zhang RJ, Lu QP. Generation of three-dimensional hepatocyte/gelatin structures with rapid prototyping system. Tissue Eng 2006;12:83-90.

[56] Xu W, Wang XH, Yan YN, Zhang W, Xiong Z, Lin F, Wu RD, Zhang RJ. Rapid prototyping three-dimensional cell/gelatin/fibrinogen constructs for medical regeneration. J Bioact Compat Polym 2007;22 (4):363-377.

[57] Zhang T, Yan YN, Wang XH, Xiong Z, Lin F, Wu RD, Zhang R.J. Three-dimensional gelatin and gelatin/hyaluronan hydrogel structures for traumatic brain injury. J Bioact Compat Polym 2007;22(1):19-29.

[58] Xu W, Wang XH, Yan YN, Zhang RJ. Rapid Prototyping of Polyurethane for the Creation of Vascular Systems. J Bioact Compat Polym 2008;23:103-114. (Featured by Nature China on May 3, 2008).

[59] Li SJ, Yan YN, Xiong Z, Weng CY, Zhang RJ, Wang XH. Gradient hydrogel construct based on an improved cell assembling system. J Bioact Compat Polym 2009;24 (S1): 84-99.

[60] Li SJ, Xiong Z, Wang XH, Yan YN, Liu HX, Zhang RJ. Direct fabrication of a hybrid cell/hydrogel construct via a double-nozzle assembling technology. J Bioact Compat Polym 2009;24:249-264.

[61] Cui TK, Yan YN, Zhang RJ, Liu L, Xu W, Wang XH. Rapid prototyping of a double layer polyurethane-collagen conduit for peripheral nerve regeneration. Tissue Eng Part C Methods 2009;15:1-9.

[62] Cui T K, Wang XH, Yan YN, Zhang RJ. Rapid prototyping a new polyurethane-collagen conduit and its Schwann cell compatibility. J Bioact Compat Polym 2009; 24(S1): 5-7.

[63] Wang XH, Cui T K, Yan YN, Zhang RJ. J Bioact Compat Polym 2009;24(2):109-127.

[64] He K, Wang XH. Rapid prototyping of tubular polyurethane and cell/hydrogel construct. J Bioact Compat Polym 2011;26(4):363-374.

[65] Lee W, Debasitis JC, Lee VK, Lee J-H, Fischer K, Edminster K, Park J-K, Yoo S-S. Multi-layered culture of human skin fibroblasts and kerainocytes through three-dimensional freeform fabrication. Biomaterials 2009;30(8):1587-1595.

[66] Norotte C, Marga FS, Niklason LE, Forgacs G. Scaffold-free vascular tissue engineering using bioprinting. Biomaterials 2009; 30(23):5910-5917.

[67] Nahmias Y, Schwartz RE, Verfaillie CM, Odde DJ. Laser-guided direct writing for three-dimensional tissue engineering. Biotech Bioeng 2005; 92(2):129-136.

[68] Leong KF, Cheah CM, Chua CK. Solid freeform fabrication of three-dimensional scaffolds for engineering replacement tissues and organs. Biomaterials 2003;24(13): 2363-2378.

[69] Yeong W-Y, Chua C-K, Leong K-F, Chandrasekaran M. Rapid prototyping in tissue engineering: challenges and potential. Trends Biotechnol 2004;22(12)643-652.

[70] Hutmacher DW, Sittinger M, Risbud MV. Scaffold-based tissue engineering: rationale for cimputer-aided design and solid free-form fabrication systems. Trends Biotechnol 2004;22(7):354-362.

[71] Hollister SJ. Porous scaffold design for tissue engineering. Nature Mater 2005;4:518524.

[72] Kou XY, Tan ST. Heterogeneous object modeling: a review. Computer-Aided Design 2007a; 39:284-301.

[73] Peltola SM, Melchels FPW, Grijpma DW, Kellomaki M. A review of rapid prototyping techniques for tissue engineering purposes. Ann Med 2008; 40:268-280.

[74] Uetla BR, Storti D, Anderson RC, Ganter M. A review of process development steps for new material-systems in three dimensional printing (3DP). J Manufacturig Process 2008;10:96-104.

[75] Grayson WL, Chao PH, Marolt D, Kaplan DL, Vunjak-Novakovic G. Engineering custom-designed osteochondral tissue grafts. Trends Biotechnol 2008;26:181-189.

[76] Bibb R, Eggbeer D, Evans P. Rapid prototyping technologies in soft tissue facial prosthetics: current state of the art. Rapid Prototyping J 2010;16(2):130-137.

[77] Melchels FPW, Feijen J, Grijpma DW. A review on stereolithography and its applications in biomedical engineering. Biomaterials 2010; 31(24):6121-6130.

[78] Neugebauer J, Stachulla G, Ritter L, Dreiseidler T, Mischkowski RA, Keeve E, Zöller JE. Computer-aided manufacturing technologies for guided implant placement. Expert. Rev. Med. Devices 2010;7(1):113-129.

[79] Dhandayuthapani B, Yoshida Y, Maekawa T, Kumar DS. Polymeric scaffolds in tissue engineering application: a review. In J Polym Science 2011, doi: 10.1155/2011/290602.

[80] Sui SC, Wang XH, Liu PY, Yan YN, Zhang RJ. Cryopreservation of cells in 3D constructs based on controlled cell assembly processes. J Bioact Compat Polym 2009;24(5):473-487.

[81] Wang XH, and Xu HR. Incorporation of DMSO and dextran-40 into a gelatin/alginate hydrogel for controlled assembled cell cryopreservation, Cryobiology 2010;61:345-351.

[82] Wang XH, Paloheimo K-S, Xu HR, Liu C. Cryopreservation of Cell/Hydrogel Constructs Based on a New Cell-assembling Technique. J BioactCompat Polym 2010;25(6): 634-653.

[83] Wang XH, Mäkitie AA, Paloheimo K-S, Tuomi J, Paloheimo M, Sui SC, Zhang QQ. Characterization of a PLGA sandwiched cell/fibrin construct and induction of the adipose stem cells (ADSCs) into smooth muscle cells. Materials Science and Engineering C 2011;31:801-808.

[84] Wang XH, Sui SC, Liu C. Optimizing the step-by-step forming processes for fabricating a poly(DL-lactic-co-glycolic acid)-sandwiched cell/hydrogel construct. J Appl Polym Sci 2011;120:1199-1207.

[85] Wang XH, Mäkitie AA, Paloheimo K-S, Tuomi, J., Paloheimo, M. A tubular PLGA-sandwiched cell/hydrogel fabrication technique based on a step-by-step mold/extraction process. Advances in Polymer Technology. 2011;30:163-173.

[86] Wang XH, Sui SC. Pulsatile culture of a PLGA sandwiched cell/hydrogel construct fabricated by a step-by step mold/extraction method. Artificial Organs 2011;35(6): 645-655.

[87] Yao R, Zhang RJ, Wang XH. Design and evaluation of a cell microencapsulating device for cell assembly technoloty. J Bioact Compat Polym 2009;24(1):48-62.

[88] Yao R, Zhang RJ, Yan YN, Wang XH. In vitro angiogenesis of 3D tissue engineered adipose tissue. J Bioact Compat Polym 2009;24(1):5-24.

[89] Xu ME, Yan YN, Liu HX, Yao R, Wang XH. Control adipose-derived stromal cells differentiation into adipose and endothelial cells in a 3-D structure established by cell-assembly technique. J Bioact Compat Polym 2009;24(S1):31-47.

[90] Xu ME, Wang XH, Yan YN, Yao R, Ge YK. An cell-assembly derived physiological 3D model of the metabolic syndrome, based on adipose-derived stromal cells and a gelatin/alginate/fibrinogen matrix. Biomaterials 2010;31(14):3868-3877.

[91] Yin DZ, Wang XH, Yan YN, Zhang RJ. Preliminary Studies on Peripheral Nerve Regeneration Using a New Polyurethane Conduit. J Bioact Compat Polym. 2007;22:143-159.

[92] Yan YN, Wang XH, Yin DZ, Zhang RJ. A New Polyurethane/Heparin Vascular Graft for Small-caliber Vein Repair. J Bioact Compat Polym. 2007;22:323-341.

[93] Pouton CW, Akhtar S. Biosynthetic polyhydroxyalkanoates and their potential in drug delivery. Advanced Drug Delivery Reviews. 1996;18(2):133-162.

[94] Kim SS, Utsunomiya H, Koski JA, Wu BM, Cima MJ, Sohn J, Mukai K, Griffith LG, Vacanti JP. Survival and function of hepatocytes on a novel three-dimensional synthetic biodegradable polymer scaffold with an intrinsic network of channels. Annals of Surgery 1998;228:8-13.

[95] Krupnick AS, Kreisel D, Engels FH, Szeto WY, Plappert T, Popma SH, Flake AW, Rosengard BR. A novel small animal of left ventricular tissue engineering. J Heart Lung Transpl 2002;21(2):233-243.

Healing Mechanism and Clinical Application of Autogenous Tooth Bone Graft Material

Young-Kyun Kim, Jeong Keun Lee,
Kyung-Wook Kim, In-Woong Um and
Masaru Murata

Additional information is available at the end of the chapter

1. Introduction

Autogenous bone, allogenic bone, xenogenic bone, and alloplastic materials are bone graft materials that are presently used in dental clinics. According to bone healing mechanism, they can be categorized into materials that induce osteogenesis, osteoinduction, and osteoconduction. Among the many different types of bone graft materials, autogenous bone is the most ideal since it is capable of osteogenesis, osteoinduction, and osteoconduction. Its advantage is the rapid healing time without immune rejection. As its biggest shortcomings, however, the harvest amount is limited, bone resorption after graft is unavoidable, and second defect is generated in the donor area. Therefore, to overcome such shortcomings, allogenic bone and synthetic bone were developed and used in clinics, and efforts have been made to develop more ideal bone substitution materials [1]. Lately, researchers and clinicians have become interested in the use of human dentin from extracted teeth in the context of autogenous bone grafts [2,3]. Dentin has inorganic and organic components that are very similar to those of human bone. In dentin, the inorganic content is 70 ~ 75%, whereas the organic content is about 20%. In alveolar bone, the inorganic content is 65%, and the organic content is 25%. At least 90% of organic content of dentin is type I collagen, which plays an important role in bone formation and mineralization. Dentin also contains bone morphogenetic proteins (BMP), which promote the differentiation of mesenchymal stem cells into chondrocytes and consequently enhance bone formation. In addition, both alveolar bone and teeth are derived from neural crest cells [4-6]. Thus, studies have been done to use fresh tooth in the form of demineralized dentin matrix (DDM) as a biocompatible autogenous bone graft material in alveolar bone repair. Butler, et al [7] and Conover and Urist, et al [8] successfully extracted bone BMP from rabbit DDM, and Bessho, et al [9] secured new bone formation *in situ* by BMP from human DDM. Furthermore, Ike and Urist [10] used dentin root matrix as a carrier of recombinant human bone morphogenetic protein (rhBMP). Starting in 1993, we developed bone graft materials using human teeth with which we conducted experimental studies [11-22]. In 2008, we developed an autogenous tooth bone graft material (AutoBT; Korea Tooth Bank Co., Seoul, Korea) from extracted teeth prepared as powder and grafted it to the donor patient himself. The mineral components of autogenous tooth bone graft materials have 4 stages (types) of calcium phosphate (HA, TCP, OCP, and ACP). Under scanning electron microscopic examination, HA crystalline structures and collagen fibers around the dentinal tubules were detected. Short-term clinical studies reported that, even when wounds became dehiscent, the bone graft materials were not infected, and good secondary healing was achieved [3,23].

2. Osteoinduction of AutoBT

Many researchers have examined tooth dentin as a potential carrier for human proteins and as grafting material because its biological composition is very similar to that of alveolar bone [9, 24-28]. Both tooth and alveolar bone are derived from neural crest cells and are made up of the same Type I collagen. Furthermore, dentin contains BMPs, which induce bone formation and noncollagenous proteins such as osteocalcin, osteonectin, and dentin phosphoprotein [29, 30]. Since its investigation by Urist in 1965, BMP has been widely studied and used in clinical applications [31]. As a result, Yeoman and Urist, et al (1967) and Bang and Urist, et al (1967) showed the osteoinductivity of rabbit DDM by BMP [32, 33]. Bessho, et al extracted BMP from bone matrix, dentin matrix, and wound tissue after extracting teeth from rabbits. Each BMP was confirmed to have induced the formation of new bone when xenogenic implantation was performed [9]. Bessho, et al extracted human dentin matrix containing 4mol/L guanidine HC1 and refined it into liquid chromatography and found out based on SDS-PAGE and IEF that purified BMP is homogenous, inducing the formation of new bone within 3 weeks of implantation in muscle pouches in Wistar rats. Dentin matrix-derived BMP is not exactly same as bone matrix-derived BMP, but they are very similar. In other words, two types of BMP exhibit the same action in the body [34]. The organic component accounts for about 20% of dentin weight and mostly consists of type I collagen. Moreover, it was proven to have BMP promoting cartilage and bone formation, and differentiating undifferentiated mesenchymal stem cells into chondrocytes and osteogenic cells [30, 35-37]. Noncollagenous proteins of dentin such as osteocalcin, osteonectin, phosphoprotein, and sialoprotein are known to be involved in bone calcification [38,39].

Patterns of matrix protein in teeth must have osteoinductive potential even though it does not perfectly match the protein in alveolar bone. Moreover, the apatite in teeth has long been known to play the role of protecting proteins [40]. According to Boden, et al, LIM mineralization protein 1 (LMP-1) is an essential positive regulator of osteoblast differentiation and maturation and bone formation [41]. Wang, et al found that LIM-1 was expressed primarily in predentin, odontoblasts, and endothelial cells of the blood vessels of teeth [42].

Many researchers have observed that alveolar bone formation occurs around bone graft materials as a result of experiments on animals [43-47]. Chung registered the patent for the technology of extracting proteins from teeth in 2002 and 2004; this carries an important, serving as evidence that teeth contain bone morphogenic protein [48,49]. Ike and Urist suggested that root dentin prepared from extracted teeth may be recycled for use as carrier of rhBMP-2 because it induces new bone formation in the periodontium [10]. Murata, et al reported that demineralized dentin matrix (DDM) does not inhibit BMP-2 activity but shows better release profile of BMP-2. Human recycled DDM is an unique, absorbable matrix with osteoinductivity, and DDM should be an effective graft material as a carrier of BMP-2 and a scaffold for bone-forming cells for bone engineering [2].

Lee [50] performed quantitative analysis of proliferation and differentiation of the MG-63 cell line on the bone grafting material using human tooth. This study demonstrated that the cellular adhesion and proliferation activity of the MG-63 cell on partially demineralized dentin matrix (PDDM) were comparable to control with enhanced osteogenic differentiation (Figure 1). Kim & Choi [51] reported a case on tooth autotransplantation with autogenous tooth bone graft. The extracted right mandibular third molar of a 37-year-old man was transplanted into the first molar area, and a bone graft procedure using autogenous tooth-bone graft material was performed for the space between the root and the alveolar socket. Reattachment was achieved (Figure 2). Therefore, the autogenous tooth bone graft material is considered reasonable for bone inducement and healing in the autotransplantation of teeth.

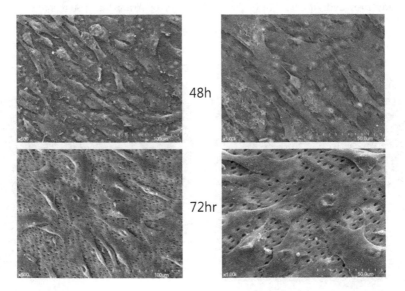

Figure 1. MG-63 cells adhered to PDDM, and they were spread out. This means excellent biocompatibility between cells and PDDM. (Lee H.J. Quantitative Analysis of Proliferation and Differentiation of MG-63 Cell Line on the Bone Grafting Material Using Human Tooth. PhD Thesis. School of Dentistry, Seoul National University, 2011.)

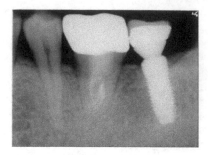

Figure 2. Periapical radiograph 2 years after autotransplantation.

Recently, we conducted a study to demonstrate the osteoinductivity of AutoBT when fabricated from bio-recycled dysfunctional teeth after patented processing. A total of 46 extracted dysfunctional teeth samples were collected from actual patients. *In vivo* study was done on 15 athymic mice by inserting AutoBT in dorsal subcutaneous muscular tissues. Samples were then biopsied in 2, 5, and 8 weeks. For additional analyses, Bradford assay, SDS-PAGE, and western blotting were performed *in vitro*. Histologic analyses *in vivo* showed new active bone formation as early as 2 weeks later (Figure 3,4,5). The Bradford assay indicated the existence of noncollagenous proteins in AutoBT. Nonetheless, rhBMP-2 was not extractable from AutoBT according to electrophoresis and immunoblotting analyses (Figure 6). In conclusion, this study provided an evidence of osteoinductivity of AutoBT th rough noncollagenous proteins.

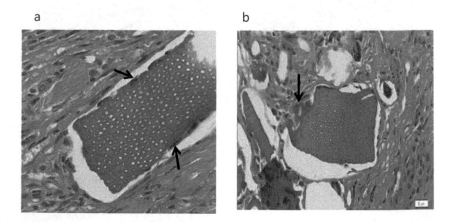

Figure 3. Histologic analyses of 2-week biopsy sample. a) The new cell lining and attachment to AutoBT powder and b) Newly deposited osteoid formations were observed. (H&E staining, X 200).

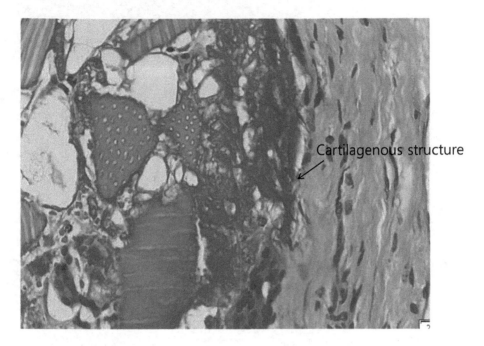

Figure 4. Cartilages were formed at the periphery of AutoBT in 5-week biopsy sample (H&E staining X 200).

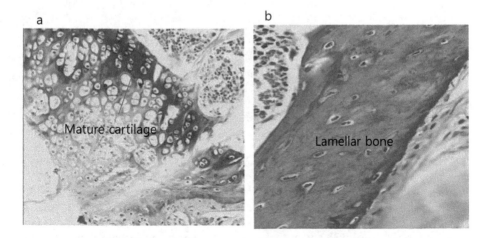

Figure 5. a) Endochondral ossification and b) lamellar bone formation were identified 8 weeks after the insertion of AutoBT powder in the intramuscular pouch of athymic mice (H&E, staining, X 200)

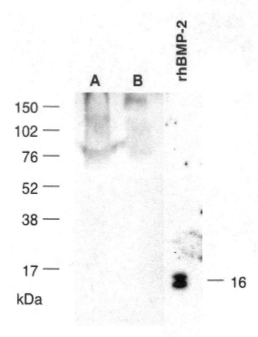

Figure 6. SDS-PAGE of purified fractions from AutoBT powder fabricated from a dried tooth in 25 ºC (A) and from wisdom tooth in fresh state (B).

3. Osteoconduction of AutoBT

The analytic results showed that AutoBT consisted of low-crystalline hydroxyapatite (HA) and possibly other calcium phosphate minerals (ß-tricalcium phosphate (ß-TCP), ACP, and OCP), similar to the minerals of human bone tissues. Note, however, that the level of HA crystallization and the amount of HA differed greatly depending on the area of the tooth. The XRD pattern was much stronger in the crown portion with enamel than in the root portion (Figure 7). Likewise, the dental crown portion consisted of high-crystalline calcium phosphate minerals (mainly HA) with higher Ca/P ratio, whereas the root portion was mainly made up of low-crystalline calcium phosphates with relatively low Ca/P ratio [3, 23]. Kim, et al [52] performed the study to evaluate the surface structures and physicochemical characteristics of a novel autogenous tooth bone graft material currently in clinical use. The material's surface structure was compared with a variety of other bone graft materials via scanning electron microscope (SEM). The crystalline structure of the autogenous tooth bone graft material from the crown (AutoBT crown) and root (AutoBT root), xenograft (BioOss), alloplastic material (MBCP), allograft (ICB), and autogenous mandibular cortical bone were compared using x-ray diffraction (XRD) analysis. The solubility of each material was measured with the Ca/P dissolution test. The result of the SEM analysis showed that the pattern associated with AutoBT was similar to that from autogenous cortical bone (Figure 8). In the XRD analysis, AutoBT root and allograft showed a low crystalline structure similar to that of autogenous cortical bone (Figure 9). In the CaP dissolution test, the amount of calcium and phosphorus dissolution in AutoBT was significant from the beginning, displaying a pattern similar to that of autogenous cortical bone (Tables 1, 2). In conclusion, autogenous tooth bone graft materials can be considered to have physicochemical characteristics similar to those of autogenous bone.

Day	MBCP	ICB	BioOss	AutoBT Crown	AutoBT Root	Auto Bone
3 d	54.2	97.7	35.5	230.7	280.0	246.8
7 d	48.6	71.7	33.6	162.7	255.2	189.2
14 d	62.7	97.6	35.1	144.5	180.6	180.6

m/z: mass-to-charge ratio

Table 1. Ca (m/z; 42.959) ion dissolution (Kim Y.K., et al. Autogenous teeth used for bone grafting: a comparison to traditional grafting materials. Oral Surg. Oral Med. Oral Pathol. Oral Radiol., 2013, in press)

Day	MBCP	ICB	BioOss	AutoBT Crown	AutoBT Root	Auto Bone
3 d	301.7	217.8	174.0	269.8	269.4	260.5
7 d	311.4	191.2	151.7	282.8	230.2	282.8
14 d	302.5	165.4	148.7	253.8	229.0	245.3

m/z: mass-to-charge ratio

Table 2. P (m/z; 30.994) ion dissolution (Kim Y.K., et al. Autogenous teeth used for bone grafting: a comparison to traditional grafting materials. Oral Surg. Oral Med. Oral Pathol. Oral Radiol., 2013, in press)

In an in vitro dissolution test, AutoBT showed excellent biodegradability, whereas apatite re-precipitation was actively visible immediately after transplantation. We conjecture that this material plays an effective role in inducing bone regrowth [52]. Priya, et al [53] reported that the extensive dissolution of calcium phosphate composites, which release calcium and phosphorus ions, induces the re-precipitation of the apatite onto the surfaces. According to them, the combination of dissolution and re-precipitation was the mechanism behind apatite formation. Apatite layer formation was expected to encourage the osseointegration of bioceramic composites.

Both the organic and inorganic compositions differ between the crown and root of autogenous tooth bone graft materials. Thus, when the material is grafted, crown and root show different healing mechanisms. Apatites present in bone tissues form a ceramic/high-molecular weight

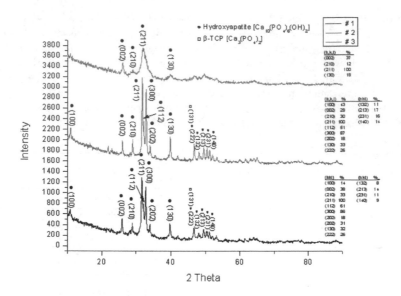

Figure 7. X-ray diffraction patterns of human tooth. (#1: root portion, #2: crown portion, 3: whole tooth) (Kim Y.K., et al. Development of a novel bone grafting material using autogenous teeth. Oral Surg. Oral Med. Oral Pathol. Oral Radiol. Endod., 2010.)

nanocomplex pattern [54]. In particular, apatites present in human bone tissues have low crystallinity and crystal size that are several tens of nanometers. On the other hand, hydroxyapatites prepared via the sintering process at high temperatures have high crystallinity. Grain growth occurs during the sintering process, resulting in sizes that are at least ten times larger than those apatites present in bone tissues [55]. The biodegradation of large particles with high crystallinity is almost impossible. Their osteoconduction capacity is very low, and osteoclasts cannot degrade them. Low-crystalline carbonic apatites show the best osteoconduction effects [56,57].

Nampo, et al introduced alveolar bone repair using extracted teeth for the graft material. DSP is a dentin-specific noncollagenous protein involved in the calcification of dentin. Based on immunohistochemical staining with anti-DSP antibody, the positive reaction was localized to the dentin of the extracted tooth fragments; thus suggesting that dentin has high affinity for and marked osteoconductive effect on the jaw bone [58].

Kim, et al reported bone healing capacity of demineralized dentin matrix materials in a minipig cranium defect [59]. A defect was induced in the cranium of mini-pigs, and those without defect were used as control. In the experimental group, teeth extracted from the mini-pig were manufactured into autogenous tooth bone graft material and grafted to the defect. The minipigs were sacrificed at 4, 8, and 12 weeks to evaluate histologically the bone healing ability and observe the osteonectin gene expression pattern with RT-PCR. At 4 weeks, the inside of the bur hole showed fibrosis, and there was no sign of bone formation in the control group. On the other

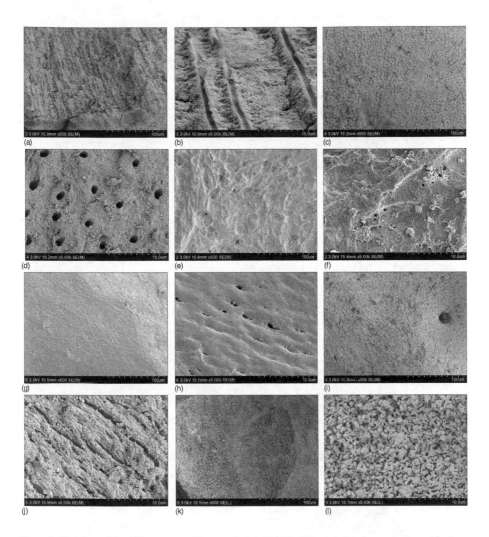

Figure 8. SEM views of the different types of bone graft materials. (Kim Y.K., et al. Autogenous teeth used for bone grafting: a comparison to traditional grafting materials. Oral Surg. Oral Med. Oral Pathol. Oral Radiol., 2013, in press) a): AutoBT crown (x500), b): AutoBT crown (x5,000), c): AutoBT root (x500), d): AutoBT root (x5,000), e): Autogenous cortical bone (x500), f): Autogenous cortical bone (x5,000), g): ICB (x500), h): ICB (x5,000), i): BioOss (x500), j): BioOss (x5,000), k): MBCP (x500), l): MBCP (x5,000)

hand, bone formation surrounding the tooth powder granule was observed at 4 weeks in the experimental group wherein the bur hole was filled with tooth powder. There was practically no osteonectin expression in the control group, whereas active osteonectin expression was observed from 4 to 12 weeks in the experimental group. In this study, excellent osteoconductive healing of autogenous tooth bone graft material was confirmed (Figure 10, 11).

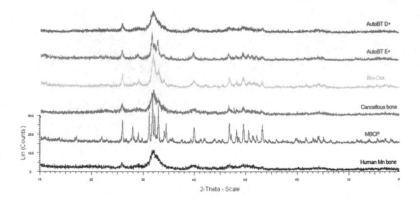

Figure 9. Results of the X-ray diffraction analysis. AutoBT D+: AutoBT root, AutoBT E+: AutoBT crown, Cancellous bone: ICB. (Kim Y.K., et al. Autogenous teeth used for bone grafting: a comparison to traditional grafting materials. Oral Surg. Oral Med. Oral Pathol. Oral Radiol., 2013, in press)

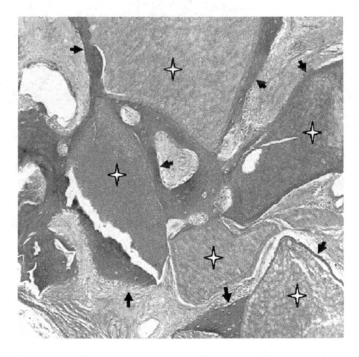

Figure 10. Experimental group of 8 weeks. New bone is actively formed around the tooth powder granules. Asterisks and arrows indicate graft tooth granule materials and new bone formation around the tooth granules, respectively. Hematoloxylin and eosin staining (×100). (Kim J.Y., et al. Bone healing capacity of demineralized dentin matrix materials in a mini-pig cranium defect. J. Korean Dent. Sci., 2012.)

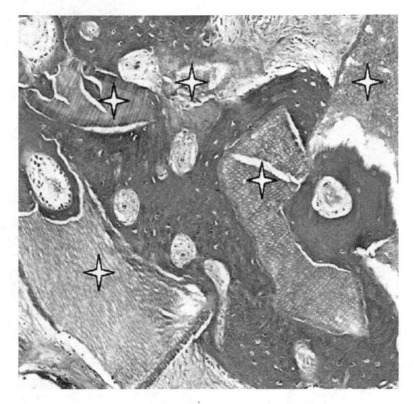

Figure 11. Experimental group of 12 weeks. Extensive new bone formation was noted around the bone powder granules in the bur hole. Asterisks indicate tooth powder materials. Hematoloxylin and eosin staining (×100). (Kim J.Y., et al. Bone healing capacity of demineralized dentin matrix materials in a mini-pig cranium defect. J. Korean Dent. Sci., 2012.)

4. Clinical application of AutoBT

Kim, et al developed a novel bone grafting material using autogenous teeth (AutoBT) in 2008 and provided the basis for its clinical application. Having organic and inorganic mineral components, AutoBT is prepared from autogenous grafting material; thus eliminating the risk of immune reaction that may lead to rejection. AutoBT was used at the time of implant placement -- simultaneously with guided bone regeneration -- and excellent bone healing by osteoinduction and osteoconduction was confirmed [3]. In a total of 6 patients, guided bone regeneration was performed simultaneously at the time of implant placement, and tissue samples were then harvested at the time of the second surgery with the patient's consent. In the histomorphometric analysis of the samples collected from 6 patients during the 3 ~ 6 months' healing period, new bone formation was detected in 46 ~ 87% of the area of interest, and excellent bone remodeling was achieved (Table 3) (Figure 12). Clinically available AutoBT consists of powder, chips, and block (Figure 13).

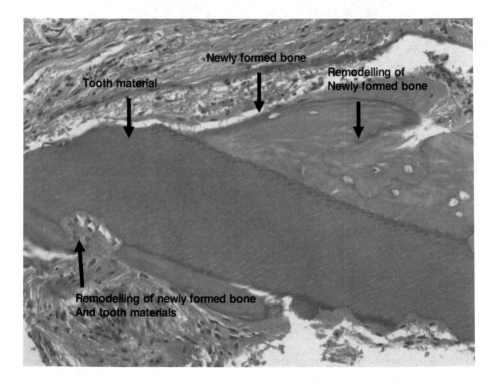

Figure 12. Newly formed bone and tooth materials showing remodeling were identified around the implant chip and at the periphery of the implant chip, respectively (H&E staining, X 100). (Kim Y.K., et al. Development of a novel bone grafting material using autogenous teeth. Oral Surg. Oral Med. Oral Pathol. Oral Radiol. Endod., 2010.)

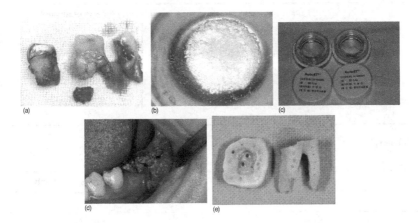

Figure 13. Three types of AutoBT can be fabricated from extracted teeth. a): Extracted teeth. Foreign body such as prosthetic crown, cements, calculus, and soft tissue are removed. AutoBT is then fabricated through pulverization, defatting, demineralization, and lyophilization. b): AutoBT one-powder. Crown and root portion are mixed. c): AutoBT crown and root powder. d): AutoBT chips. e): AutoBT block.

Case	Age/Sex	Site	Healing period	WB:LB:IM ratio	New bone-forming area (%)
1	40/M	#24	3	43:11:46	74
2	28/F	#17	4	85:14:1	87
3	47/F	#17	6	56:39:5	46
4	50/M	#24	5	84:12:4	73
5	43/F	#36	3	51:1:48	52
6	61/M	#25-27	6	65:0:35	68

WB: woven bone; LB: lamellar bone; IM: residual implant material

Table 3. Histomorphometric finding (Kim Y.K., et al. Development of a novel bone grafting material using autogenous teeth. Oral Surg. Oral Med. Oral Pathol. Oral Radiol. Endod., 2010.)

Lee and Kim [60]performed a retrospective study to evaluate the clinical efficacy of AutoBT. This study included 37 patients (54 implants) into which AutoBT was grafted between Oct. 2008 and Dec. 2009. The mean follow-up period was 31 months. Postoperative complications and marginal bone status around the implants were evaluated using medical records and dental radiography. Wound dehiscence and hematoma developed in 7 patients (8 implants). Osseointegration failure in 2 patients (4 implants) was recorded. These complications were well managed through conservative treatment and re-implantation. Mean peri-implant marginal bone loss 1 year after implant placement was 0.33±0.63mm. Autogenous tooth bone graft was confirmed to be a safe procedure, showing excellent bone healing through a 2-year retrospective study (Tables 4, 5, 6).

Type	Number of implants
GBR	29 (53.7%)
Sinus graft (lateral approach)	14 (25.9%)
Sinus lifting (crestal approach)	7 (13.0%)
Ridge augmentation	4 (7.4%)
Total	54 (100%)

Table 4. Types of surgery

Type	Number of patients
Powder	32 (86.5%)
Block	2 (5.4%)
Powder + Block	3 (8.1%)
Total	37 (100%)

Table 5. Types of AutoBT

Type	Number of implants
Wound dehiscence	7
Hematoma	1
Osseointegration failure	4
Total	12

Table 6. Types of complications

5. Sinus bone graft

If there is any material whose resorption speed is not too high and whose bone healing process approximates that of autogenous bone graft, it may be useful in maxillary sinus bone grafting. Likewise, more excellent clinical achievement may be expected when these materials are used in mixture with other bone substitutes with slow resorption properties [61,62,63]. With evidence presented in the foregoing paragraphs, AutoBT® developed by the author, et al was proven to exhibit bone healing ability through osteoinduction and osteoconduction, demonstrating a histological healing process similar to that of free bone grafting being resorbed over 3~6 months [3]. Accordingly, AutoBT® is regarded as a possible substitute when autogenous bone is needed for sinus bone graft, and it may wield a useful effect on increasing the volume of bone graft materials and minimizing repneumatization (Figure 14).

A retrospective study on sinus bone graft was performed. One hundred implants in 51 patients were selected, with the patients receiving maxillary sinus augmentation and implant placement using autogenous tooth graft materials at Chosun University Dental Hospital and Seoul National University Bundang Hospital (SNUBH) between July 2009 and November 2010. In cases of using autogenous tooth bone graft alone or together with other graft material, the implant survival rate was 96.15%. Based on the histomorphologic examination, autogenous tooth bone graft materials showed gradual resorption and new bone formation through osteoconduction and osteoinduction. The results suggest that autogenous tooth bone graft materials are appropriate for use in maxillary sinus augmentation [64].

Lee, et al [65] conducted a study to evaluate histomorphometrically and compare the efficiency of various bone graft materials and autogenous tooth bone graft material used in the sinus bone graft procedure. The subjects were 24 patients who had been treated with sinus bone graft using the lateral approach from October 2007 to September 2009 at SNUBH. The average age was 52.51 ± 11.86 years. All cases were taken after 4 months of procedure and divided into 3 groups according to bone graft material: Group 1 for autogenous tooth bone graft material (AutoBT), Group 2 for OrthoblastII (Integra Lifescience Corp., Irvine, US)+Biocera (Osscotec, Cheonan, Korea), and Group 3 for DBX (Synthes, West Chester, PA, USA), BioOss (Geistlich Pharm AG, Wolhusen, Switzerland). A total of 37 implant placement areas was included and evaluated (7 in group 1, 10 in group 2, 20 in group 3). The evaluation of new bone formation, ratio of woven bone to lamellar bone, and ratio of new bone to graft material was performed on each tissue section. The Kruskal-Wallis test was used for statistical analysis (SPSS Ver. 12.0, USA). New bone formation was 52.5 ± 10.7 % in group 1, 52.0 ± 23.4% in group 2, and 51.0 ± 18.3% in group 3 (Table 7) (Figure 15-18). There were no statistically significant differences between groups, however. The ratio of woven bone to lamella bone was 82.8 ± 15.3% in group 1, 36.7 ± 59.3% in group 2, and 31.0 ± 51.2% in group 3. The ratio of new bone to graft material was 81.3 ± 10.4% in group 1, 72.5 ± 28.8% in group 2, and 80.3 ± 24.0% in group 3. After a 4-month healing period, all groups showed favorable new bone formation and around the graft material and implant. Within the limitation of our study, autogenous tooth bone graft material may be used as a novel bone graft material for sinus bone graft. Kim, et al and Lee, et al performed sinus bone graft and guided bone regeneration using autogenous tooth bone from humans and took the tissue specimen 2 months and 4 months later for histomorphometric analysis. They found favorable new bone formation as a result and suggested that autogenous tooth bone graft materials could be used in various bone grafts [65,66].

Group	New bone formation
I	52.5 ± 10.7%
II	52.0 ± 23.4%
III	51.0 ± 18.3%

*Kruskal-Wallis test: P-value>0.05

Table 7. Histomorphometric data on new bone formation (Mean±SD)

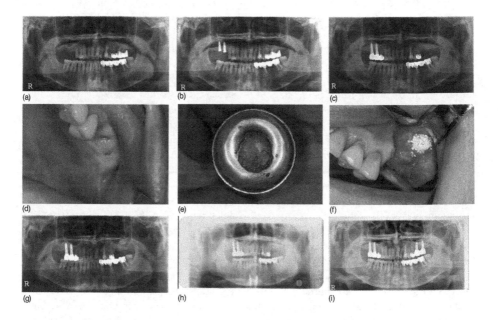

Figure 14. A case of sinus bone graft performed by the mixture of AutoBT, autogenous maxillary tuberosity bone and synthetic bone. a) Panoramic radiography of a 64-year-old man at the first examination. b) Radiography after placing implants simultaneously with the sinus bone graft on the right side. c) Panoramic radiography after 2 weeks of maxillary left 1st molar extraction. The prosthodontic therapy for the upper right maxillary bone was completed, and the extracted tooth was replaced with bone graft materials. d) Intraoral photography before operation. e) View of mixture of AutoBT and maxillary tuberosity bone. f) Grafted in the mixture with a synthetic bone, OSTEON (GENOSS, Suwon, Korea). g) Panoramic radiography after sinus bone graft. h) Panoramic radiography taken in a private dental clinic after 3 months of bone grafting. Performing implant placement in a private dental clinic was decided due to the medical costs. i) Panoramic radiography one year after final prosthetic delivery. The bone materials grafted on the maxillary sinus are maintained stably.

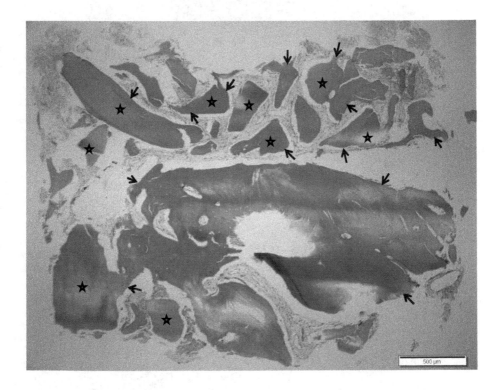

Figure 15. Overview of biopsy of Group I (Auto BT°). New bone formation (arrows) was identified around the graft material (asterisks). (Hematoxylin & Eosin stain, x40. scale bar measures 500um)

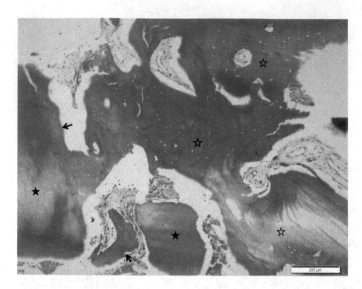

Figure 16. Histomorphometric image of Group I (Auto BT*). New bone formation (arrows) was identified around the graft material (asterisks). Confluent new bone formation was observed (open asterisk) (Hematoxylin & Eosin stain, x200. scale bar measures 200um)

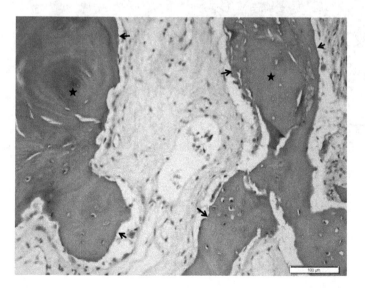

Figure 17. Microphotograph 4 months after Orthoblast/Biocera transplantation (Group II). Higher magnification demonstrated new bone formation (arrows) around the implant chips (asterisks). (Hematoxylin & Eosin stain, x200. scale bar measures 100um)

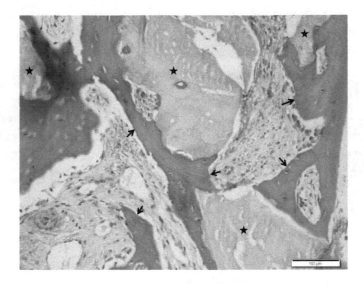

Figure 18. Microphotograph 4 months after DBX/BioOss transplantation (Group III). Higher magnification demonstrated new bone formation (arrows) around the implant chips (asterisks). (Hematoxylin & Eosin stain, x200. scale bar measures 100um)

6. Guided bone regeneration

Bone dehiscence or bone fenestration often develops after dental implant placement, and guided bone regeneration using bone graft materials has become a popular method. The most ideal material for guided bone regeneration is autogenous bone, but autogenous bone graft has limited sources and high risk of complications at the donor site and causes high resorption after bone graft. Therefore, alternative bone materials have been developed and used clinically, such as allogenic bone, xenogenic bone, and synthetic bone. Note, however, that they are often mixed with autogenous bone to maximize their advantages.

Autogenous teeth bone graft materials have very good osteoinductive and osteoconductive properties due to the organic and inorganic contents of the teeth, such as collagen, bone growth factors, and various forms of calcium phosphate. In our study, we achieved 46~74% new bone formation in 3~6 months compared with the results of Babbush [3,67]. Considering the histological healing of the sites where autogenous teeth bone graft materials were applied, bone graft materials were replaced with new bone following resorption, and new bone directly fused with the remaining autogenous teeth bone graft materials. A healing process associated with excellent osteoinduction and osteoconduction was observed in every sample, including abundant lamella bone; thus indicating that rapid bone reconduction was occurring [50,51,59,65,66]. Kim, et al [68] installed implants combined with guided bone regeneration using autogenous tooth bone graft material in 6 patients. In the 6 months' histological examination after operation, excellent osteoconductive bone healing was noted. A clinically favorable outcome was obtained (Figure 19~21).

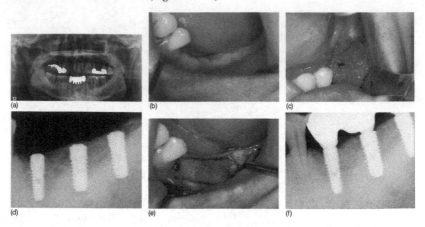

Figure 19. Guided bone regeneration using AutoBT powder (Kim Y.K., et al. Guided bone regeneration using autogenous teeth: case reports. J. Korean Assoc. Oral Maxillofac. Surg., 2011.) a): Initial panoramic radiography of a 44-year-old male patient. b): Preoperative intraoral view. Teeth were extracted 2 months ago. c): Implants were placed, and dehiscence defects were covered with autogenous tooth bone graft material. d): Periapical radiography 6 months after implant placement. e): Secondary surgery was performed, and flap was elevated. Excellent bone healing was observed. f): Periapical radiography 6 months after the final prosthetic delivery.

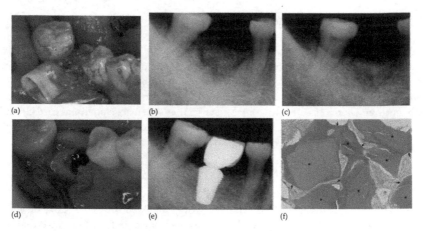

Figure 20. GBR was performed on the right mandibular 1st molar area of a 49-year-old female patient. (Kim Y.K., et al. Guided bone regeneration using autogenous teeth: case reports. J. Korean Assoc. Oral Maxillofac. Surg., 2011.) a): Autogenous tooth bone graft material and collagen membrane (BioGuide) were used. b): Periapical radiography 3 weeks after bone graft. c): Periapical radiography 6 months after bone graft. The alveolar crestal level was stable. d): Implant was installed 6 months after bone graft. Bone quality was type I. e): Periapical radiography after the final prosthetic delivery. f): Microphotograph 6 months after AutoBT transplantation. Higher magnification demonstrated new bone formation (arrows) around the implant chips (asterisks). Hematoxylin & Eosin stain, x100.

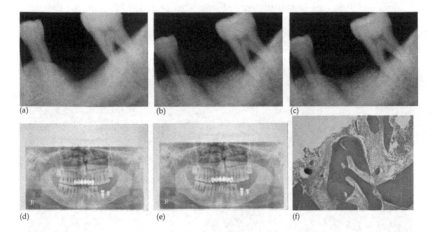

Figure 21. GBR was performed on the mandibular left 1st molar. (Kim Y.K., et al. Guided bone regeneration using autogenous teeth: case reports. J. Korean Assoc. Oral Maxillofac. Surg., 2011.) a): Periapical radiography of a 50-year-old male patient 2 months after the extraction of the mandibular left 1st molar. b): Periapical radiography 2 weeks after autogenous tooth bone graft. c): Periapical radiography 5 months after autogenous tooth bone graft. Alveolar crestal bone level was stable. d): Implant was placed 6 months after bone graft. The adjacent 2nd molar was extracted. e): Second surgery was performed at the #36 area. Additional implant was placed at the #37 area. f): Periapical radiography after the final prosthetic delivery. g): Microphotograph 6 months after AutoBT transplantation. Higher magnification demonstrated new bone formation around the implant chips. Hematoxylin & Eosin stain, x200

7. Ridge augmentation (Figure 22)

Autogenous bone grafting produces the best results in case a large volume of bone increase is required, as in the reconstruction of a site with lots of bone defects or ridge augmentation. The autograft may be taken from the endochondral bone such as ilium, rib, tibia, etc., and from the intramembranous bone such as calvaria, facial bone, etc. Alveolar ridge augmentation is a method of augmenting the height or width of the alveolar ridge by implementing bone grafting on the upper part or lateral part of the ridge in particulate or block type in case bone volume is insufficient vertically or horizontally; vertical and horizontal augmentation may be done simultaneously, but it may also be carried out individually. Since it is a kind of onlay graft, bone resorption occurs considerably after grafting, and dehiscence on the upper soft tissue easily arises [69]. Meanwhile, as for the autogenous bone graft, there may be some complications on the donor site, and doing the grafting takes time. Likewise, there are several problems such as limit to the volume of collection. Consequently, patients and clinical doctors are inclined to avoid it in many cases. As substitutes for autograft, bone graft materials such as allograft, xenograft, synthetic bone, etc., were developed, but the single use of each is not recommended in the method of augmenting bone tissue vertically or horizontally [69,70]. For the vertical or horizontal ridge augmentation, AutoBT may be a substitute method for autogenous bone graft and may be very useful in clinical practices when used in mixture with other graft materials in case of insufficient volume. Kim, et al. [71,72] reported the successful

case of alveolar ridge augmentation using various autogenous tooth bone graft materials.

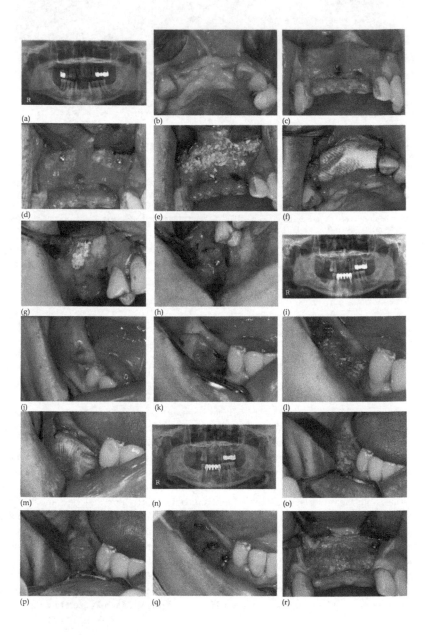

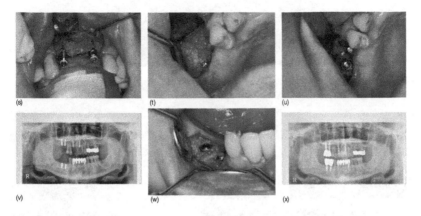

Figure 22. Placement of implants after the ridge augmentation of the maxillary anterior and maxillary/mandibular posterior area. a): Panoramic radiography at the first examination. Alveolar resorption was in considerable progress on the whole. b): Intraoral photograph taken just before the ridge augmentation of the maxillary anterior area. One month passed after extraction. c): View of the elevated mucoperiosteal flap. The labial side concavity is observed. d): View of fixation with titanium screws after applying the AutoBT block on the labial side. e): View of grafting the AutoBT powder additionally. f): Sutured after covering the resorbable collagen membrane (Ossix plus). g): View of the sinus bone graft on the right side using the AutoBT powder. h): View of fixation with titanium screws after vertical ridge augmentation with the AutoBT block. i): Panoramic radiography after grafting the bone on the maxillary anterior area and the right posterior area. j): Intraoral photograph prior to the right mandibular posterior bone grafting. One month passed after extraction. k): View of the elevated mucoperiosteal flap. The vertical bone defects on the ridge is observed. l): After applying the AutoBT block on the #45 area, the AutoBT powder was grafted on the surrounding sites. The AutoBT block was hydrated in saline solution for 15 ~ 30 minutes and operated. m): After covering the Ossix plus, the wound was closed. n): Panoramic radiography after bone graft. o): View of the elevated mucoperiosteal flap on the #45 and 46 sites after 2 months of ridge augmentation. Some Ossix plus that were not resorbed is observed. p): After removing Ossix plus, very excellent bone healing was observed. q): View of #45 and 46 implant placement. r):View of the elevated mucoperiosteal flap on the maxillary anterior area 4 months after bone grafting. Good bone healing is observed. There was not much bone resorption when the state of titanium screws was examined. s): After removing the titanium screws, the implants were placed. t): Exposed #15 and 16 areas. The titanium screws fixing the block is observed, and bone healing was very good. u): View of implants placed on the site. v): Panoramic radiography after the #12, 21, 15, and 16 implants were placed. w): View of the #45 and 46 implants exposed while doing the secondary surgery after 2 months. x): Panoramic radiography 6 months after the final prosthetic delivery.

8. Extraction socket preservation or reconstruction (Figure 23)

The resorption of the residual alveolar bone in the vicinity of extraction sockets reportedly occurs primarily during the initial period after tooth extraction; in cases wherein teeth are infected with periodontal diseases, it shows more severe resorption [73]. Severe resorption of the alveolar bone may cause aesthetic problems in the anterior teeth. In addition, normal, natural healing may be difficult since the soft tissues may fall down into the defective area if there is progressive periodontal disease or periapical inflammatory lesion, or in case of serious defects of the surrounding bone wall after tooth extraction. Therefore, the preservation or reconstruction of the extraction sockets should be considered positively in case of serious defects after tooth extraction [74]. Ridge preservation methods using various bone graft materials were introduced and reported to be effective in preventing vertical and horizontal ridge resorption [75-77]. Kim, et al [78] reported an actual case of extraction socket preservation and reconstruction using autogenous tooth bone powder and block. They reported good healing of extraction socket after 3~3.5 months, and they could successfully perform the placement of implants.

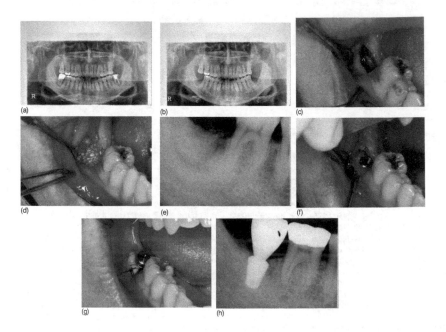

Figure 23. Extraction socket graft and delayed implant placement were performed on a 48-year-old male patient. (Kim Y.K., et al. Extraction socket preservation and reconstruction using autogenous tooth bone graft. J. Korean Assoc. Maxillofac. Plast. Reconstr. Surg., 2011.). a): Initial panoramic radiographic view, Periapical radiolucent lesion was observed at #37, 47 area. Radiolucent lesion was extended to the vicinity of the inferior alveolar canal. b):. Panoramic radiograph 3 months after extraction. c): The mucoperiosteal flap was elevated for implant placement 3 months after #47 extraction. The healing of extraction socket was poor. It was impossible to install the implants because of inadequate stability. d): Autogenous tooth bone graft powder was grafted into the socket. e): Postoperative periapical radiograph. f): Implant was installed 3 months after socket graft. Primary implant stability was excellent. g): Second surgery was performed 2.5 months after implant placement. h): Periapical radiograph 14 months after the final prosthetic delivery.

9. Conclusion

It is obvious that autogenous tooth bone graft materials(AutoBT) are safer than allogeneic and xenogeneic bon egraft materials; the fact that they are compared with the healing performance of free autogenous bone graft in histological view is clear evidence. AutoBT can be used safely in a variety of bone reconstructive procedures such as sinus bone graft, GBR, ridge augmentation and extraction socket graft.

Author details

Young-Kyun Kim[1], Jeong Keun Lee[2], Kyung-Wook Kim[3], In-Woong Um[4] and
Masaru Murata[5]

1 Department of Oral and Maxillofacial Surgery, Section of Dentistry, Seoul National University Bundang Hospital, Seongnam, Korea

2 Department of Dentistry Oral & Maxillofacial Surgery, Ajou University School of Medicine, Suwon, Korea

3 Department of Oral and Maxillofacial Surgery, College of Dentistry, Dankook University, Cheonan, Korea

4 Director, Korea Tooth Bank, R&D Institute, Seoul, Korea

5 Division of Oral and Maxillofacial Surgery, University of Hokkaido, Hokkaido, Japan

References

[1] Misch, C. E, & Dietsh, F. Bone-grafting materials in implant dentistry. Implant Dent (1993). , 2(3), 158-167.

[2] Murata, M, Akazawa, T, Mitsugi, M, Um, I. W, Kim, K. W, & Kim, Y. K. Human Dentin as Novel Biomaterial for Bone Regeneration. In: Rosario Pignatello R. (ed.) Biomaterials- Physics and Chemistry, InTech; (2011). , 127-140.

[3] Kim, Y. K, Kim, S. G, Byeon, J. H, Lee, H. J, Um, I. U, Lim, S. C, & Kim, S. Y. Development of a novel bone grafting material using autogenous teeth. Oral Surg Oral Med Oral Pathol Oral Radiol Endod. (2010). , 109(4), 496-503.

[4] Nanci, A. Ten Cate's Oral Histology, 7[th]edi. Elsevier Inc. (2008). , 202-211.

[5] Min, B. M. Oral Biochemistry. Daehan Narae Pub Co. Seoul.(2007). , 22-26.

[6] Bhaskar, S. N. Orban's Oral histology and embryology. 9th edition. Mosby Co. USA. (1980).

[7] Butler, W. T, Mikulski, A, & Urist, M. R. Noncollagenous proteins of a rat dentin matrix possessing bone morphogenetic activity. J Dent Res (1977). , 56(3), 228-232.

[8] Bang, G. Induction of heterotopic bone formation by demineralized dentin in guinea pigs: antigenicity of the dentin matrix. J Oral Pathol (1972). , 1(4), 172-185.

[9] Bessho, K, Tagawa, T, & Murata, M. Purification of rabbit bone morphogenetic protein derived from bone, dentin, and wound tissue after tooth extraction. J Oral Maxillofac Surg (1990). , 48(2), 162-169.

[10] Ike, M, & Urist, M. R. Recycled dentin root matrix for a carrier of recombinant human bone morphogenetic protein. J Oral Implantol (1998). , 24(3), 124-132.

[11] Kim, Y. K, Yeo, H. H, Ryu, C. H, Lee, H. B, Byun, U. R, & Cho, J. E. An experimental study on the tissue reaction of toothash implanted in mandible body of the mature dog. J Korean Assoc Maxillofac Plast Reconstr Surg (1993). , 15, 129-136.

[12] Kim, Y. K, Yeo, H. H, Yang, I. S, Seo, J. H, & Cho, J. O. Implantation of toothash combined with plaster of paris: Experimental study. J Korean Assoc Maxillofac Plast Reconstr Surg (1994). , 16, 122-129.

[13] Kim, Y. K. The experimental study of the implantation of toothash and plaster of Paris and guided tissue regeneration using Lyodura. J Korean Assoc Oral Maxillofac Surg (1996). , 22, 297-306.

[14] Kim, Y. K, & Yeo, H. H. Transmitted electronic microscopic study about the tissue reaction after the implantation of toothash. J Korean Assoc Oral Maxillofac Surg (1997). , 23, 283-289.

[15] Kim, Y. K, Kim, S. G, Lee, J. G, Lee, M. H, & Cho, J. O. An experimental study on the healing process after the implantation of various bone substitutes in the rats. J Korean Assoc Oral Maxillofac Surg (2001). , 27, 15-24.

[16] Kim, Y. K, Kim, S. G, & Lee, J. H. Cytotoxicity and hypersensitivity test of toothash. J Korean Maxillofac Plast Reconstr Surg (2001). , 23, 391-395.

[17] Kim, S. G, Yeo, H. H, & Kim, Y. K. Grafting of large defects of the jaws with a particulate dentin-plaster of Paris combination. Oral Surg Oral Med Oral Pathol Oral Radiol Endod (1999). , 88(1), 22-25.

[18] Kim, S. G, Kim, H. K, & Lim, S. C. Combined implantation of particulate dentine, plaster of Paris, and a bone xenograft (Bio-Oss) for bone regeneration in rats. J Craniomaxillofac Surg (2001). , 29(5), 282-288.

[19] Kim, S. G, Chung, C. H, Kim, Y. K, Park, J. C, & Lim, S. C. Use of particulate dentin-plaster of Paris combination with/without platelet-rich plasma in the treatment of bone defects around implants. Int J Oral Maxillofac Implants (2002). , 17(1), 86-94.

[20] Kim, S. Y, Kim, S. G, Lim, S. C, & Bae, C. S. Effects on bone formation in ovariectomized rats after implantation of toothash and plaster of Paris mixture. J Oral Maxillofac Surg (2004). , 62(7), 852-857.

[21] Park, S. S, Kim, S. G, Lim, S. C, & Ong, J. L. Osteogenic activity of the mixture of chitosan and particulate dentin. J Biomed Mater Res A (2008). , 87(3), 618-623.

[22] Kim, W. B, Kim, S. G, Lim, S. C, Kim, Y. K, & Park, S. N. Effect of Tisseel on bone healing with particulate dentin and plaster of Paris mixture. Oral Surg Oral Med Oral Pathol Oral Radiol Endod (2010). ee40., 34.

[23] Kim, Y. K, Kim, S. G, Oh, J. S, Jin, S. C, Son, J. S, Kim, S. Y, & Lim, S. Y. Analysis of the inorganic component of autogenous tooth bone graft material. J Nanosci Nanotechnol. (2011). , 11(8), 7442-7445.

[24] Bang, G, & Urist, M. R. Bone induction in excavation chambers in matrix of decalcified dentin. Arch Surg (1967). , 94(6), 781-789.

[25] Butler, W. T, Mikulski, A, & Urist, M. R. Noncollagenous proteins of a rat dentin matrix processing bone morphogenetic activity. J Dent Res (1977). , 56(3), 228-232.

[26] Conover, M. A, & Urist, M. R. Transmembrane bone morphogenesis by implanted of dentin matrix. J Dent Res (1979).

[27] Conover, M. A, & Urist, M. R. Dentin matrix morphogenetic protein. The Chemistry and Biology of Mineralized Connective Tissues. Northwestern University. New York;Elsevier-North Holland Inc.; (1981). , 597-606.

[28] Ike, M, & Urist, M. R. Recycled dentin toot matrix for a carrier of recombinant human bone morphogenetic protein. J Oral Implantol (1998). , 24(3), 124-132.

[29] Morotome, Y, Goseki-sone, M, Ishikawa, I, & Oida, S. Gene expression of growth and differentiation factors-5,-6, and-7 in developing bovine tooth at the root forming stage. Biochem Biophys Res Commun (1988). , 244(1), 85-90.

[30] Urist, M. R, & Strates, B. S. Bone morphogenetic protein. J Dent Res (1971). , 50, 1393-406.

[31] Urist, M. R. Bone: formation by autoinduction. Science (1965). , 150(3698), 893-899.

[32] Yeomans, D. J, & Urist, M. R. Bone induction by decalcified dentin implanted into oral osseous and muscle tissues. Arch Oral Biol (1967). , 12(8), 999-1008.

[33] Bang, G, & Urist, M. R. Bone induction in excavation chambers in matrix of decalcified dentin. Arch Surg (1967). , 94(6), 781-789.

[34] Bessho, K, Tanaka, N, Matsumoto, J, Tagawa, T, & Murata, M. Human dentin-matrix-derived bone morphogenetic protein. J Dent Res (1991). , 70, 171-175.

[35] Turnbull, R. S, & Freeman, E. Use of wounds in the parietal bone of the rat for evaluating bone marrow for grafting into periodontal defects. J Periodontal Res (1974). , 9(1), 39-43.

[36] Inoue, T, Deporter, D. A, & Melcher, A. H. Induction of cartilage and bone by dentin demineralized in citric acid. J Periodontal Res (1986). , 21(3), 243-255.

[37] Kawai, T, & Urist, M. R. A bovine tooth derived bone morphogenetic protein. J Dent Res (1989). , 68(6), 1069-1074.

[38] Feng, J. Q, Luan, X, Wallace, J, Jing, D, Ohshima, T, Kulkarni, A. B, Souza, D, & Kozak, R. N. CA, MacDougall Ml. Genomic organization, chromosomal mapping, and promoter analysis of the mouse dentin sialophosphoprotein (Dspp) gene, which codes for both dentin sialoprotein and dentin phosphoprotein. J Biol Chem (1998). , 273(16), 9457-9464.

[39] Ritchie, H. H, Ritchie, D. G, & Wang, L. H. Six decades of dentinogenesis research. Historical and prospective views on phosphophoryn and dentin sialprotein. Eur J Oral Sci (1998). Suppl , 1, 211-220.

[40] Schmidt-schultz, T. H, & Schultz, M. Intact growth factors are conserved in the extracellular matrix of ancient human bone and teeth: a storehouse for the study of human evolution in health and disease. Biol Chem (2005). , 386(8), 767-776.

[41] Boden, S. D, Liu, Y, Hair, G. A, Helms, J. A, Hu, D, Racine, M, Nanes, M. S, & Titus, L. LMP-1, aLIM-domain protein, mediates BMP-6 effects on bone formation. Endocrinology (1998). , 139(12), 125-134.

[42] Wang, X, Zhang, Q, Chen, Z, & Zhang, L. Immunohistochemical localization of LIM mineralization protein 1 in pulp-dentin complex of human teeth with normal and pathologic conditions. J Endod (2008). , 34(2), 143-147.

[43] Al-talabani, N. G, & Smith, C. J. Continued development of 5-day old tooth-germs transplanted to syngeneic hamster (Mesocricetus Auratus) cheek pouch. Arch Oral Biol (1978). , 23(12), 1069-1076.

[44] Steidler, N. E, & Reade, P. C. An histological study of the effects of extra-corporeal time on murine dental isografts. Arch Oral Biol (1979). , 24(2), 165-169.

[45] Barrett, A. P, & Reade, P. C. Changes in periodontal fibre organization in mature bone/tooth isografts in mice. J Oral Pathol (1981). , 10, 276-283.

[46] Barrett, A. P, & Reade, P. C. The relationship between degree of development of tooth isografts and the subsequent formation of bone and periodontal ligament. J Periodontal Res (1981). , 16, 456-465.

[47] Barrett, A. P, & Reade, P. C. A histological investigation of isografts of immature mouse molars to an intrabony and extrabony site. Arch Oral Biol (1982). , 27, 59-63.

[48] Chung, P. H. Method for extracting tooth protein from extracted tooth. Korea Intellectual Property Rights Information Service. Patent. Application (2002). (10-2002)

[49] Chung, P. H. Tooth protein extracted from extracted tooth and method for using the same. Korea Intellectual Property Rights Information Service. Patent. Application (2004). (10-2004)

[50] Lee, H. J. Quantitative analysis of proliferation and differentiation of MG-63 cell line on the bone grafting material using human tooth. PhD thesis. School of Dentistry, Seoul National University; (2011).

[51] Kim, Y. K, & Choi, Y. H. Tooth autotransplantation with autogenous tooth-bone graft: A case report. J Korean Dent Sci (2011). , 4(2), 79-84.

[52] Kim, Y. K, Kim, S. G, Yun, P. Y, et al. Autogenous teeth used for bone grafting: A comparison to traditional grafting materials. Oral Surg Oral Med Oral Pathol Oral Radiol. (2013). in press.

[53] Priya, A, Nath, S, Biswas, K, & Bikramjit, B. In vitro dissolution of calcium phosphate-mullite composite in simulated body fluid. J Mater Sci Mater Med (2010). , 21, 1817-1828.

[54] Glimcher, M. J. Molecular biology of mineralized tissues with particular reference to bone. Rev Mod Phys (1959). , 31, 359-393.

[55] Lee, S. H. Low Crystalline hydroxyl carbonate apatite. J Korean Dental Assoc (2006). , 44, 524-533.

[56] Lu, J, Descamps, M, Dejou, J, Koubi, G, Hardouin, P, Lemaitre, J, & Proust, J. P. The biodegradation mechanism of calcium phosphate biomaterials in bone. J Biomed Mat Res Appl Biomater (2002). , 63(4), 408-412.

[57] Fulmer, M. T, & Ison, I. C. Hanker mayer CR, Constantz BR, Ross J. Measurements of the solubilities and dissolution rates of several hydroxyapatites. Biomaterials (2002). , 23(3), 751-755.

[58] Nampo, T, Watahiki, J, Enomoto, A, Taguchi, T, Ono, M, Nakano, H, Tamamoto, G, Irie, T, Tachikawa, T, & Maki, K. A new method for alveolar bone repair using extracted teeth for the graft material. J Periodontol (2010). , 81(9), 1264-1272.

[59] Kim, J. Y, Kim, K. W, Um, I. W, Kim, Y. K, & Lee, J. K. Bone healing capacity of demineralized dentin matrix materials in a mini-pig cranium defect. J Korean Dent Sci (2012). , 5(1), 21-8.

[60] Lee, J. Y, & Kim, Y. K. Retrospective cohort study of autogenous tooth bone graft. Oral Biol Res (2012). , 36(1), 39-43.

[61] Hatano, N, Shimizu, Y, & Ooya, K. A clinical long-term radiographic evaluation of graft height changes after maxillary sinus floor augmentation with a 2:1 autogenous bone/xenograft mixture and simultaneous placement of dental implants. Clin Oral Impl Res. (2004). , 15(3), 339-345.

[62] Velich, N, Nemeth, Z, Toth, C, & Szabo, G. Long-term results with different bone substitutes used for sinus floor elevation. J Craniofacial Surg (2004). , 15(1), 38-41.

[63] Garg, A. K. Current concepts in augmentation grafting of the maxillary sinus for placement of dental implants. Dent Implantol Update. (2001). , 12(3), 17-22.

[64] Jeong, K. I, Kim, S. G, Kim, Y. K, Oh, J. S, Jeong, M. A, & Park, J. J. Clinical Study of Graft Materials Using Autogenous Teeth in Maxillary Sinus ugmentation. Implant Dent (2011). , 20(6), 471-475.

[65] Lee, J. Y, Kim, Y. K, Kim, S. G, & Lim, S. C. Histomorphometric study of sinus bone graft using various graft material. J Dental Rehabilitation and Applied Science (2011). , 27, 141-147.

[66] Kim, S. G, Kim, Y. K, Lim, S. C, Kim, K. W, & Um, I. W. Histomorphometric analysis of bone graft using autogenous tooth bone graft. Implantology (2011). , 15, 134-141.

[67] Babbush, C. Histologic evaluation of human biopsies after dental augmentation with a demineralized bone matrix putty. Implant Dent (2003). , 12, 325-332.

[68] Kim, Y. K, Lee, H. J, & Kim, K. W. Kim SGm Um IW. Guided bone regeneration using autogenous teeth: case reports. J Korean Assoc Oral Maxillofac Surg (2011). , 37, 142-147.

[69] Kim, Y. K, & Kim, S. G. Lee BG: Bone Graft and Implant. Clinical application of a variety of bone graft, Seoul: Narae Pub Co; (2007). , 2-2, 86-134.

[70] Kim, M. J, Kim, Y. K, & Kim, S. G. A variety of grafting biomaterial used in dental surgery, Seoul: Narae Pub Co.; (2004). , 19-24.

[71] Kim, Y. K, & Yi, Y. J. Horizontal Ridge Augmentation using Ridge expansion and Autogenous Tooth Bone Graft: A Case Report. J Dent Rehabil Appl Sci, (2011). , 2011(1), 109-115.

[72] Kim, Y. K, & Um, I. W. Vertical and horizontal ridge augmentation using autogenous tooth bone graft materials: A case report. J Korean Assoc Maxillofac Plast Reconstr Surg (2011). , 33(2), 166-170.

[73] Becker, W, Urist, M, Becker, B. E, et al. Clinical and histological observation of sites implanted with intraoral autologous bone grafts or allografts. 15 human case reports. J Periodontol (1996). , 67, 1025-1033.

[74] Kim, Y. K, & Um, I. W. Autogenous tooth bone graft. Seoul: Charmyun: (2011). , 192-211.

[75] Kim, Y. K, Yun, P. Y, Lee, H. J, Ahn, J. Y, & Kim, S. G. Ridge preservation of the molar extraction socket using collagen sponge and xenogeneic bone grafts. Implant Dent (2011). , 20(4), 267-272.

[76] Sclar, A. The Bio-Col technique. In: Bowyers LC, ed. Soft Tissue and Esthetic Considerations in Implant Therapy. Chicago, IL: Quintessence; (2003). , 2003, 163-187.

[77] Iasella, J. M, Greenwell, H, Miller, R. L, Hill, M, Drisko, C, Bohra, A. A, & Scheetz, J. P. Ridge preservation with freeze-dried bone allograft and a collagen membrane compared to extraction alone for implant site development: A clinical and histologic study in humans. J Periodontol. (2003). , 74(7), 990-999.

[78] Kim, Y. K, Kim, S. G, Kim, K. W, & Um, I. W. Extraction socket preservation and reconstruction using autogenous tooth bone graft. J Korean Assoc Maxillofac Plast Reconstr Surg (2011). , 33, 264-269.

Chapter 8

Mesenchymal Stem Cells from Extra-Embryonic Tissues for Tissue Engineering – Regeneration of the Peripheral Nerve

Andrea Gärtner, Tiago Pereira, Raquel Gomes,
Ana Lúcia Luís, Miguel Lacueva França,
Stefano Geuna, Paulo Armada-da-Silva and
Ana Colette Maurício

Additional information is available at the end of the chapter

1. Introduction

Recent advances in Regenerative Biology and Regenerative Medicine are impressive and in the last years the scientific community has witnessed the emergence of many new concepts and discoveries. Until a few years ago, biological tissues were regarded as unable of extensive regeneration, but nowadays organs and tissues like the brain, spinal cord or cardiac muscles appear as capable to be reconstructed, based on "stem cells" [1].

Stem cell research has sparked an international effort due to the variety of possible uses in clinical procedures to treat diseases and improve health and life expectancy. Stem cell research has crossed a century journey and has evolved greatly even in its own defini‐ tion. In 1967, Lajtha defined that adult stem cells could only be found in regenerative organs, such as blood, intestine, cartilage, bone and skin. Nowadays, these cells are con‐ sidered to exist even in tissues with no commitment to regeneration such as the central nervous system [1, 2].

2. Stem cells

Stem cells are undifferentiated cells, with endless self-renewal sustained proliferation *in vitro* and multilineage differentiation capacity [3]. This *in vitro* multilineage differentiation capacity has targeted these cells with extreme importance for use in tissue and cell-based therapies.

The first stem cell appearance is in the early zygotic cells, which are totipotent and give rise to the blastocyst. They are capable to differentiate into all cell and tissue types. With differentiation, cells become less capable of self-renewal and differentiation in other cell type becomes more limited [1]. Stem cells can be loosely classified into 3 broad categories based on their growth behavior and isolation time during ontogenesis: embryonic, fetal and adult.

Embryonic stem cells (ESCs) were first observed in a pre-implantation embryo by Bongso and colleagues in 1994 [4]. Since then, many cell lines and a multiplicity of tissues have been successfully derived from ESCs and tested in several animal disease models [5-7]. Nevertheless, post-transplantation immune-rejection has been a major problem. Many studies are being conducted to avoid this major issue. This could be resolved by personalizing tissues through somatic nuclear transfer (NT) or induced pluripotent stem cells (iPSC) techniques [8], but the teratoma development in animals is still a concern and a serious problem [9]. In order to overcome the limitations placed by ESCs and iPSCs, a variety of adult stem cell populations have been recently isolated and characterized for their potential clinical use. While still multipotent, adult stem cells have long been considered restricted, giving rise only to progeny of their resident tissues [9]. *In vivo*, adult stem cells exist in a quiescent state, located in almost all tissues, until mediators activate them to restore and repair injured tissues. These cells are surrounded by mature cells that have reached the end line in terms of differentiation and proliferation [10]. Stem cell research focuses on the development of cell and tissue differentiation, so as characterization techniques, for tissue and cell identification with marker patterns. Such protocols are essential for regenerative therapies [11].

2.1. Mesenchymal stem cells

The development of cell-based therapies for cartilage [12] and skin [13] reconstruction marks the beginning of a new age in tissue regeneration. Mesenchymal stem cells (MSCs) have become one of the most interesting targets for tissue regeneration due to their high plasticity, proliferative and differentiation capacity together with their attractive immunosuppressive properties. MSCs present low immunogenicity and high immunosuppressive properties due to a decreased or even absence of Human Leucocyte Antigen (HLA) class II expression [14]. Research in this field has brought exciting promises in many disorders and therefore in tissue regeneration. Currently the differentiation potential of MSCs in multilineage end-stage cells is already proven, and their potential for treatment of cardiovascular [15], neurological [16], musculoskeletal [17, 18], and cutaneous [19] diseases is now well established. Fibroblast colony-forming units or marrow stromal cells, currently named MSCs, were first isolated in 1968 from rat bone marrow [20]. These cells were clonogenic, formed colonies when cultured, and were able to differentiate *in vitro* into bone, cartilage, adipose tissue, tendon, muscle and fibrous tissue. Since then many other tissues have been used to isolate these cells. MSCs can be obtained from many different tissues, including bone marrow, adipose tissue, skeletal muscle, umbilical cord matrix and blood, placental tissue, amniotic fluid, synovial membranes, dental pulp, fetal blood, liver, and lung [21]. The concept of MSCs is based on their ability to differentiate into a variety of mesodermal tissues and was first proposed by Caplan in 1991 [22] and further validated by additional research in 1999 [23]. Due to the many different methods and approaches used for MSCs culture, the Mesenchymal and Tissue Stem Cell Committee, of the International Society for Cellular Therapy (ISCT), recommended several standards do define MSCs [24]. Therefore, MSCs are defined as presenting: i) plastic adherent ability; ii) absence of definitive hematopoietic lineage markers, such as CD45, CD34, CD14, CD11b, CD79α, CD19 and class-II Major Histocompatibility Complex (MHC) molecules, specially HLA-DR; and expression of nonspecific markers CD105, CD90 and CD73 iii) ability to differentiate into mesodermal lineage cells, osteocytes, chondrocytes and adipocytes. Along with mesodermal differentiation, it has been demonstrated the capacity of MSCs to differentiate into ectodermal cell lines, as neurons [25, 26], keratocytes [27] and keratinocytes [28], so as endodermal cell line, like hepatocytes [29, 30] and pancreatic β-cells [31]. Moreover, they also possess anti-inflammatory and immunomodulation properties and trophic effects [32, 33]. Increasing evidence now demonstrates that the therapeutic effects of MSCs do not lay only on the ability to repair damage tissue, but also on the capacity of modulating surrounding environment, by secretion of multiple factors and activation of endogenous progenitor cells [34, 35]. Compared with ESCs and other tissue specific stem cells, MSCs are more advantageous. Moreover some studies have demonstrated that MSCs have a higher chromosomal stability and lower tendency to form tumors and teratomas, compared to other stem cells [36, 37].

Although they present similar biological characteristics, it cannot be ignored the existing of some disparities, as differences in, expansion potential under same culture conditions and age-related functional properties [38]. Compared to ESCs, MSCs isolated from the umbilical cord matrix (Wharton's jelly) have many advantages, such as shorter population doubling time, easy culture in plastic flasks, good tolerance towards the immune system, so that transplantation into non-immunesuppressed animals does not induce acute rejection, anticancer properties, [9] and most important absence of tumorigenic activity. As well as ESCs, these cells are originated from the inner cell mass of the blastocyst but with a major difference: they do not raise ethical controversies, since they are collected from tissues usually discarded at birth [39].

2.1.1. MSCs sources and validation of transport and processing protocols

Bone marrow, adipose tissue, umbilical cord blood and umbilical cord matrix have been considered the main sources of MSCs for tissue engineering purposes. Among these sources, bone marrow represents the main source of MSCs for cell therapy. However, the proliferative capacity [40-43], differentiation potential and clonal expandability [44] of MSCs derived from bone marrow decrease significantly with age, gender and seeding density, and the number of cells per marrow aspirate is usually quite low [3, 45]. It is still a mystery if MSCs ageing is due to factors intrinsic or extrinsic to the cells. Many possible reasons have been described in an attempt to explain MSCs ageing. Possible extrinsic factors include: reduced synthesis of proteoglycans and glycosaminoglycans reducing proliferation and viability [46], and production of glycosylated end products, inducing apoptosis and reactive oxygen species [47]. Intrinsic factors causing MSCs ageing might include: cell senescence-associated β-galactosidase and higher expression of p53 and pathway genes p21 and BAX, resulting in blunted proliferation potential [43]. Regarding seeding density, many authors suggest that lower seeding densities induce faster proliferation rates [48, 49]. This has been explained by contact inhibition in higher seeding densities [49], and higher nutrient availability per cell in lower seeding densities [49]. Use of bone marrow MSCs has disadvantages; donors are submitted to invasive harvest of bone marrow. This raises the need to find alternative sources of MSCs for autologous and allogenic use. Candidate tissue sources should provide MSCs displaying high proliferative and differentiation potency [50].

Extra-embryonic tissues are a good alternative to adult donor. This tissues, such as, amnion, microvillus, Wharton's jelly and umbilical cord perivascular cells, are routinely discarded at child-birth, so little ethical and religious controversy attends the harvesting of the resident stem cell populations. The comparatively large volume of extra-embryonic tissues increases the chance of isolating suitable amounts of stem cells, despite the complex and expensive procedures needed for their isolation. Some protocols use enzymatic digestion while others use enzyme-free tissue explant methods that require longer culture time [51]. There are also MSCs in cord blood (CB), but many studies report low frequency of these cells and unsuccessful isolation. However, Zhang and colleagues were able to isolate MSCs from CB with a 90% successful rate when CB volume was $\geq$ 90ml and a transport time until storage was $\leq$ 2 hours [51].

In recent years, MSCs derived from umbilical cord matrix Wharton's jelly, have attracted much interest. Wharton's jelly is a mature mucous tissue and the main component of the umbilical cord, connecting the umbilical vessels to the amniotic epithelium. Umbilical cord derives from extra-embryonic or embryonic mesoderm; at birth it weighs about 40g and measures approximately 30-65cm in length and 1.5cm in width [52]. Anyway, individual differences are observed within newborn babies. Fong and colleagues characterized Wharton's Jelly stem cells and found the presence of both embryonic and MSCs, targeting this source as unique and of valuable use for clinical applications. MSCs from the Wharton's jelly can be cultured with little or even no major loss trough at least 50 passages [53].

CB and more recently, umbilical cord tissue (UCT) have been stored cryopreserved in private and public cord blood and tissue banks worldwide in order to obtain hematopoietic and MSCs and, although guidelines exist (Netcord – Foundation for the Accreditation of Cellular Therapy), standardized procedures for CB and UCT transport from the hospital / clinic to the laboratory, storage, processing, cryopreservation and thawing are still awaited.

These may be critical in order to obtain higher viable stem cells number after thawing and limit microbiological contamination.

Our research group focused in determining whether UCT storage and transport from the hospital / clinical to the laboratory at room temperature (RT) or refrigerated (4-6°C) and immersed in several sterile saline solutions affects the UCT integrity in order to be cryopreserved. The umbilical cord contains two arteries and one vein, which are surrounded by mucoid connective tissue, and this is called the Wharton's jelly. The cord is covered by an epithelium derived from the enveloping amnion. The interlaced collagen fibers and small, woven bundles are arranged to form a continuous soft skeleton that encases the umbilical vessels. In the Wharton's jelly, the most abundant glycosaminoglycan is hyaluronic acid, which forms a hydrated gel around the fibroblasts and collagen fibrils and maintains the tissue architecture of the umbilical cord by protecting it from pressure [54].

One centimeter-long fragments of umbilical cords (N = 12) were collected from healthy donors after written informed consent and following validated procedures according to the clinical and technical guidelines of the Private Bank Biosckin, Molecular and Cell Therapies, SA (authorized for processing and cryopreserving CB and UCT units by the Portuguese Minister of Health, ASST – Autoridade para os Serviços de Sangue e de Transplantação). The 1 cm fragments were immersed for 168 hours in 4 different sterile saline solutions at RT (22-24°C) and refrigerated (4-6°C): NaCl 0.9% (Labesfal, Portugal), AOSEPT®-PLUS (Ciba Vision, Portugal), Dulbecco's Phosphate-Buffered Saline without calcium, magnesium and phenol red (DPBS, Gibco, Invitrogen, Portugal) and Hank's Balanced Salt Solution (HBSS, Gibco, Invitrogen, Portugal). The preservative-free, aqueous AOSEPT® PLUS solution contains hydrogen peroxide 3%, phosphonic acid (stabiliser), sodium chloride, phosphate (buffer system), and poloxamer (surfactant), and is usually used to transport and wash contact lenses. After 168 hours, the fragments were collected in 4% of paraformaldehyde and processed for light microscopy. The samples were fixed in 4% paraformaldehyde for 4 hours and then washed and conserved in phosphate buffer saline (PBS) until embedding. The specimens were dehydrated and embedded in paraffin and cut at 10 µm perpendicular to the main umbilical cord axis. For light microscope analysis, sections were stained with haematoxylin and eosin (HE) and observed with a Leica DM400 microscope equipped with a Leica DFC320 digital camera. The UCT integrity was evaluated through the following parameters:

i.   detachment of vessels and retraction of vascular structures;

ii.   loss of detail and integrity of the endothelium;

iii.   connective tissue degradation;

iv.   autolysis of fat (impossible to assess, due to histological technique); and

v.   loss of detail and integrity of the mesothelium.

It was concluded that the best transport solutions were HBSS or DPBS at a temperature of 4-6°C since those maintained the histological structure of UC evaluated through those 5 parameters previously referred (Figure 1 and Figure 2).

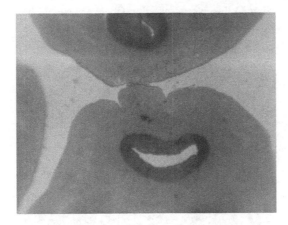

Figure 1. Cross section of an umbilical cord transported immersed in DPBS at the refrigerated temperature of 4-6°C. Samples were stained with haematoxylin and eosin (HE). Magnification: 10X.

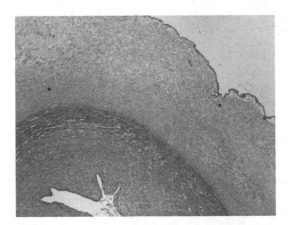

Figure 2. Cross section of an umbilical cord transported immersed in DPBS at the refrigerated temperature of 4-6°C. Samples were stained with haematoxylin and eosin (HE). The UCT integrity was quality evaluated through the following parameters: i) detachment of vessels and retraction of vascular structures; ii) loss of detail and integrity of the endothelium; iii) connective tissue degradation; iv) autolysis of fat (impossible to assess, due to histological technique); and v) loss of detail and integrity of the mesothelium. Magnification: 40X.

As a matter of fact, the UC immersed for 168 hours in DPBS and HBSS at refrigerated temperature presented integrity of the histological structure comparable to a UC collected and processed for histological analysis immediately after birth (Figure 3). With DPBS, a slight retraction of the vessels was noted, which is advantageous since the vessels are stripped and discarded before cryopreservation of the UCT. It was concluded that the transport of the UC from the hospital / clinic to the cryopreservation laboratory should be performed with the UC immersed in DPBS or HBSS at refrigerated temperatures.

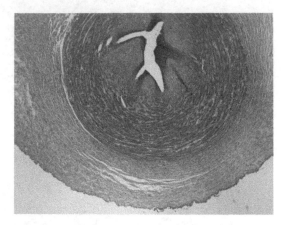

Figure 3. Cross section of an umbilical cord collected and processed for histological analysis immediately after birth under optimal conditions according to Netcord guidelines. Stained with haematoxylin and eosin (HE). Magnification: 40X.

The isolation and culture of MSCs from the Wharton's jelly was performed by our research group in order to obtain undifferentiated MSCs and *in vitro* differentiated into neural-like cells to be tested in axonotmesis and neurotmesis lesions of the rat sciatic nerve. The isolation has been performed by enzyme-free tissue explant and enzymatic isolation. Despite our standard approaches, we are aware that there are still significant variations that exist between laboratory protocols, which must be taken into account when comparing results using other methodologies. There is a wide range of individual differences among donor tissues also and our protocols usually use 15 - 20 cm of UC. While most UC samples will provide a reasonable number of MSCs using the provided protocols, some samples may result in sub-optimal cell isolation and expansion. The reasons behind this phenomenon still remain to be clarified, but as we have previously mentioned, the temperature and the time of transport from the hospital / clinic to the cryopreservation laboratory is crucial.

Irrespective of the specific protocol, the washing procedure of the umbilical cord fragments is crucial in order to avoid microbiological contamination of the cultures. After obtaining the written informed consent from the parents, fresh human umbilical cords are obtained after birth and collected in HBSS or DPBS at 4-6°C, as it was previously described. After washing the umbilical cord unit 4 times in rising DPBS, disinfection is performed in 75% ethanol for 30 seconds. Finally, and before the dissection step, umbilical cord unit is washed in DPBS. The vessels are usually stripped with UC unit still immersed in DPBS. Once washing step in MSCs isolation and culture is essential to achieve good UCT units for cryopreservation and future clinical use, washing protocol was validated. DPBS from the first washing step (used immediately after collection for transportation of the unit to the laboratory – *washing step 1 solution*) and

DPBS used in washing step after disinfection in 75% ethanol (*washing step 6 solution*) from 14 umbilical cord units (N = 14) collected from healthy donors and transported from the hospital/clinic at 4-6°C in less than 96 hours were tested for microbiological contamination using BacT/ALERT® (bioMérieux). Each unit was tested for aerobic and anaerobic microorganisms and fungi using 10 ml of the *washing step 1 solution* and *washing step 6 solution* which were aseptically introduced into the BacT/ALERT® testing flasks. All procedures were performed in a laminar flow tissue culture hood under sterile conditions. All the units that presented microbial contamination in DPBS obtained from the first washing step (*washing step 1 solution*) presented no contamination in the analysis performed to DPBS from the last washing step immediately performed before MSCs isolation or UCT cryopreservation (*washing step 6 solution*). The following microorganisms were identified in the DPBS solution from the first washing step: *Staphylococcus lugdunensis* (N = 2); *Staphylococcus epidermidis* (N = 1); *Staphylococcus coagulase* (N = 2); *Escherichia coli* (N = 4); *Enterococcus faecalis* (N = 1); and *Streptococcus sanguinis* (N = 1). The DPBS solution from the first washing step (*washing step 1 solution*) from 3 units was negative for microbial contamination (N = 3). These results permitted us to conclude that the washing protocol was 100% efficient in what concerns microbiological elimination (including aerobic and anaerobic bacteria, yeast and fungi).

Once the transport and washing protocols were validated, it was important to isolate and expand *in vitro* the MSCs from the UCT units for pre-clinical trials.

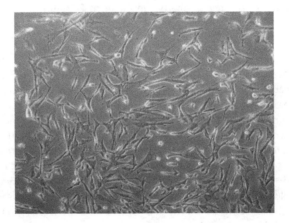

Figure 4. MSCs isolated from Wharton's jelly using the "enzymatic protocol" exhibiting a mesenchymal-like shape with a flat polygonal morphology. Magnification: 100x.

In the "enzymatic procedure" we use collagenase type I (Sigma-Aldrich). With the written informed consent from the parents, fresh human umbilical cords were obtained after birth and stored in HBSS (Gibco, Invitrogen, Portugal) for 1–48 hours before tissue processing to obtain MSCs. After removal of blood vessels, the mesenchymal tissue is scraped off from the Wharton's jelly with a scalpel and centrifuged at 250 g for 5 minutes at room temperature and the pellet is washed with serum-free Dulbecco's modified Eagle's medium (DMEM,

Gibco, Invitrogen, Portugal). Next, the cells are centrifuged at 250 g for 5 minutes at room temperature and then treated with collagenase (2 mg/ml) for 16 hours at 37°C,washed, and treated with 2.5% trypsin-EDTA solution (Sigma-Aldrich) for 30 minutes at 37°C with agitation. Finally, the cells are washed and cultured in DMEM (Gibco, Invitrogen, Portugal) supplemented with 10% fetal bovine serum (FBS), glucose (4.5 g/l), 1% (w/v) penicillin and streptomycin (Sigma), and 2.5 mg/ml amphotericin B (Sigma) in 5% CO_2 in a 37°C incubator (Nuaire). Around 2×10^5 cells are plated into each T75 flask in 10 ml culture medium. Cells are allowed to attach and grow for 3 days. To remove the non-adherent cells or fragments, the flasks are gently washed using pre-warmed DPBS after which 10 ml of pre-warmed culture medium is added. The culture medium is changed every third day (or twice per week). Confluence (80-90%) is normally reached at day 12–16, and the cells are removed with pre-warmed trypsin-EDTA solution (4 ml per flask), for 10 min at 37°C. The cells are plated onto poly-l-lysine coated glass coverslips (in 6- or 24-well tissue culture plates) or on biomaterials used in the nerve reconstruction. Normally, 5000 cells/cm^2 are plated on the coverslips or on the membranes (Figure 4).

In our "enzyme-free tissue explant protocol" for isolation of MSCs, enzymatic digestion is not employed. The mesenchymal tissue (Wharton's jelly) is diced into cubes of about 0.5 cm^3 and the remaining vessels are removed by dissection. Using a sterile scalp, the cubes are diced in 1-2 mm fragments and transferred to a Petri dish pre-coated with poly-l-lysine (Sigma) with Mesenchymal Stem Cell Medium (PromoCell, C-28010) supplemented with 1% (w/v) penicillin and streptomycin (Sigma), and 2.5 mg/ml amphotericin B (Sigma) and cultured in 5% CO_2 in a 37°C incubator (Nuaire). Some tissue fragments will allow cell migration from the explants in 3-4 days incubation. Confluence is normally obtained 15-21 days after.

The laboratory's processing and cryopreservation protocols of the UCT units following the technical procedures of Biosckin, Molecular and Cell Therapies S.A. (BSK.LCV.PT.7) were validated for the ability of isolating and expanding *in vitro* MSCs after cryopreserved UCT thawing. The protocols of processing and cryopreservation of the UCT are protected by a Confidentiality Agreement between Biosckin, Molecular and Cell Therapies S.A. and all the involved researchers. Briefly, the UCT collected from healthy donors (N = 60), and according to Netcord guidelines and following the Portuguese law 12/2009 (*Diário da República, lei 12/2009 de 26 de Março de 2009*) is diced into cubes of about 0.5 cm^3 and the remaining vessels are removed by dissection. In order to ensure the viability of the UCT after parturition and limit the microbiological contamination of the samples, the umbilical cords were transported from the hospital / clinic to the laboratory at refrigerated temperatures monitored by a datalloger in less than 72 hours. The UCT units from 15-20 centimeters-long umbilical cords and after the blood vessels dissection are treated and processed for cryopreservation using a cryoprotective solution (freezing medium). The UCT units are transferred to a computer-controlled slow rate freezer (Sylab, Consensus, Portugal) and a nine-step freezing program is used to set up the time, temperature, and rates specifically optimized for the human umbilical cord-MSCs cooling. To thaw frozen cells, the cryovials are transferred directly to a 37°C water bath. Upon thawing in less than a minute, the cell suspension is centrifuged at $150 \times g$ for 10 min, and the supernatant is gently removed and the cell pellet is resuspended in culture medium. It was possible to obtain MSCs in culture from 52 out of 60 thawed UCT units.

In some UCT cryopreserved units (N = 8) it was not possible to isolate MSCs due to increase number of erythrocytes' lysis or microbiological contamination during cell culture. The MSCs morphology was observed in an inverted microscope (Zeiss, Germany) at different points of expansion. The MSCs exhibited a mesenchymal-like shape with a flat and polygonal morphology. The MSCs obtained were characterized by flow cytometry (FACSCalibur®, BD Biosciences) analysis for a comprehensive panel of markers, such as PECAM (CD31), HCAM (CD44), CD45, and Endoglin (CD105). In the presence of neurogenic medium, the MSCs were able to, became exceedingly long and there was a formation of typical neuroglial-like cells with multi-branches and secondary branches. These results permitted to conclude that the processing and cooling protocols used for UCT units' cryopreservation were adequate to preserve the UCT viability since it was possible to isolate and expand MSCs after appropriate thaw and in presence of adequate cell culture conditions.

An established and ready-to-use Human MSC cell line was also employed for promoting axonotmesis and neurotmesis lesions regeneration. Human MSCs from Wharton's jelly umbilical cord were purchased from PromoCell GmbH (C-12971, lot-number: 8082606.7). Cryopreservated cells are cultured and maintained in a humidified atmosphere with 5% CO_2 at 37°C. Mesenchymal Stem Cell Medium (PromoCell, C-28010) is replaced every 48 hours. At 80-90% confluence, cells are harvested with 0.25% trypsin with EDTA (Gibco) and passed into a new flask for further expansion. MSCs at a concentration of 2500 cells/ml are cultured on poli-D-lysine coverslips (Sigma) or on biomaterials membranes and after 24 hours cells exhibit 30-40% confluence. Differentiation into neuroglial-like cells is induced with MSC neurogenic medium (Promocell, C-28015). Medium is normally replaced every 24 hours during 3 days. The formation of neuroglial-like cells can be observed after 24 hours in an inverted microscope (Zeiss, Germany) (Figure 5 and Figure 6).

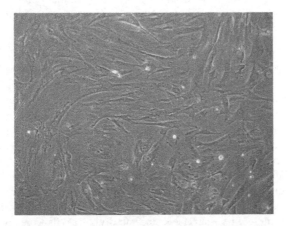

Figure 5. MSC cell line from Wharton's jelly (PromoCell) exhibiting a mesenchymal-like shape with a flat polygonal morphology. Magnification: 100x.

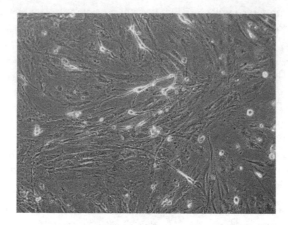

Figure 6. MSC cell line from Wharton's jelly (PromoCell) after 72h of incubation in neurogenic medium. The cells became exceedingly long and there is a formation of typical neuroglial-like cells with multibranches. Magnification: 100x.

This established human MSC cell line is preferred for *in vivo* testing in rats, since the number of MSCs obtained is higher in a shorter culture time, it is not dependent on donors availability and ethic committee authorization, and the protocol is much less time consuming which is advantageous for pre-clinical trials with a large number of experimental animals. As a matter of fact, there is no need of administrating immunosuppressive treatment to the experimental animals during the entire healing period after the surgical procedure. The phenotype of MSCs was assessed by PromoCell. Rigid quality control tests are performed for each lot of PromoCell MSCs isolated from Wharton's jelly of umbilical cord. MSCs are tested for cell morphology, adherence rate and viability. Furthermore, each cell lot is characterized by flow cytometry analysis for a comprehensive panel of markers.

The MSCs isolated with the two protocols described (from fresh and the cryopreserved UCT units) and from the established Promocell cell line exhibited a mesenchymal-like shape with a flat and polygonal morphology. During expansion the cells became long spindle-shaped and colonized the whole culturing surface. After 96 hours of culture in neurogenic medium, cells changed in morphology. The cells became exceedingly long and there was a formation of typical neuroglial-like cells with multi-branches and secondary branches. Giemsa-stained cells of differentiated MSC cell line at passage 5 were analyzed for cytogenetic characterization. However, no metaphases were found, therefore the karyotype could not be established. The karyotype of undifferentiated HMSCs was determined previously and no structural alterations were found demonstrating absence of neoplastic characteristics in these cells, as well as chromosomal stability to the cell culture procedures [55, 56]. The differentiated MSCs karyotype could not be established, since no dividing cells were obtained at passage 5, which can be in agreement with the degree of differentiation. The karyotype analysis of undifferentiated MSCs previously determined, excluded the presence of neoplastic cells, thus supporting the suitability of our cell culture and differentiation procedures. This concern also resulted from our previous experience with N1E-115 neoplastic cell line and the negative results we obtained in the treatment of axonotmesis and neurotmesis injuries [57-59]. Nevertheless, undifferentiated MSCs from the Wharton's jelly culture (obtained from either protocol or from the Promocell cell line) showed normal morphology when inspected with an inverted microscope (Figure 7).

The differentiation was tested based on the expression of typical neuronal markers such as GFAP, GAP-43 and NeuN by neural-like cells attained from MSCs. Undifferentiated MSCs were negatively labeled to GFAP, GAP-43 and NeuN. After 96 hours of differentiation the attained cells were positively stained for glial protein GFAP and for the growth-associated protein GAP-43. All nucleus of neural-like cells were also labeled with the neuron specific nuclear protein called NeuN showing that differentiation of MSCs in neural-like cells was successfully achieved for MSCs obtained from UCT (fresh and cryopreserved) and for the Promocell MSC cell line (Figure 8) [55].

2.1.2. Differentiation into neuroglial-like cells

MSCs express nestin, a maker for neural and other stem cells [60, 61] and can be differentiated in adipose tissue, bone, cartilage, skeletal muscle cells, cardiomyocyte-like cells, and neuroglial-like cells [54, 55, 60, 62], presenting great potential to biomedical engineering applications. These cells fit into the category of primitive stromal cells and because they are abundant and inexpensive, they might be very useful for regenerative medicine and biotechnology applications.

By employing neuron-conditioned media, sonic hedgehog and fibroblast growth factor 8, MSCs isolated from the Wharton's jelly can be induced toward dopaminergic neurons. These cells have been transplanted into hemiparkinsonian rats where they prevented the progressive degeneration/behavioral deterioration seen in these rats [63]. Rat MSCs isolated from the Wharton's jelly when transplanted into brains of rats with global cerebral ischemia significantly reduced neuronal loss, apparently due to a rescue phenomenon [64]. Neuronal differentiation of human MSCs could also provide cells to replace neurons lost due to neurodegenerative diseases. Recent studies showed that transplanted MSCs-derived neurons become electrophysiologically integrated within the host neural tissue [65]. However, all these therapeutic applications need uniform and reproducible regulation.

A consequence of cell metabolism during *in vitro* expansion is that culture conditions are constantly changing. The comprehension and optimization of the expansion and differentiation process will contribute to maximization of cell yield, reduced need of cell culture, and a decrease in total processing costs [66, 67]. Elucidation of regulatory mechanisms of MSCs differentiation will allow optimization of *in vitro* culture and their clinical use in the treatment of neural-related diseases. Research is being performed to optimize expansion process parameters in order to grow MSCs in a controlled, reproducible, and cost-effective way [68]. Metabolism is certainly one of these parameters.

3. Regeneration and in vivo testing

With the world wide global increase in life expectancy, a variety of disabling diseases with large impact on human population are arising. This includes cardiovascular, neurological, musculoskeletal, and malignancies. Therefore, it is imperative that new and more effective treatment methods are developed to correct for these changes. Further research with experimental animal systems is required to translate to in vivo cell-based therapy that has been extensively investigated in vitro [1]. Stem cell biology is probably the golden key for cell therapies and regenerative medicine. Regeneration is the physical process where remaining tissues organize themselves to replace missing or injured tissues *in vivo* [39].

It has been speculated that once MSCs have the potential to differentiate into several tissues, they might be responsible for turnover and maintenance of adult tissues, just like hematopoietic stem cells have this role in blood cells [69]. First, it was believed that after injection of MSCs, these were able to migrate to the damaged site and to differentiate into ones with the appropriate function for repairing, so MSCs could mediate tissue repair through there multilineage capacity replacing damaged cells. Subsequent studies have suggested that the mechanism used by MSCs for tissue repairing is not really this way. This new idea was reinforced by the confirmation that this cells homed to damaged site, particularly to spots of hypoxia, inflammation and apoptosis [70, 71].

Recent studies demonstrated that transplanted MSCs modified the surrounding tissue microenvironment, promoting repair with functional improvement by secretion factors (known as paracrine effect), stimulation of preexisting stem cells in the original tissue and decreasing of inflammation and immune response [72]. Other studies have demonstrated that MSC-conditioned media by itself could have therapeutic effects. All this data suggest that MSC apply a reparative effect on injured side through its paracrine effects [73].

It is necessary to overcome some barriers before a cell-based therapy becomes routine in clinics, including the cell number and the administration way of treatment. MSCs are difficult to be maintained stable in culture for long time, but due to their short doubling time, if at the outset many cells are harvested they may be properly scaled up in primary culture, never forgetting the ideal seeding number [39].

MSCs are an attractive candidate for cell-based regenerative therapy; the evidence is that currently there are 139 trial registries for MSC therapy 27 of which are based on umbilical cord MSCs [74].

3.1. Nerve regeneration

After Central Nervous System (CNS) lesions, Peripheral Nervous System (PNS) injuries are the ones with minor successes in terms of functional recovery. These kinds of injuries are frequent in clinical practice. About two centuries ago it was assumed that these nerves would never regenerate. Indeed, scientific and clinical knowledge greatly increased in this area. Nevertheless, a full understanding of axonal recovery and treatment of nerve defects, especially complete functional achievement and organ reinnervation after nerve injury, still remains the principle challenge of regenerative biology and medicine [75, 76].

3.1.1. Nerve repair

Many peripheral nerve injuries can only be dealt through reconstructive surgical procedures. Despite continuous refinement of microsurgery techniques, peripheral nerve repair still stands as one of the most challenging tasks in neurosurgery, as functional recovery is rarely satisfactory in these patients [76]. Direct repair should be the procedure of choice whenever tension-free suturing is possible; however, patients with loss of nerve tissue, resulting in a nerve gap, are considered for a nerve graft procedure. In these cases, the donor nerves used for grafting are commonly expendable sensory nerves. This technique, however, has some disadvantages, with the most prominent being donor site morbidity, that may lead to a secondary sensory deficit and occasionally neuroma and pain. In addition, no donor and recipient nerve diameters often occurs which might be the basis for poor functional recovery. Alternatives to peripheral nerve grafts include cadaver nerve segments allografts, end-to-side neurorrhaphy, and entubulation by means of autologous non-nervous tissues, such as vein and muscles [76]. One advantage of these allografts compared with the autografts is the absence of donor site morbidity and theoretically the unlimited length of tissue available [77]. Experimental work from a number of laboratories has emphasized the importance of entubulation for peripheral nerve repair to manage nerve defects that cannot be bridged without tension (neurotmesis with loss of nerve tissue). Nerves will regenerate from the proximal nerve stump towards the distal one, whereas neuroma formation and ingrowth of fibrous tissue into the nerve gap are prevented [78]. The reliability of animal models is crucial for PN research, including therapeutic strategies using biomaterials and cellular systems. As a matter of fact, rodents, particularly the rat and the mouse, have become the most frequently used animal models for the study of peripheral nerve regeneration because of the widespread availability of these animals as well as the distribution of their nerve trunks which is similar to humans [79]. Because of its PN size, the rat sciatic nerve has been the most commonly experimental model used in studies concerning the PN regeneration and possible therapeutic approaches [80]. Functional recovery after PN injury is frequently incomplete, even with adequate microsurgery, so, many research and clinical studies have been performed including biomaterials for tube-guides. Since the 80's, Food and Drug Administration (FDA) has approved a variety of these biomaterials both natural and synthetic. The ideal biomaterial nerve graft should increase number, length and speed of axon regeneration [77]. It should be:

i.   biocompatible, not toxic neither present undesired immunologic response;

ii.   permeable enough to permit nutrient and oxygen diffusion and allows cell support systems;

iii.   flexible and soft to avoid compression;

iv.   biodegradable, the ideal rate is to remain intact during axon regeneration across nerve gap and after degrade softly and

v.   technically reproducible, transparent, easy to manipulate, and sterilize [81].

Currently 3 types of materials are available for nerve reconstruction: non-resorbable, natural resorbable and synthetic resorbable. Polyvinil alcohol hydrogel (PVA) is an example of a non-absorbable biomaterial. It combines water in similar proportions to human tissue, with PVA providing a stable structure easy to sterilize, which is a main advantage of this materials, but has some limitations such as: nerve compression and suture tension after regeneration due to its non-resorbable nature [77]. Collagen type I from humans or animals, is an example of a natural resorbable device, which has some advantages such as:

i.   easy to isolate and purify,

ii.   good adhesiveness for supporting cell survival an proliferation,

iii.   has been proven to be highly biocompatible and support nerve regeneration *in vivo*.

On the other hand, offers some immune response requiring the use of immunosuppressive drugs or pre-treatment of the material before clinical use [77]. Poly (DL-lactide-ε-caprolactone) (PLC) a synthetic resorbable material is the only transparent device approved by FDA, important characteristic for the surgeon that facilitates the insertion of the nerve stumps across the nerve gap, but, on the other hand it is not flexible [77]. Chitosan, PLC, collagen, poly(L-lactide) and poly(glycolide) copolymers (PLGA) and others, some of them, previously studied by our group [57, 58, 82] were associated to cellular systems, which are able to differentiate into neuroglial-like cells or capable of modulating the inflammatory process, improved nerve regeneration, in terms of motor and sensory recovery, and also shortening the healing period after axonotmesis and neurotmesis, avoiding regional muscular atrophy [57, 58, 82].

Researches with acellular nerve allografts, as alternative for repairing peripheral nerve defects have been reported. These nerve allografts remove the immunoreactive SCs and myelin however preserve the internal structure of original nerve, containing vital components such as collagen I, laminin and growth factors essential for repairmen of the lesions [83]. Acellular grafts remain insufficient, due to the increasing extent of nerve damages. Also, viable cells are necessary for debris removal and environmental regeneration reestablishment [83].

Cell transplantation, such as Schwann cells (SCs) transplantation has been proposed as a method of improving peripheral nerve regeneration [84]. SCs are peripheral glial cells that enwrap axons to form myelin with a central role in neuronal function. When there is damage in PNS, SCs are induced to mislay myelin, proliferate and segregate numerous factors, including cytokines responsible for reproducing a microenvironment suitable for supporting axon regeneration [85, 86]. They also have a vital participation in endogenous repair, reconstructing myelin, which are essential for functional recovery [85, 86]. SCs, MSCs, ESCs, marrow stromal cells are the most studied support cells candidates. SCs transplantation enhance axon outgrowth both *in vitro* [87] and *in vivo* [88]. Although to achieve an adequate amount of autologous SC, a donor nerve is necessary and a minimum of 4-8 weeks for *in vitro* expansion. Umbilical cord MSCs may be the perfect cell model as supplement for nerve grafts, once they are easily obtained, with no ethical controversy and can differentiate into neuglial-like cells [83]. Matuse and collaborators induced MSCs from the umbilical cord into SCs capable of supporting peripheral nerve regeneration and myelin reconstruction *in vivo*. They transplanted these SCs into injured sciatic nerve, and proved that these cells maintained their differentiated phenotype *in vivo*, and contributed for axonal regeneration and functional recovery [89].

In our studies we aimed to explore the therapeutic value of human umbilical cord matrix (Wharton's jelly) derived MSCs, undifferentiated and differentiated in neuroglial-like cells, both *in vitro* and *in vivo*, associated to a variety of biomaterials such as, Poly (DL-lactide-ε-caprolactone) PLC (Vivosorb®) membrane, and Chitosan type III on rat sciatic nerve axonotmesis and neurotmesis experimental model. For cell transplantation into injured nerves (with axonotmesis and neurotmesis injuries), there are two main techniques. The cellular system may be directly inoculated into the neural scaffold which has been interposed between the proximal and distal nerve stumps or around the crush injury (in neurotmesis and axonotmesis injuries, respectively); or the cells can be pre-added to the neural scaffold via inoculation or co-culture (in most of the cellular systems, it is allowed to form a monolayer) and then the biomaterial with the cellular system is implanted in the injured nerve [82].

Our PLC studies [55] demonstrated that this biomaterial does not interfere negatively with the nerve regeneration process, in fact, the information on the effectiveness of PLC membranes and tube-guides for allowing nerve regeneration was already provided experimentally and with patients [82]. PLC becomes hydrophilic by water uptake, which increases the permeability of the polymer. This is essential for the control of nutrient and other metabolite transportation to the surrounding healing tissue. A few weeks after implantation, the mechanical power gradually decreases and there is a loss of molecular weight as a result of the hydrolysis process. Nearly in 24 months, PLC degrades into lactic acid and hydroxycaproic acid which are both safely metabolized into water and carbon dioxide and/or excreted through the urinary tract. In contrast to other biodegradable polymers, PCL has the advantage of not creating an acidic and potentially disturbing micro-environment, which is favorable to the surrounding tissue [90]. Chitosan has attracted particular attention in medical areas due to its biocompatibility, biodegradability, and low toxicity, low cost, improvement of wound-healing and antibacterial properties. Moreover, the potential use of chitosan in nerve regeneration has been demonstrated both *in vitro* and *in vivo* [57, 91]. Chitosan is a partially deacetylated polymer of acetyl glucosamine obtained after the alkaline deacetylation of chitin [57, 82]. While chitosan matrices have low mechanical strength under physiological conditions and are unable to maintain a predefined shape after transplantation, their mechanical properties can be improved by modification with a silane agent, namely γ-glycidoxypropyltrimethoxysilane (GPTMS), one of the silane-coupling agents which has epoxy and methoxysilane groups. The epoxy group reacts with the amino groups of chitosan molecules, while the methoxysilane groups are hydrolyzed and form silanol groups. Finally, the silanol groups are subjected to the construction of a siloxane network due to the condensation. Thus, the mechanical strength of chitosan can be improved by the cross-linking between chitosan, GPTMS and siloxane network. By adding GPTMS and employing a freeze-drying technique, we have previously obtained chitosan type III membranes (hybrid chitosan membranes) with pores of about 110 μm diameter and about 90% of porosity, and which were successful in improving sciatic nerve regeneration after axonotmesis and neurotmesis [56, 57, 82].

The induction of a crush injury in rat sciatic nerve provides a very realistic and useful model of damage for the study of the role of numerous factors in regenerative processes [57]. Focal crush causes axonal interruption but preserves the connective sheaths (axonotmesis). After axonotmesis injury regeneration is usually successful, after a short (1-2 day) latency, axons regenerate at a steady rate towards the distal nerve stump, supported by the reactive SCs and the preserved endoneural tubules enhance axonal elongation and facilitate adequate re-innervation [92]. Our research group has been testing the efficacy of combining biomaterials and cellular systems in the treatment of sciatic nerve crush injury [57-59, 82, 90, 91, 93-95]. Following transection, axons show staggered regeneration and may take substantial time to actually cross the injury site and enter the distal nerve stump [60]. Although delayed axonal elongation might be caused by growth inhibition originating from the distal nerve itself, growth-stimulating influences may overcome axons stagger. More robust and fast nerve regeneration is expected to result in better reinnervation and functional recovery. As a potential source of growth promoting signals, MSCs transplantation is expected to have a positive outcome. Our results showed that the use of either undifferentiated or differentiated HMSCs enhanced the recovery of sensory and motor function in axonotmesis lesion of the rat sciatic nerve [56]. Neurotmesis must be surgically treated by direct end-to-end suture of the two nerve stumps or by a nerve graft harvested from elsewhere in the body in case of tissue loss. To avoid secondary damage due to harvesting of the nerve graft, a tube-guide can be used to bridge the nerve gap. Acutely after sciatic nerve transection there is a complete loss of both motor and thermal sensory function. Sensory and motor deficit then progressively decrease along the post-operative. From a morphological point of view, nerve regeneration occurs if Wallerian degeneration is efficient and is substituted by re-growing axons and the accompanying viable SCs [96, 97]. The axon regeneration pattern is improved by using appropriate biomaterials for the tube-guide design, like chitosan type III and PLC and cellular systems like MSCs from the Wharton jelly [57, 90, 91, 95]. The surgical technique and the time for the reconstructive surgery is also crucial for the nerve regeneration after neurotmesis [57, 90, 91, 95].

3.2. Assessment of nerve regeneration in the sciatic nerve rat model

Although both morphological and functional data have been used to assess neural regeneration after induced crush injuries, the correlation between these two types of assessment is usually poor [94, 98-100]. Classical and newly developed methods of assessing nerve recovery, including histomorphometry, retrograde transport of horseradish peroxidase and retrograde fluorescent labeling [79] do not necessarily predict the reestablishment of motor and sensory functions [100-103]. Although such techniques are useful in studying the nerve regeneration process, they generally fail in assessing functional recovery [100]. In this sense, research on peripheral nerve injury needs to combine both functional and morphological assessment. The use of biomechanical techniques and rat's gait kinematic evaluation is a progress in documenting functional recovery [104]. Indeed, the use of biomechanical parameters has given valuable insight into the effects of the sciatic denervation/reinnervation, and thus represents an integration of the neural control acting on the ankle and foot muscles, which is very useful and accurate to evaluate different therapeutic approaches [103-105].

3.2.1. Functional Assessment

After injury and treatment of animals, follow-up results are very important for analysis of functional recovery. Animals are tested preoperatively (week 0), and every week during 12 and 20 weeks, for axonotmesis and neurotmesis of the rat sciatic nerve, respectively. Motor performance and nociceptive function are evaluated by measuring extensor postural thrust (EPT) and withdrawal reflex latency (WRL), respectively [55, 58, 94]. For EPT test, the affected and normal limbs are tested 3 times, with an interval of 2 minutes between consecutive tests, and the 3 values are averaged to obtain a final result. The normal (unaffected limb) EPT (NEPT) and experimental EPT (EEPT) values are incorporated into an equation (Equation (1)) to derive the percentage of functional deficit, as described in the literature [106]:

$$\% \text{ Motor deficit} = \left[(\text{NEPT} - \text{EEPT}) \ / \ \text{NEPT}\right] \times 100 \tag{1}$$

The nociceptive withdrawal reflex (WRL) was adapted from the hotplate test developed by Masters et al. [107]. Normal rats withdraw their paws from the hotplate within 4s or less. The cutoff time for heat stimulation is set at 12 seconds to avoid skin damage to the foot.

For Sciatic Functional Index (SFI), animals are tested in a confined walkway that they cross, measuring 42 cm long and 8.2 cm wide, with a dark shelter at the end. Several measurements are taken from the footprints:

i.   distance from the heel to the third toe, the print length (PL);

ii.   distance from the first to the fifth toe, the toe spread (TS); and

iii.   distance from the second to the fourth toe, the intermediary toe spread (ITS).

In the static evaluation (SSI) only the parameters TS and ITS, are measured. For SFI and SSI, all measurements are taken from the experimental (E) and normal (N) sides. Prints for measurements are chosen at the time of walking based on precise, clear and completeness of footprints. The mean distances of three measurements are used to calculate the following factors (dynamic and static):

$$\text{Toe spread factor} \ (\text{TSF}) \ = \ (\text{ETS} - \text{NTS}) \ / \ \text{NTS} \tag{2}$$

$$\text{Intermediate toe spread factor} \ (\text{ITSF}) \ = \ (\text{EITS} - \text{NITS}) \ / \ \text{NITS} \tag{3}$$

$$\text{Print length factor } (PLF) = (EPL - NPL) / NPL \tag{4}$$

SFI is calculated as described by Bain et al. [108] according to the following equation:

$$SFI = -38.3(EPL - NPL) / NPL + 109.5(ETS - NTS) / NTS + 13.3(EIT - NIT) / NIT - 8.8$$
$$= (-38.3 \times PLF) + (109.5 \times TSF) + (13.3 \times ITSF) - 8.8 \tag{5}$$

For SFI and SSI, an index score of 0 is considered normal and an index of -100 indicates total impairment. When no footprints are measurable, the index score of -100 is given [109]. In each walking track 3 footprints are analyzed by a single observer, and the average of the measurements is used in SFI calculations.

Ankle kinematics analysis is carried out prior nerve injury, at week-2 and every 4 weeks during the 12 or the 20-week follow-up time, for axonotmesis and neurotmesis lesions, respectively. The motion capture is performed with 2 digital high speed cameras (Oqus, Qualysis®) at a rate of 200 images per second, and Qualisys Track Manager software (QTM, Qualysis®). The cameras operate on a infra-red light frequency ensuring a high level of accuracy on the determination of reflective marker position and a position residual of less than 2.7 mm was obtained. Cameras are usually positioned to not recorder significant signal deflection during the test and four reflective markers were placed at the skin of the rat right hindlimb at the proximal edge of the tibia, the lateral malleolus and the fifth metatarsal head. Advanced analysis of the 2-D movement (sagittal plan) data is performed with Visual3D software (C-Motion®, Inc). The rats' ankle angle is determined using the scalar product between a vector representing the foot and a vector representing the lower leg. With this model, positive and negative values of position of the ankle joint ($\theta°$) indicate dorsiflexion and plantarflexion, respectively. For each step cycle the following time points are identified: midswing, midstance, initial contact (IC) and toe-off (TO) [104, 109-113] and are time normalized for 100% of step cycle. The normalized temporal parameters are averaged over all recorded trials. Angular velocity of the ankle joint ($\Omega°/s$) is also determined where negative values correspond to dorsiflexion. A total of 6 walking trials for each animal with stance phases lasting between 150 and 400 ms are considered for analysis, since this corresponds to the normal walking velocity of the rat (20–60 cm/s) [104]. Animals walk on a Perspex track with length, width and height of respectively 120, 12, and 15 cm. In order to ensure locomotion in a straight direction, the width of the apparatus is adjusted to the size of the rats during the experiments.

3.2.2. Morphologic Assessment

Nerve samples are processed for quantitative morphometry of myelinated nerve fibers [114]. Fixation is usually carried out using 2.5% purified glutaraldehyde and 0.5% saccarose in 0.1M Sorensen phosphate buffer for 6-8 hours and resin embedding is obtained following Glauerts' procedure (Scipio et al., 2008). Series of 2-μm thick semi-thin transverse sections are cut using a Leica Ultracut UCT ultramicrotome (Leica Microsystems, Wetzlar, Germany) and stained by Toluidine blue. Stereology is carried out on a DM4000B microscope equipped with a DFC320 digital camera and an IM50 image manager system (Leica Microsystems, Wetzlar, Germany). Systematic random sampling and D-disector is always adopted using a protocol previously described [115, 116]. Fiber density and total number of myelinated fibers is estimated together with fiber and axon diameter and myelin thickness.

3.3. Results

3.3.1. Differentiation and metabolism of MSCs from Wharton's jelly

In our experimental studies we expanded undifferentiated MSCs from human umbilical cord Wharton's jelly that exhibited a normal star-like shape with a flat morphology in culture (Figures 4 and 5). To prevent the possibility of eventual mutations due to expansion artifacts, a total of 20 Giemsa-stained metaphases of these cells, were analyzed for numerical aberrations. Sporadic, non-clonal aneuploidy was found in 3 cells (41-45 chromosomes). The other 17 metaphases had 46 chromosomes (Figure 7). The karyotype was determined in a completely analyzed G-banding metaphase. No structural alterations were found. The karyotype analysis to the MSCs cell line derived from Human Wharton jelly demonstrated that this cell line has not neoplastic characteristics and is stable during the cell culture procedures in terms of number and structure of the somatic and sexual chromosomes [55].

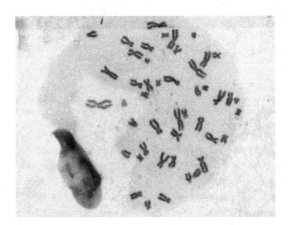

Figure 7. Selected metaphases from undifferentiated MSC cells isolated from Wharton's jelly, showing the normal number of chromosomes (46, XY). Magnification: 1000X.

We differentiated MSC from Wharton's Jelly into neuroglial-like cells. After 96 hours of incubation in neurogenic medium, we observed a morphological change. The cells became exceedingly long and there was a formation of typical neural-like cells with multi-branches and secondary branches (Figure 6). The differentiation was tested based on the expression of typical neuronal markers such as GFAP, GAP-43 and NeuN by neural-like cells attained from HwMSCs. Undifferentiated MSCs were negatively labeled to GFAP, GAP-43 and NeuN (Figure 8A,C,E). After 96 hours of differentiation the attained cells were positively stained for glial protein GFAP (Figure 8B) and for the growth-associated protein GAP-43 (Figure 8D). All nucleus of neural-like cells were also labeled with the neuron specific nuclear protein called NeuN (Figure 8F) showing that differentiation of MSCs in neural-like cells were successfully achieved [55].

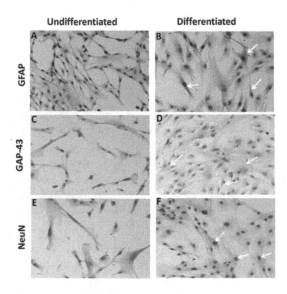

Figure 8. Undifferentiated MSC cells from the Wharton's jelly presenting a negative staining for: (A) GFAP which is a glial cell marker; (C) GAP-43 which is related with axonal outgrowth and (E) NeuN which is a marker for nucleus of neurons. Neuroglial-like cells obtained from HMSCs in vitro differentiated with neurogenic medium exhibiting a positive staining for: (B) GFAP; (D) GAP-43 and (F) NeuN. Magnification: 200x [55].

The *in vitro* expansion and differentiation of MSCs for clinical cell-based therapy is a very expensive and long process that needs standardization. Although pre-clinical and clinical data demonstrated the safety and effectiveness of MSCs therapy in some pathologies such as neurological, there are still questions surrounding the mechanism of action. In our research work we aimed to disclose the possible role of metabolism not only in the MSCs maintenance and expansion but also during the differentiation in neural-like cells [55]. MSCs maintenance and differentiation, to neural-like cells, depends on metabolic modulation. *In vitro*, glucose is the most widely used substrate for the generation ATP which is essential for cell growth and maintenance. It has been proposed that cells undergoing high proliferation rates depend on glycolysis to generate ATP, known as Warburg effect, although this pathway is less effective than the oxidative phosphorylation in terms of ATP production [117]. Our results showed that during expansion, the undifferentiated MSCs consume glucose and produce high concentration of lactate as a metabolic sub product which is consistent with the

Warburg effect and glycolysis stimulation. MSCs do not require oxidative phosphorylation to survive as alternative, hypoxia extends the lifespan, increases their proliferative ability and reduces differentiation [118]. The morphologic and biochemical characteristics of neu-ral-like cells are already described but the mechanism by which stem cells differentiate into neural-like cells is still unknown. In our research work, MSCs that undergone differentiation into neural-like cells, consumed significantly less glucose and produced significantly less lactate than MSCs that undergone only expansion. These major differences allow us to con-clude that during MSCs differentiation in neural-like cells the glycolytic process, which proved to be the crucial metabolic mechanism during MSCs expansion, is switched to oxida-tive metabolism [55].

Our results show clear evidences that MSCs expansion is dependent of glycolysis while their differentiation in neural-like cells requires the switch of the metabolic profile to oxida-tive metabolism. Also important may be the role of oxidative stress during this process. This work is a first step to identify key metabolic-related mechanisms responsible for human MSCs from the Wharton's jelly expansion and differentiation [55].

The lack of standardization of MSCs isolated from the Wharton's jelly culture conditions has limited some progress in scientific and clinical research. Understanding these MSCs metabo-lism during expansion, as well as determining molecular and biochemical mechanisms for differentiation is of great significance to develop new effective stem cell-based therapies.

4. Biomaterial and cellular system association – discussion and final remarks

Using the rat model, we recently tested *in vivo* the efficacy of biomaterials and cellular sys-tem association in treatment of sciatic nerve axonotmesis and neurotmesis injury. Following transection, axons show staggered regeneration and may take substantial time to cross the injured site and enter the distal nerve stump [119]. However delayed axonal elongation might be caused by growth inhibition originated from the distal nerve itself, growth-stimu-lating influences may overcome axons stagger. As a potential source of growth promoting signals, MSCs transplantation is expected to give a positive outcome. Our results showed that the use of either undifferentiated or differentiated MSCs in axonotmesis lesion boosted the recovery of sensory and motor function. In both cell-enriched experimental groups we observed that the myelin sheath was thicker, this suggests that MSCs might apply their posi-tive effects on SCs, the key element in Wallerian degeneration and the following axonal re-generation [120]. Also results from *in vivo* testing previously performed by our research group showed that infiltration of MSCs from the Wharton's jelly, or the combination of chi-tosan type III membrane enwrapment and MSCs enrichment after nerve crush injury pro-vide an advantage to post-traumatic nerve regeneration [56, 57]. Chitosan type III was developed as a hybrid of chitosan by adding GPTMS. A synergistic effect of an extra perme-ability and physicochemical properties of chitosan type III and the presence of silica ions may be responsible for the good results in post-traumatic nerve regeneration promotion observed in the sciatic nerve after axonotmesis and neurotmesis [57, 91]. The substantial improvement of axonal regeneration found in sciatic nerve crush enwrapped by chitosan type III membranes and for bridging nerve gaps after neurotmesis [57, 91], suggests that this biomaterial may not just work as a simple mechanical device but instead may induce nerve regeneration. The neuroregenerative properties of chitosan type III may be explained by the effect on SCs proliferation, axon elongation and myelinization [55, 91]. Our data also showed that PLC does not deleteriously interfere with the nerve regeneration process, as a matter of fact, the information on the effectiveness of PLC membranes and tube-guides for allowing nerve regeneration was already provided experimentally and with patients [82]. The MSCs from the Wharton's jelly may be a valuable source in the repair of the peripheral nervous system with capacity to differentiate into neuroglial-like cells. The transplanted MSCs are also able to promote local blood vessel formation and release the neurotrophic factors brain-derived neurotrophic factor (BDNF) and glial cell line-derived neurotrophic factor (GDNF) [55]. Previous results obtained by our research group using N1E-115 cells *in vitro* differentiated into neuroglial-like cells to promote regeneration of axonotmesis and neurotmesis lesions in the rat model showed that there was no significant effect in promoting axon regeneration and, when N1E-115 cells were cultured inside a PLGA scaffold used to bridge a nerve defect, they can even exert negative effects on nerve fiber regeneration. The presence of transplanted N1E-115 cells in nerve scaffolds competing for the local blood supply of nutrients and oxygen and by space-occupying effect could have hindered the positive effect of local neurotrophic factor release leading a negative outcome on nerve regeneration. Thus, N1E-115 cells did not prove to be a suitable candidate cellular system for treatment of nerve injury after axonotmesis and neurotmesis and their application is limited only to research purposes as a basic scientific step for the development of other cell delivery systems, due to its neoplastic origin [57-59, 91, 93]. The MSCs isolated from the Wharton's jelly through PLC and chitosan type III membranes might be a potentially valuable tool to improve clinical outcome especially after trauma to sensory nerves, such as digital nerves. The results from our experimental work [55, 56] showed that the use of either undifferentiated or neuroglial-like differentiated MSCs enhanced the recovery of sensory and motor function of the rat sciatic nerve. The observation that in both cell-enriched experimental groups myelin sheath was thicker, suggest that MSCs might exert their positive effects on SCs, the key element in Wallerian degeneration and the following axonal regeneration [120]. In addition, these cells represent a non-controversial source of primitive mesenchymal progenitor cells that can be harvested after birth, cryogenically stored, thawed, and expanded for therapeutic uses, including nerve injuries like axonotmesis and neurotmesis. The time and temperature of the transport (and the saline solution used) of the UC units from the hospital / clinic to the laboratory is crucial for a successful outcome considering MSCs isolation and proliferation from fresh and cryopreserved UCT. It is highly recommend that the transport from the clinic or hospital to the laboratory should be refrigerated, and the UC units should be immediately immersed in a sterile saline solution like HBSS or DPBS.

Acknowledgements

The authors would like to gratefully acknowledge the valuable support by Dr. José Manuel
Correia Costa, from Laboratório de Parasitologia, Instituto Nacional de Saúde Dr. Ricardo
Jorge (INSRJ), Porto, Portugal; and Biosckin, Molecular and Cell Therapies SA support for
the umbilical cord units supply used in the experimental work and for the access of the authors to the GMP classified cell culture room and all the equipment used in cell culture and
flow citometry analysis (Scientific Protocol between Porto University and Biosckin, Molecular and Cell Therapies SA). This work was supported by Fundação para a Ciência e Tecnologia (FCT), Ministério da Ciência e Ensino Superior (MCES), Portugal, through the financed
research project PTDC/DES/104036/2008, and by QREN N° 1372 para Criação de um Núcleo
I&DT para Desenvolvimento de Produtos nas Áreas de Medicina Regenerativa e de Terapias Celulares – Núcleo Biomat & Cell. A Gärtner has a Doctoral Grant from Fundação para
a Ciência e Tecnologia (FCT), Ministério da Ciência e Ensino Superior (MCES), Portugal,
SFRH/BD/70211/2010.

Author details

Andrea Gärtner[1,2], Tiago Pereira[1,2], Raquel Gomes[1,2], Ana Lúcia Luís[1,2],
Miguel Lacueva França[1,2], Stefano Geuna[4], Paulo Armada-da-Silva[3*] and
Ana Colette Maurício[1,2]

*Address all correspondence to: ana.colette@hotmail.com

1 Instituto de Ciências Biomédicas Abel Salazar (ICBAS), Universidade do Porto (UP), Portugal

2 Centro de Estudos de Ciência Animal (CECA), Instituto de Ciências e Tecnologias Agrárias e Agro-Alimentares (ICETA), Universidade do Porto (UP), Portugal

3 Faculdade de Motricidade Humana (FMH), Universidade Técnica de Lisboa (UTL), Portugal

4 Department of Clinical and Biological Sciences, University of Turin, Italy

References

[1] Triffitt, J. T. (2002). Stem cells and the philosopher's stone. *Journal of cellular biochemistry Supplement*, 38, 13-9, 2002/06/06.

[2] Lajtha, L. G. (1967). Stem cells and their properties. *Proceedings Canadian Cancer Conference*, 7, 31-9, 1967/01/01.

[3] Fossett, E., & Khan, W. S. (2012). Optimising human mesenchymal stem cell numbers for clinical application: a literature review. *Stem cells international*, 2012, 465259, 2012/03/27.

[4] Bongso, A., Fong, C. Y., Ng, S. C., & Ratnam, S. (1994). Isolation and culture of inner cell mass cells from human blastocysts. *Human reproduction (Oxford, England)*, 9(11), 2110-7, 1994/11/01.

[5] Shim, J. H., Kim, S. E., Woo, D. H., Kim, S. K., Oh, C. H., Mc Kay, R., et al. (2007). Directed differentiation of human embryonic stem cells towards a pancreatic cell fate. *Diabetologia*, 50(6), 1228-38, 2007/04/26.

[6] Yang, D., Zhang, Z. J., Oldenburg, M., Ayala, M., & Zhang, S. C. (2008). Human embryonic stem cell-derived dopaminergic neurons reverse functional deficit in parkinsonian rats. *Stem Cells*, 26(1), 55-63, 2007/10/24.

[7] Mohib, K., & Wang, L. (2012). Differentiation and characterization of dendritic cells from human embryonic stem cells. *Current protocols in immunology / edited by John E Coligan [et al]*, Chapter 22:Unit 22F 11, 12/08/03.

[8] Takahashi, K., & Yamanaka, S. (2006). Induction of pluripotent stem cells from mouse embryonic and adult fibroblast cultures by defined factors. *Cell*, 126(4), 663-76, 2006/08/15.

[9] Fong-Y, C., Chak-L, L., Biswas, A., Tan-H, J., Gauthaman, K., Chan-K, W., et al. (2010). Human Wharton's Jelly Stem Cells Have Unique Transcriptome Profiles Compared to Human Embryonic Stem Cells and Other Mesenchymal Stem Cells. *Stem Cell Reviews and Reports*, 7(1), 1-16.

[10] Jones, E. A., Kinsey, S. E., English, A., Jones, R. A., Straszynski, L., Meredith, D. M., et al. (2002). Isolation and characterization of bone marrow multipotential mesenchymal progenitor cells. *Arthritis and rheumatism*, 46(12), 3349-60, 2002/12/17.

[11] Wohlers, I., Stachelscheid, H., Borstlap, J., Zeilinger, K., & Gerlach, J. C. (2009). The Characterization Tool: A knowledge-based stem cell, differentiated cell, and tissue database with a web-based analysis front-end. *Stem Cell Res*, 3(2-3), 88-95, 2009/06/13.

[12] Brittberg, M., Lindahl, A., Nilsson, A., Ohlsson, C., Isaksson, O., & Peterson, L. (1994). Treatment of deep cartilage defects in the knee with autologous chondrocyte transplantation. *The New England journal of medicine*, 331(14), 889-95, 1994/10/06.

[13] Gentzkow, G. D., Iwasaki, S. D., Hershon, K. S., Mengel, M., Prendergast, J. J., Ricotta, J. J., et al. (1996). Use of dermagraft, a cultured human dermis, to treat diabetic foot ulcers. *Diabetes care*, 19(4), 350-4, 1996/04/01.

[14] Le Blanc, K., & Ringden, O. (2005). Immunobiology of human mesenchymal stem cells and future use in hematopoietic stem cell transplantation. *Biol Blood Marrow Transplant*, 11(5), 321-34, 2005/04/23.

[15] Leri, A., Kajstura, J., Anversa, P., & Frishman, W. H. (2008). Myocardial regeneration and stem cell repair. *Current problems in cardiology*, 33(3), 91-153, 2008/02/05.

[16] Sanchez-Ramos, J. R. (2002). Neural cells derived from adult bone marrow and umbilical cord blood. *J Neurosci Res*, 69(6), 880-93, 2002/09/03.

[17] Wakitani, S., Imoto, K., Yamamoto, T., Saito, M., Murata, N., & Yoneda, M. (2002). Human autologous culture expanded bone marrow mesenchymal cell transplantation for repair of cartilage defects in osteoarthritic knees. *Osteoarthritis and cartilage OARS, Osteoarthritis Research Society*, 10(3), 199-206, 2002/03/01.

[18] Wang, L., Ott, L., Seshareddy, K., Weiss, M. L., & Detamore, MS. (2011). Musculoskeletal tissue engineering with human umbilical cord mesenchymal stromal cells. *Regen Med*, 6(1), 95-109, 2010/12/24.

[19] Chen, J. S., Wong, V. W., & Gurtner, G. C. (2012). Therapeutic potential of bone marrow-derived mesenchymal stem cells for cutaneous wound healing. *Frontiers in immunology*, 3, 192, 2012/07/13.

[20] Friedenstein, A. J., Petrakova, K. V., Kurolesova, A. I., & Frolova, G. P. (1968). Heterotopic of bone marrow. Analysis of precursor cells for osteogenic and hematopoietic tissues. *Transplantation*, 6(2), 230-47, 1968/03/01.

[21] Phinney, D. G., & Prockop, D. J. (2007). Concise review: mesenchymal stem/multipotent stromal cells: the state of transdifferentiation and modes of tissue repair--current views. *Stem Cells*, 25(11), 2896-902, 2007/09/29.

[22] Caplan, A. I. (1991). Mesenchymal stem cells. *Journal of orthopaedic research : official publication of the Orthopaedic Research Society*, 9(5), 641-50, 1991/09/01.

[23] Pittenger, M. F. (1999). Multilineage Potential of Adult Human Mesenchymal Stem Cells. *Science*, 284(5411), 143-7.

[24] Dominici, M., Le Blanc, K., Mueller, I., Slaper-Cortenbach, I., Marini, F., Krause, D., et al. (2006). Minimal criteria for defining multipotent mesenchymal stromal cells. The International Society for Cellular Therapy position statement. *Cytotherapy*, 8(4), 315-7, 2006/08/23.

[25] Ahmadi, N., Razavi, S., Kazemi, M., & Oryan, S. (2012). Stability of neural differentiation in human adipose derived stem cells by two induction protocols. *Tissue & cell*, 44(2), 87-94, 2011/12/20.

[26] Chen, J., Liu, R., Yang, Y., Li, J., Zhang, X., Wang, Z., et al. (2011). The simulated microgravity enhances the differentiation of mesenchymal stem cells into neurons. *Neurosci Lett*, 505(2), 171-5, 2011/10/22.

[27] Du, Y., Roh, D. S., Funderburgh, M. L., Mann, M. M., Marra, K. G., Rubin, J. P., et al. (2010). Adipose-derived stem cells differentiate to keratocytes in vitro. *Molecular vision*, 16, 2680-9, 2010/12/24.

[28] Jin, G., Prabhakaran, M. P., & Ramakrishna, S. (2011). Stem cell differentiation to epidermal lineages on electrospun nanofibrous substrates for skin tissue engineering. *Acta Biomater*, 7(8), 3113-22, 2011/05/10.

[29] Al, Battah. F., De Kock, J., Vanhaecke, T., & Rogiers, V. (2011). Current status of human adipose-derived stem cells: differentiation into hepatocyte-like cells. *Scientific World Journal*, 11, 1568-81, 12/01/10.

[30] Ayatollahi, M., Soleimani, M., Tabei, S. Z., & Kabir, Salmani. M. (2011). Hepatogenic differentiation of mesenchymal stem cells induced by insulin like growth factor-I. *World journal of stem cells*, 3(12), 113-21, 2012/01/10.

[31] Bhandari, D. R., Seo, K. W., Sun, B., Seo, M. S., Kim, H. S., Seo, Y. J., et al. (2011). The simplest method for in vitro beta-cell production from human adult stem cells. *Differentiation; research in biological diversity*, 82(3), 144-52, 2011/07/26.

[32] Ankrum, J., & Karp, J. M. (2010). Mesenchymal stem cell therapy: Two steps forward, one step back. *Trends in molecular medicine*, 16(5), 203-9, 2010/03/26.

[33] Nauta, A. J., & Fibbe, W. E. (2007). Immunomodulatory properties of mesenchymal stromal cells. 2007/08/01. *Blood*, 110(10), 3499-506.

[34] Togel, F., Weiss, K., Yang, Y., Hu, Z., Zhang, P., & Westenfelder, C. (2007). Vasculotropic, paracrine actions of infused mesenchymal stem cells are important to the recovery from acute kidney injury. *American journal of physiology Renal physiology*, 292(5), F1626-35, 2007/01/11.

[35] Zhang, M., Mal, N., Kiedrowski, M., Chacko, M., Askari, A. T., Popovic, Z. B., et al. (2007). SDF-1 expression by mesenchymal stem cells results in trophic support of cardiac myocytes after myocardial infarction. *FASEB journal : official publication of the Federation of American Societies for Experimental Biology*, 21(12), 3197-207, 2007/05/15.

[36] Rao, M. S. (2006). Are there morally acceptable alternatives to blastocyst derived ESC? *J Cell Biochem*, 98(5), 1054-61, 2006/04/07.

[37] Vilalta, M., Degano, I. R., Bago, J., Gould, D., Santos, M., Garcia-Arranz, M., et al. (2008). Biodistribution, long-term survival, and safety of human adipose tissue-derived mesenchymal stem cells transplanted in nude mice by high sensitivity non-invasive bioluminescence imaging. *Stem Cells Dev*, 17(5), 993-1003, 2008/06/10.

[38] Si, Y. L., Zhao, Y. L., Hao, H. J., Fu, X. B., & Han, W. D. (2011). MSCs: Biological characteristics, clinical applications and their outstanding concerns. *Ageing research reviews*, 10(1), 93-103, 2010/08/24.

[39] Bongso, A., Fong-Y, C., & Gauthaman, K. Taking stem cells to the clinic: Major challenges. *Journal of Cellular Biochemistry*, 105(6), 1352-60.

[40] Baxter, MA, Wynn, R. F., Jowitt, S. N., Wraith, J. E., Fairbairn, L. J., & Bellantuono, I. (2004). Study of telomere length reveals rapid aging of human marrow stromal cells following in vitro expansion. *Stem Cells*, 22(5), 675-82, 2004/09/03.

[41] Mareschi, K., Ferrero, I., Rustichelli, D., Aschero, S., Gammaitoni, L., Aglietta, M., et al. (2006). Expansion of mesenchymal stem cells isolated from pediatric and adult donor bone marrow. *J Cell Biochem*, 97(4), 744-54, 2005/10/18.

[42] Stolzing, A., Jones, E., Mc Gonagle, D., & Scutt, A. (2008). Age-related changes in human bone marrow-derived mesenchymal stem cells: consequences for cell therapies. *Mechanisms of ageing and development*, 129(3), 163-73, 2008/02/05.

[43] Zhou, S., Greenberger, J. S., Epperly, M. W., Goff, J. P., Adler, C., Leboff, MS, et al. (2008). Age-related intrinsic changes in human bone-marrow-derived mesenchymal stem cells and their differentiation to osteoblasts. *Aging Cell*, 7(3), 335-43, 2008/02/06.

[44] Dexheimer, V., Mueller, S., Braatz, F., & Richter, W. (2011). Reduced reactivation from dormancy but maintained lineage choice of human mesenchymal stem cells with donor age. *PLoS One*, 6(8), e22980, 11/08/19.

[45] Gronthos, S., Zannettino, A. C., Hay, S. J., Shi, S., Graves, S. E., Kortesidis, A., et al. (2003). Molecular and cellular characterisation of highly purified stromal stem cells derived from human bone marrow. *Journal of cell science*, 116(Pt 9), 1827-35, 2003/04/01.

[46] Bi, Y., Stuelten, C. H., Kilts, T., Wadhwa, S., Iozzo, R. V., Robey, P. G., et al. (2005). Extracellular matrix proteoglycans control the fate of bone marrow stromal cells. *The Journal of biological chemistry*, 280(34), 30481-9, 2005/06/21.

[47] Kume, S., Kato, S., Yamagishi, S., Inagaki, Y., Ueda, S., Arima, N., et al. (2005). Advanced glycation end-products attenuate human mesenchymal stem cells and prevent cognate differentiation into adipose tissue, cartilage, and bone. *Journal of bone and mineral research : the official journal of the American Society for Bone and Mineral Research*, 20(9), 1647-58, 2005/08/02.

[48] Both, S. K., van der Muijsenberg, A. J., van Blitterswijk, C. A., de Boer, J., & de Bruijn, J. D. (2007). A rapid and efficient method for expansion of human mesenchymal stem cells. *Tissue Eng*, 13(1), 3-9, 2007/05/24.

[49] Colter, D. C. (2000). Rapid expansion of recycling stem cells in cultures of plastic-adherent cells from human bone marrow. *Proceedings of the National Academy of Sciences*, 97(7), 3213-8.

[50] Romanov, Y. A., Svintsitskaya, V. A., & Smirnov, V. N. (2003). Searching for alternative sources of postnatal human mesenchymal stem cells: candidate MSC-like cells from umbilical cord. *Stem Cells*, 21(1), 105-10, 2003/01/17.

[51] Zhang, X., Hirai, M., Cantero, S., Ciubotariu, R., Dobrila, L., Hirsh, A., et al. (2011). Isolation and characterization of mesenchymal stem cells from human umbilical cord blood: Reevaluation of critical factors for successful isolation and high ability to proliferate and differentiate to chondrocytes as compared to mesenchymal stem cells fro. *Journal of Cellular Biochemistry*, 112(4), 1206-18.

[52] Conconi, M. T., Di Liddo, R., Tommasini, M., Calore, C., & Parnigotto, P. P. (2011). Phenotype and Differentiation Potential of Stromal Populations Obtained from Various Zones of Human Umbilical Cord: An Overview. *Open Tissue Engineering & Regenerative Medicine Journal*, 4, 6-20.

[53] Fong, C. Y., Richards, M., Manasi, N., Biswas, A., & Bongso, A. (2007). Comparative growth behaviour and characterization of stem cells from human Wharton's jelly. *Reprod Biomed Online*, 15(6), 708-18, 2007/12/08.

[54] Wang, H. S., Hung, S. C., Peng, S., Huang, T. C. C., , C., Wei, H. M., Guo, Y. J., et al. (2004). Mesenchymal Stem Cells in the Wharton's Jelly of the Human Umbilical Cord. *Stem Cells*, 22(7), 1330-7.

[55] Gärtner, A., Pereira, T., Armada-da-Silva, P., Amorim, I., Gomes, R., Ribeiro, J., et al. Use of poly(DL-lactide-ε-caprolactone) membranes and Mesenchymal Stem Cells for promoting nerve regeneration in an axonotmesis rat model: in vitro and in vivo analysis. *Differentiation; research in biological diversity.Submitted.*

[56] Gärtner, A., Pereira, T., Simões, MJ, Armada da Silva, P., França, M. L., Sousa, R., et al. Use of hybrid chitosan membranes and human mesenchymal stem cells from the Wharton jelly of umbilical cord for promoting nerve regeneration in an axonotmesis rat model. *Neural Regeneration Research.In Press.*

[57] Amado, S., Simoes, MJ, Armada da Silva, P. A., Luis, A. L., Shirosaki, Y., Lopes, MA, et al. (2008). Use of hybrid chitosan membranes and N1E-115 cells for promoting nerve regeneration in an axonotmesis rat model. *Biomaterials*, 29(33), 4409-19, 2008/08/30.

[58] Luis, A. L., Rodrigues, J. M., Geuna, S., Amado, S., Shirosaki, Y., Lee, J. M., et al. (2008). Use of PLGA 90:10 scaffolds enriched with in vitro-differentiated neural cells for repairing rat sciatic nerve defects. *Tissue engineering Part A*, 14(6), 979-93, 2008/05/02.

[59] Luis, A. L., Rodrigues, J. M., Geuna, S., Amado, S., Simoes, MJ, Fregnan, F., et al. (2008). Neural cell transplantation effects on sciatic nerve regeneration after a standardized crush injury in the rat. *Microsurgery*, 28(6), 458-70, 2008/07/16.

[60] Fu, Y.-S, Shih, Y.-T, Cheng, Y.-C, & Min, M.-Y. (2004). Transformation of Human Umbilical Mesenchymal Cells into Neurons in vitro. *Journal of Biomedical Science*, 11(5), 652-60.

[61] Weiss, M. L., Medicetty, S., Bledsoe, A. R., Rachakatla, R. S., Choi, M., Merchav, S., et al. (2006). Human Umbilical Cord Matrix Stem Cells: Preliminary Characterization and Effect of Transplantation in a Rodent Model of Parkinson's Disease. *Stem Cells*, 24(3), 781-92.

[62] Conconi, M. T., Burra, P., Di Liddo, R., Calore, C., Turetta, M., Bellini, S., et al. (2006). CD105(+) cells from Wharton's jelly show in vitro and in vivo myogenic differentiative potential. *Int J Mol Med*, 18(6), 1089-96, 2006/11/08.

[63] Fu, Y. -S, Cheng, Y. -C, Lin, M. -Y, Cheng, A., Chu, H. -MP., Chou, S. -C, et al. (2006). Conversion of Human Umbilical Cord Mesenchymal Stem Cells in Wharton's Jelly to Dopaminergic Neurons In Vitro: Potential Therapeutic Application for Parkinsonism. *Stem Cells*, 24(1), 115-24.

[64] Jomura, S., Uy, M., Mitchell, K., Dallasen, R., Bode, C. J., & Xu, Y. (2007). Potential treatment of cerebral global ischemia with Oct-4+ umbilical cord matrix cells. *Stem Cells*, 25(1), 98-106, 2006/09/09.

[65] Levy, Y. S., Bahat-Stroomza, M., Barzilay, R., Burshtein, A., Bulvik, S., Barhum, Y., et al. (2008). Regenerative effect of neural-induced human mesenchymal stromal cells in rat models of Parkinson's disease. *Cytotherapy*, 10(4), 340-52, 2008/06/25.

[66] Gong, Z., Calkins, G., Cheng, E. C., Krause, D., & Niklason, L. E. (2009). Influence of culture medium on smooth muscle cell differentiation from human bone marrow-derived mesenchymal stem cells. *Tissue Eng Part A*, 15(2), 319-30, 2009/01/01.

[67] Kirouac, D. C., & Zandstra, P. W. (2008). The systematic production of cells for cell therapies. *Cell Stem Cell*, 3(4), 369-81, 08/10/23.

[68] Semenov, O. V., Koestenbauer, S., Riegel, M., Zech, N., Zimmermann, R., Zisch, A. H., et al. (2010). Multipotent mesenchymal stem cells from human placenta: critical parameters for isolation and maintenance of stemness after isolation. *American journal of obstetrics and gynecology*, e1-e13, 2009/12/29.

[69] Caplan, A. I. (2009). Why are MSCs therapeutic? New data: new insight. *The Journal of Pathology*, 217(2), 318-24.

[70] Barry, F. P., & Murphy, J. M. (2004). Mesenchymal stem cells: clinical applications and biological characterization. *Int J Biochem Cell Biol*, 36(4), 568-84, 2004/03/11.

[71] Joyce, N., Annett, G., Wirthlin, L., Olson, S., Bauer, G., & Nolta, J. A. (2010). Mesenchymal stem cells for the treatment of neurodegenerative disease. *Regen Med*, 5(6), 933-46, 2010/11/19.

[72] Dimmeler, S., Burchfield, J., & Zeiher, A. M. (2008). Cell-based therapy of myocardial infarction. *Arteriosclerosisthrombosis, and vascular biology*, 28(2), 208-16, 2007/10/24.

[73] Strioga, M., Viswanathan, S., Darinskas, A., Slaby, O., & Michalek, J. (2012). Same or Not the Same? Comparison of Adipose Tissue-Derived Versus Bone Marrow-Derived Mesenchymal Stem and Stromal Cells. *Stem Cells Dev*, 2012/04/04.

[74] Health USNIo. (2012). ClinicalTrials.gov. http://clinicaltrials.gov/, [3 August].

[75] Battiston, B., Geuna, S., Ferrero, M., & Tos, P. (2005). Nerve repair by means of tubulization: Literature review and personal clinical experience comparing biological and synthetic conduits for sensory nerve repair. *Microsurgery*, 25(4), 258-67.

[76] Mackinnon, S. E., Doolabh, V. B., Novak, C. B., & Trulock, E. P. (2001). Clinical outcome following nerve allograft transplantation. *Plast Reconstr Surg*, 107(6), 1419-29, 2001/05/04.

[77] Kehoe, S., Zhang, X. F., & Boyd, D. (2012). FDA approved guidance conduits and wraps for peripheral nerve injury: a review of materials and efficacy. *Injury*, 43(5), 553-72, 2011/01/29.

[78] Siemionow, M., Bozkurt, M., & Zor, F. (2010). Regeneration and repair of peripheral nerves with different biomaterials: Review. *Microsurgery*, 30(7), 574-88.

[79] Mackinnon, S. E., Hudson, A. R., & Hunter, D. A. (1985). Histologic assessment of nerve regeneration in the rat. *Plast Reconstr Surg*, 75(3), 384-8, 1985/03/01.

[80] Ronchi, G., Nicolino, S., Raimondo, S., Tos, P., Battiston, B., Papalia, I., et al. (2009). Functional and morphological assessment of a standardized crush injury of the rat median nerve. *Journal of Neuroscience Methods*, 179(1), 51-7.

[81] de Ruiter, G. C., Malessy, M. J., Yaszemski, M. J., Windebank, A. J., & Spinner, R. J. (2009). Designing ideal conduits for peripheral nerve repair. *Neurosurg Focus*, 26(2), E5, 2009/05/14.

[82] Maurício, A. C., Gärtner, A., Armada-da-Silva, P., Amado, S., Pereira, T., Veloso, A. P., et al. (2011). Cellular Systems and Biomaterials for Nerve Regeneration in Neurotmesis Injuries. *Pignatello R, editor. Biomaterials Applications for Nanomedicine*, 978-9-53307-661-4, Available from: InTech.

[83] Wang, Y., Zhao, Z., Ren, Z., Zhao, B., Zhang, L., Chen, J., et al. (2012). Recellularized nerve allografts with differentiated mesenchymal stem cells promote peripheral nerve regeneration. *Neurosci Lett*, 514(1), 96-101, 2012/03/13.

[84] Madduri, S., & Gander, B. (2010). Schwann cell delivery of neurotrophic factors for peripheral nerve regeneration. *J Peripher Nerv Syst*, 15(2), 93-103, 2010/07/16.

[85] Hall, S. (2001). Nerve repair: a neurobiologist's view. *Journal of hand surgery (Edinburgh, Scotland)*, 26(2), 129-36, 2001/04/03.

[86] Torigoe, K., Tanaka, H. F., Takahashi, A., Awaya, A., & Hashimoto, K. (1996). Basic behavior of migratory Schwann cells in peripheral nerve regeneration. *Exp Neurol*, 137(2), 301-8, 1996/02/01.

[87] Schlosshauer, B., Muller, E., Schroder, B., Planck, H., & Muller, H. W. (2003). Rat Schwann cells in bioresorbable nerve guides to promote and accelerate axonal regeneration. *Brain Res*, 963(1-2), 321-6, 2003/02/01.

[88] Keilhoff, G., Goihl, A., Langnase, K., Fansa, H., & Wolf, G. (2006). Transdifferentiation of mesenchymal stem cells into Schwann cell-like myelinating cells. *European Journal of Cell Biology*, 85(1), 11-24.

[89] Matsuse, D., Kitada, M., Kohama, M., Nishikawa, K., Makinoshima, H., Wakao, S., et al. (2010). Human umbilical cord-derived mesenchymal stromal cells differentiate into functional Schwann cells that sustain peripheral nerve regeneration. *J Neuropathol Exp Neurol*, 69(9), 973-85, 2010/08/20.

[90] Luis, A. L., Rodrigues, J. M., Amado, S., Veloso, A. P., Armada-Da-Silva, P. A., Rai-mondo, S., et al. (2007). PLGA 90/10 and caprolactone biodegradable nerve guides for the reconstruction of the rat sciatic nerve. *Microsurgery*, 27(2), 125-37, 2007/02/10.

[91] Simoes, MJ, Amado, S., Gartner, A., Armada-Da-Silva, P. A., Raimondo, S., Vieira, M., et al. (2010). Use of chitosan scaffolds for repairing rat sciatic nerve defects. *Ital J Anat Embryol*, 115(3), 190-210, 2011/02/04.

[92] Luis, A. L., Amado, S., Geuna, S., Rodrigues, J. M., Simoes, MJ, Santos, JD, et al. (2007). Long-term functional and morphological assessment of a standardized rat sci-atic nerve crush injury with a non-serrated clamp. *J Neurosci Methods*, 163(1), 92-104, 2007/04/03.

[93] Amado, S., Rodrigues, J. M., Luis, A. L., Armada-da-Silva, P. A., Vieira, M., Gartner, A., et al. (2010). Effects of collagen membranes enriched with in vitro-differentiated N1E-115 cells on rat sciatic nerve regeneration after end-to-end repair. *J Neuroeng Re-habil*, 7, 7, 2010/02/13.

[94] Luís, A. L., Amado, S., Geuna, S., Rodrigues, J. M., Simões, MJ, Santos, JD, et al. (2007). Long-term functional and morphological assessment of a standardized rat sci-atic nerve crush injury with a non-serrated clamp. *Journal of Neuroscience Methods*, 163(1), 92-104.

[95] Luis, A. L., Rodrigues, J. M., Lobato, J. V., Lopes, MA, Amado, S., Veloso, A. P., et al. (2007). Evaluation of two biodegradable nerve guides for the reconstruction of the rat sciatic nerve. *Biomed Mater Eng*, 17(1), 39-52, 2007/02/01.

[96] Frattini, F., Pereira, Lopes. F. R., Almeida, F. M., Rodrigues, R. F., Boldrini, L. C., Tomaz, M., et al. (2012). Mesenchymal stem cells in a polycaprolactone conduit pro-mote sciatic nerve regeneration and sensory neuron survival after nerve injury. *Tis-sue Eng Part A*, 2012/06/01.

[97] Spivey, E. C., Khaing, Z. Z., Shear, J. B., & Schmidt, C. E. (2012). The fundamental role of subcellular topography in peripheral nerve repair therapies. *Biomaterials*, 33(17), 4264-76, 2012/03/20.

[98] Dellon, A. L., & Mackinnon, S. E. (1989). Selection of the appropriate parameter to measure neural regeneration. *Ann Plast Surg*, 23(3), 197-202, 1989/09/01.

[99] Kanaya, F., Firrell, J. C., & Breidenbach, W. C. (1996). Sciatic function index, nerve conduction tests, muscle contraction, and axon morphometry as indicators of regen-eration. *Plast Reconstr Surg*, 98(7), 1264-71, discussion 72-4., 1996/12/01.

[100] Shen, N., & Zhu, J. (1995). Application of sciatic functional index in nerve functional assessment. *Microsurgery*, 16(8), 552-5, 1995/01/01.

[101] Almquist, E., & Eeg-Olofsson, O. (1970). Sensory-nerve-conduction velocity and two-point discrimmination in sutured nerves. *J Bone Joint Surg Am*, 52(4), 791-6, 1970/06/01.

[102] de Medinaceli, L., Freed, W. J., & Wyatt, R. J. (1982). An index of the functional condition of rat sciatic nerve based on measurements made from walking tracks. *Exp Neurol, 77*(3), 634-43, 82/09/01.

[103] Varejao, AS, Cabrita, A. M., Meek, M. F., Bulas-Cruz, J., Melo-Pinto, P., Raimondo, S., et al. (2004). Functional and morphological assessment of a standardized rat sciatic nerve crush injury with a non-serrated clamp. *Journal of neurotrauma, 21*(11), 1652-70, 2005/02/03.

[104] Varejao, AS, Cabrita, A. M., Meek, M. F., Bulas-Cruz, J., Filipe, V. M., Gabriel, R. C., et al. (2003). Ankle kinematics to evaluate functional recovery in crushed rat sciatic nerve. *Muscle Nerve, 27*(6), 706-14, 2003/05/27.

[105] Varejao, AS, Cabrita, A. M., Meek, M. F., Fornaro, M., Geuna, S., & Giacobini-Robecchi, M. G. (2003). Morphology of nerve fiber regeneration along a biodegradable poly (DLLA-epsilon-CL) nerve guide filled with fresh skeletal muscle. *Microsurgery, 23*(4), 338-45, 2003/08/28.

[106] Koka, R., & Hadlock, T. A. (2001). Quantification of Functional Recovery Following Rat Sciatic Nerve Transection. *Experimental Neurology, 168*(1), 192-5.

[107] Masters, D. B., Berde, C. B., Dutta, S. K., Griggs, C. T., Hu, D., Kupsky, W., et al. (1993). Prolonged regional nerve blockade by controlled release of local anesthetic from a biodegradable polymer matrix. *Anesthesiology, 79*(2), 340-6, 1993/08/01.

[108] Bain, J. R., Mackinnon, S. E., & Hunter, D. A. (1989). Functional evaluation of complete sciatic, peroneal, and posterior tibial nerve lesions in the rat. *Plast Reconstr Surg, 83*(1), 129-38, 1989/01/01.

[109] Dijkstra, J. R., Meek, M. F., Robinson, P. H., & Gramsbergen, A. (2000). Methods to evaluate functional nerve recovery in adult rats: walking track analysis, video analysis and the withdrawal reflex. *J Neurosci Methods, 96*(2), 89-96, 2000/03/18.

[110] Cappozzo, A., Della Croce, U., Leardini, A., & Chiari, L. (2005). Human movement analysis using stereophotogrammetry. Part 1: theoretical background. *Gait & posture, 21*(2), 186-96, 2005/01/11.

[111] Goulermas, J. Y., Findlow, A. H., Nester, C. J., Howard, D., & Bowker, P. (2005). Automated design of robust discriminant analysis classifier for foot pressure lesions using kinematic data. *IEEE transactions on bio-medical engineering, 52*(9), 1549-62, 2005/09/30.

[112] Johnson, A., Aibinder, W., & Deland, J. T. (2008). Clinical tip: partial plantar plate release for correction of crossover second toe. *Foot & ankle international / American Orthopaedic Foot and Ankle Society [and] Swiss Foot and Ankle Society, 29*(11), 1145-7, 2008/11/26.

[113] Varejao, AS, Cabrita, A. M., Meek, M. F., Bulas-Cruz, J., Gabriel, R. C., Filipe, V. M., et al. (2002). Motion of the foot and ankle during the stance phase in rats. *Muscle Nerve, 26*(5), 630-5, 2002/10/29.

[114] Raimondo, S., Fornaro, M., Di Scipio, F., Ronchi, G., Giacobini-Robecchi, M. G., & Geuna, S. (2009). Chapter 5: Methods and protocols in peripheral nerve regeneration experimental research: part II-morphological techniques. *Int Rev Neurobiol*, 87, 81-103, 2009/08/18.

[115] Geuna, S., Gigo-Benato, D., & Rodrigues, Ade. C. (2004). On sampling and sampling errors in histomorphometry of peripheral nerve fibers. *Microsurgery*, 24(1), 72-6, 2004/01/30.

[116] Geuna, S., Tos, P., Battiston, B., & Guglielmone, R. (2000). Verification of the two-dimensional disector, a method for the unbiased estimation of density and number of myelinated nerve fibers in peripheral nerves. *Ann Anat*, 182(1), 23-34, 2000/02/11.

[117] Vander Heiden, M. G., Cantley, L. C., & Thompson, C. B. (2009). Understanding the Warburg effect: the metabolic requirements of cell proliferation. *Science*, 324(5930), 1029-33, 2009/05/23.

[118] Fehrer, C., Brunauer, R., Laschober, G., Unterluggauer, H., Reitinger, S., Kloss, F., et al. (2007). Reduced oxygen tension attenuates differentiation capacity of human mesenchymal stem cells and prolongs their lifespan. *Aging Cell*, 6(6), 745-57, 2007/10/11.

[119] Brushart, T. M., Hoffman, P. N., Royall, R. M., Murinson, B. B., Witzel, C., & Gordon, T. (2002). Electrical stimulation promotes motoneuron regeneration without increasing its speed or conditioning the neuron. *J Neurosci*, 22(15), 6631-8, 2002/08/02.

[120] Geuna, S., Raimondo, S., Ronchi, G., Di Scipio, F., Tos, P., Czaja, K., et al. (2009). Chapter 3: Histology of the peripheral nerve and changes occurring during nerve regeneration. Int Rev Neurobiol 2009/08/18., 87, 27-46.

Special Applications of Biomaterials

Chapter 9

Dental Materials

Junko Hieda, Mitsuo Niinomi, Masaaki Nakai and Ken Cho

Additional information is available at the end of the chapter

1. Introduction

Metallic biomaterials used for dental applications, which are called dental alloys, and such alloys require a high corrosion resistance because the pH and temperature vary widely in the oral environment where foods and beverages are taken in. These alloys also require biocompatibility in order to prevent an allergic reaction to the metals. Dental alloys are mainly used to make devices for filling cavities and as substitutes for teeth that are lost because of decay and periodontal disease. A variety of dental devices have been developed, which include metallic fillers, inlays, crowns, bridges, clasps, dentures, dental implants composed of a fixture and an abutment, and fixed braces (train tracks). These forms of dental restoration, custom-shaped for an individual, are made by casting; therefore, the castability of alloys is another requirement for dental applications.

Dental alloys are mainly classified into two groups: precious and nonprecious metals. Suitable alloys are employed according to the intended use. Alloys of precious metals such as gold (Au), palladium (Pd), and silver (Ag) are usually employed because of their high corrosion resistance, biocompatibility, and castability, as compared to those of nonprecious metals. Precious alloys are grouped into high-carat alloy (high-precious or -nobility alloy) and low-carat alloy (low-precious or –nobility alloy). The high-carat alloy contains more than 75 % precious metals. Non-precious metal alloys such as stainless steels, cobalt-chromium, nickel-chromium, and titanium alloys are also commonly used.

Among the dental alloys, precious alloys are widely used. Au alloys have been commonly used in dental applications from past to the present, and many commercial variations of alloy compositions have been developed, despite their high cost. American Dental Association classifies these Au alloys on the basis of their mechanical properties. Many studies have been carried out to improve the mechanical properties of the Au alloys containing copper (Cu) (Au–Cu–Pd [1, 2], Au–Ag–Pd–In [3], Au–Cu–Zn [4], Au–Cu–Zn–Ag [5], and Au–Ag–Cu–Pd [6] alloys), with the main focus on the microstructural changes produced by heat treatment. However, recent trends have shown that low-carat dental alloys (Ag and Pd alloys) are attracting much attention as alternatives to Au alloys because of their lower price. Thus, Ag alloys such as Ag–Pd–Cu–Au [7-17], and Ag–Cu–Pd–Au [18, 19] alloys have been developed for commercial applications. The hardness of these alloys increases with aging or solution treatment, and many studies have reported on the behaviors of these alloys in response to various heat treatments and the various mechanisms. Dental casting of Ag–20Pd–14.5Cu-12Au alloy (mass%) has been developed and used widely in Japan. In general, this alloy is subjected to aging treatment (AT) at around 673 K after solution treatment (ST) at 1023 K in order to enhance its mechanical strength. Recently, it has been reported that the mechanical strength of Ag–20Pd–14.5Cu–12Au alloy is significantly enhanced when the alloy is subjected to ST at temperatures higher than 1073 K and subsequently water quenched without any AT [9-16]. The Vickers hardness of this alloy increases with an increase in the cooling rate after ST [11]. This unique hardening behavior and the increase in mechanical strength induced by the high-temperature ST have been explained in terms of the precipitation hardening caused by the precipitation of an $L1_0$-type ordered β' phase.

This chapter describes with focusing on the relationship between the unique hardening behavior exhibited by the as-solutionized dental Ag–Pd–Cu–Au alloys and the corresponding microstructural changes. Other mechanical properties (fatigue, fretting-fatigue, and friction wear properties) and corrosion properties are also described.

2. Age hardening behavior of Ag–Pd–Cu–Au alloys

Ag-Pd alloys have complete miscibility in all composition ratios. Addition of Cu leads to age hardening in these alloys. In the early researches during 1960–70s, mechanisms for age hardening of Ag-Pd-Cu alloys were proposed [20-22]. According to them, the age hardening was caused by the formation of a CuPd ordered phase ($L2_0$-type) [20], precipitation of a Cu-rich α_1 phase [21], and phase separation of α solid solution to a CuPd ordered phase ($L2_0$-type) and Ag-rich α_2 phase [22]. More recently, Au has been added to Ag-Pd-Cu alloys to increase their corrosion resistance. Therefore, since 1980 to the present, many studies have focused on the age-hardening mechanism of the Ag-Pd-Cu-Au alloys (Table 1) [8, 19, 23, 24]. Ohta et al. [23] reported that the precipitation of a $L1_0$-type face-centered tetragonal CuPd ordered platelet (β') inside the grains and discontinuous precipitation of the Ag-rich α_2 phase and CuPd ordered phase (β) in the grain boundary regions enhance the hardening of Ag-Pd-Cu-Au alloys with a low Au content (Au = 10 mass%). According to their report, TEM images of the precipitates (β and α_2) along the grain boundaries in the alloys show strain contrast and moiré fringes, which indicates that β and α_2 phases are coherent with each other. Solution hardening behavior was also found in alloys subjected to ST at 1223 K followed by slow quenching (SQ) before aging. Researches since 2000 have focused on the age hardening behavior of the Ag-Pd-Cu-Au alloys as a function of the treatment duration [8, 19]. It was found that during the early stage of the aging, diffusion and aggregation of Cu atoms from the Ag-rich α phase occur, and in the later stage, the hardness of the alloy decreases because of the coarsening of the Cu-rich lamellar precipitates [8, 19]. At a Cu concentration of 20 mass%, the CuPd ordered phase (β) does not exhibit any change after aging and thus does not contribute to the age hardening [19].

The age-hardening mechanism of Ag-Pd-Cu-Au alloys with an Au content of 20 mass% was also investigated, and it was concluded that β' and the discontinuous Ag-rich α_2 phase contribute to the age hardening of these alloys [24]. Fig.1 shows the hardness (Hv) of the precipitates measured independently inside the grains (inter grain) and along the grain boundaries (nodule) [24]. These curves indicate that there are two hardening stages of the alloys in terms of aging temperature: the formation of β' phase in the grain interior at low aging temperatures and the precipitation of the Ag-rich α_2 phase along the grain boundaries at high aging temperatures. It was also found that the Cu concentration influences the formation of β' phase in these alloys (Fig. 2) [24]. The hardness (H_v) of each alloy increases with an increase of the Cu concentration, i.e. the volume fraction of β' phase, at any temperatures.

Compositions of Ag-Pd-Cu-Au alloys (mass%)	References
Ag-20.9Pd-8.5Cu-12.5Au-2.5Zn-0.5Sn-0.1Ir	[8]
Ag-20Pd-20Cu-12Au-2(Zn, Ir, and In)	[19]
Ag-25.4Pd-21.8Cu-10Au	[23]
Ag-25.20Pd-9.88Cu-20Au, Ag-30.32Pd-9.66Cu-5.04Au, Ag-25.4Pd-12.82Cu-9.96Au, Ag-28Pd-9.12Cu-12.04Au	[24]

Table 1. Compositions of Ag-Pd-Cu-Au alloys (mass%).

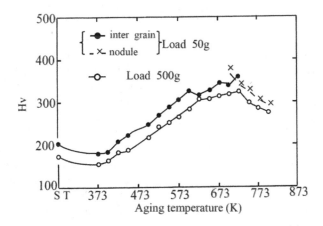

Figure 1. Anisothermal age hardening curve of Ag-25.2Pd-9.88Cu-20Au alloy.

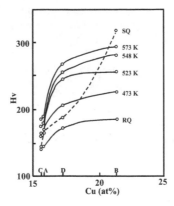

Figure 2. Effect of Cu concentration (at%) on hardness (Hv) of Ag-30.32Pd-9.66Cu-5.04Au (A), Ag-25.4Pd-12.82Cu-9.96Au (B), Ag-28Pd-9.12Cu-12.04Au (C), and Ag-25.2Pd-9.88Cu-20Au (D) alloys. SQ and RQ indicate specimens subjected to slow quenching and rapid quenching after ST, respectively.

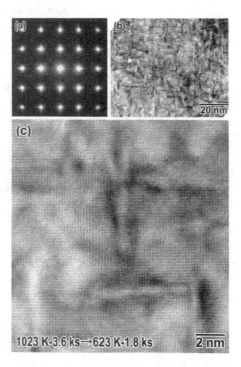

Figure 3. (a) Diffraction pattern, (b) TEM image, and (c) HRTEM image of Ag-Pd-Cu-Au alloy subjected to ST at 1023 K for 3.6 ks followed by aging treatment at 623 K for 1.8 ks.

Figure 3 shows a diffraction pattern, a transmission electron microscopy (TEM) image, and a high resolution TEM (HRTEM) image of β′ phase formed in the Ag–20Pd–14.5Cu–12Au alloy subjected to ST at 1023 K for 3.6 ks followed by AT at 623 K for 1.8 ks [25]. β′ phase is platelet shape with the size of about 10 nm long, which precipitates parallel to {200} crystal plane of matrix. A lattice constant of a-axis matches with that of the matrix, which exhibits coherent with the matrix [25].

3. Mechanical properties of Ag–20Pd–14.5Cu–12Au alloy

3.1. Unique hardening behavior

3.1.1. Precipitation of β′ phase after high temperature solution treatment

Commercial Ag–20Pd–14.5Cu–12Au dental alloy (as-received) is fabricated by a rolling process. The commercial Ag–20Pd–14.5Cu–12Au alloy has a multiphase microstructure (α_1, α_2, β). It is well known that the Ag–Pd–Cu–Au alloy exhibits age hardening behavior as described in the section 2, but the drastic increase in the hardness of Ag–20Pd–14.5Cu–12Au alloy through ST at temperatures over 1073 K subjected to water quenching has been newly reported [10]. This unique hardening behavior has been explained in terms of two hardening mechanisms: (1) solid solution hardening mechanism in which the alloying elements are dissolved into the matrix (α phase) during ST, and (2) precipitation hardening mechanism, in which $L1_0$-type ordered phases are precipitated during the quenching process after ST. Recent studies on the hardening mechanism of Ag–20Pd–14.5Cu–12Au alloy have revealed that the precipitation hardening mechanism is the probable mechanism for the unique hardening behavior exhibited [11, 26].

Conventionally, dentists have employed AT for the hardening of Ag–20Pd–14.5Cu–12Au alloy as mentioned above. Figure 4 [10] shows the effects of heat treatment (AT and ST) temperatures on the mechanical properties (tensile strength, elongation, and hardness (H_{RA})) of this alloy. The tensile strength and hardness increase until the temperature reaches 673 K, and then decrease for up to 923 K due to the removal of strain from the alloy. At temperatures higher than 923 K, this alloy exhibits a unique hardening behavior. Under AT, the tensile strength and hardness of this alloy drastically increase and the elongation decreases after treatment at 673 K. On the other hand, under ST, the tensile strength and hardness still increase but the elongation does not decrease after treatment at 1073 K. Since high temperature ST is very useful for the hardening of this alloy, this treatment will be widely adopted in the future.

The relationship between the microstructural changes in the $L1_0$-type ordered β′ phase and the hardening behavior in the solutionized alloys was investigated by changing the cooling rate. Figure 5 shows a schematic drawing of various cooling rates employed after ST [11]. The Vickers hardness of the as-received alloy and of the alloys subjected to ST followed by water quenching (WQ), air cooling (AC), and cooling in a furnace (FC) are shown in Fig. 6 [11]. ST subjected to WQ and AC leads to a significant and slight increase in the hardness of the alloy,

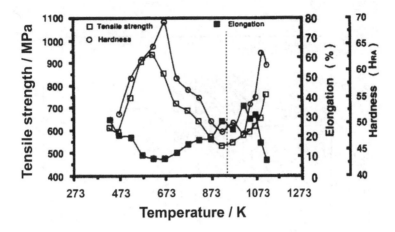

Figure 4. Effect of heat treatment temperature on mechanical properties of Ag–20Pd–14.5Cu–12Au alloy.

respectively, while ST subjected to FC decreases the hardness of the alloy. Thus, the hardness tends to decrease with a decrease in the cooling rate after ST.

Figures 7 and 8 show the microstructures of the as-received and solutionized alloy, respectively, as measured by backscattered electron (BSE) and energy dispersive X-ray spectroscopy (EDX) analysis [13]. The as-received alloy composed of a Cu-rich α_1 phase, an Ag-rich α_2 phase, and Cu–Pd intermetallic β phase, while the solutionized alloy composed of α_2 and β phases. After ST, the α_1 phase dissolved into the Ag-rich α_2 phase and the β phase remained in the matrix. The β' phase precipitated in the matrix could not be observed by BSE, but could be observed by TEM.

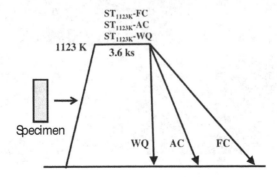

Figure 5. Schematic drawing of heat treatments with various cooling rates after ST. ST_{1123K}-WQ, ST_{1123K}-AC, and ST_{1123K}-FC indicate specimens subjected to ST at 1123 K followed by water, air, and furnace cooling, respectively.

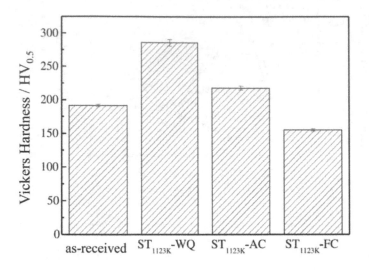

Figure 6. Vickers hardness of as-received, ST$_{1123K}$-WQ, ST$_{1123K}$-AC, and ST$_{1123K}$-FC.

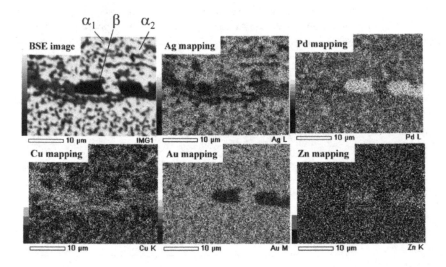

Figure 7. BSE image and elemental mappings obtained by EDX of as-received Ag–20Pd–14.5Cu–12Au alloy.

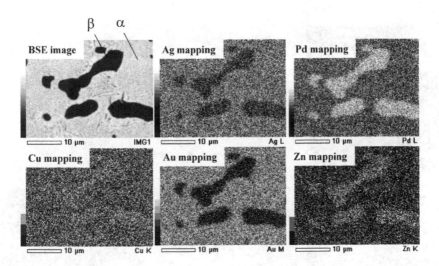

Figure 8. BSE image and elemental mappings obtained by EDX of Ag–20Pd–14.5Cu–12Au alloy subjected to ST at 1123 K for 3.6 ks.

The selected area diffraction patterns (SADP) and key diagrams obtained from TEM for the alloy subjected to ST and WQ, given in Fig. 9, show that three variants of the $L1_0$-type ordered β' phase are present when the beam direction is parallel to [100] crystal direction: one variant (P) has a c-axis parallel to the electron beam; the other two variants (N_1, N_2) have c-axes normal to the electron beam [11]. The SADPs indicate that an $L1_0$-type ordered β' phase is densely precipitated in the matrix. The dark field images using a $(001)N_1$ and $(001)N_2$ reflections (Fig. 9 (d) and (e)) show that the β' phase is 2–6 nm wide and 20–60 nm long. In the alloy subjected to ST and AC, the β' phase is 3–13 nm wide and 50–400 nm long, and in the alloy subjected to ST and FC the β' phase is 3–25 nm wide and 70–700 nm long, as confirmed by the dark field images using a $(001)N_1$ reflection. In the alloys subjected to ST followed by AC and FC, the β' phase is less densely precipitated than the alloy subjected to ST and WQ. These dark field images indicate that the size and number of the β' phase vary with the cooling rates after ST. In the solutionized alloy subjected to WQ, the size of the β' phase is small and the amount of the β' phase is large. The size of the β' phase decreased and the amount of the β' phase increased with an increase in the cooling rate after ST. The driving force behind the nucleation of the β' phase in the solutionized alloy subjected to WQ is stronger than that in the solution-ized alloy subjected to AC and FC, because the degree of undercooling in the solutionized alloy subjected to WQ is larger than that in the solutionized alloy subjected to AC and FC. The extent of nucleation of the β' phase in the solutionized alloy subjected to WQ is larger than that in the solutionized alloy subjected to AC and FC. The β' phase in the solutionized alloys subjected to AC and FC grew more coarsely than that in the solutionized alloy subjected to WQ, because the diffusion occurred more easily owing to the slow cooling process in the solutionized alloys subjected to AC and FC. Therefore, it is likely that the β' phase is formed during the cooling process and grows by diffusion.

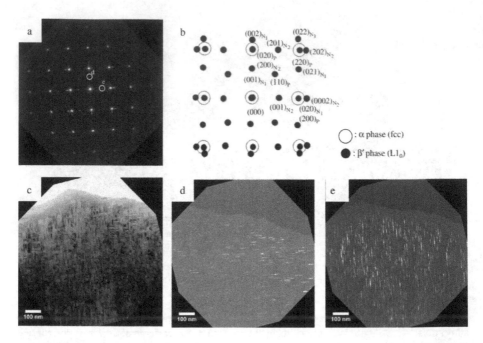

Figure 9. TEM micrographs of ST$_{1123K}$-WQ: (a) a selected area diffraction pattern, (b) a key diagram, (c) a bright-field image, and (d) and (e) dark-field images using (001)N$_1$ and (001)N$_2$ reflections, respectively. The beam direction is parallel to [100] crystal direction.

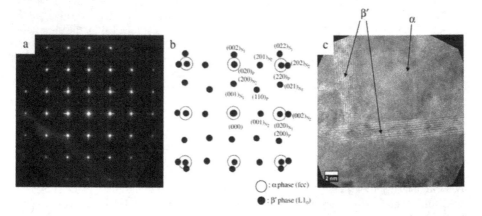

Figure 10. HRTEM micrographs of ST$_{1123K}$-WQ: (a) a selected area diffraction pattern, (b) a key diagram, and (c) a bright-field image. The beam direction is parallel to [100].

Figure 10 shows the SADP, key diagram, and HRTEM bright field image of ST_{1123K}-WQ [11]. The SADP and the key diagram in Fig. 10 (a) and (b) indicate that the FCC α phase and the three variants of the $L1_0$-type ordered β' phase are superimposed. The $L1_0$-type ordered β' phase is precipitated in the FCC matrix after ST. The streaks on the reflection spots of the $L1_0$-type ordered β' phase indicate that the shape of the β' phase is similar to a thin plate. The HRTEM bright field image in Fig. 10 (c) shows that several nanometer-sized thick plate-shaped β' phase with two variants (N_1, N_2), whose c-axes are normal to the electron beam, are precipitated in the matrix.

It is well known that it is difficult to make a single phase by quenching after high temperature ST; the supersaturated vacancies help the solutes to diffuse more easily and also help to form more clusters, G–P zones, and metastable phases during quenching after high temperature ST. The precipitated β' phase of ST_{1123K}-WQ shown in Fig.9 (d), (e) and Fig. 10 (c) is like a thin plate with a nanometer-scale thickness. These images also suggest that the formation of the β' phase is diffusion controlled. Generally, the formation of precipitates can be considered to be order–disorder transition, diffusionless transformation (martensitic transformation), or diffusional transformation. In the as-solutionized Ag–Pd–Cu–Au alloy used in this case, the dependence of microstructural changes in the precipitated β' phase on both the cooling rate after ST and the ST temperature show that the precipitated $L1_0$-type ordered β' phase is formed during the cooling process and that the growth of the β' phase is influenced by the diffusion process. The hardness increases with an increase in the cooling rate after ST, and consequently, the hardness of ST_{1123K}-WQ increases significantly by quenching after ST (Fig. 6). The fine β' phase in ST_{1123K}-WQ is densely precipitated in the matrix. The hardness of ST_{1123K}-AC increased only slightly, while the hardness of ST_{1123K}-FC decreases, as only coarse β' phases are precipitated in the matrix of ST_{1123K}-AC and ST_{1123K}-FC. Thus, the increase in hardness may be strongly affected by the presence of finely precipitated β' phase. The coherent precipitation of β' phases with long and short axes of around 100 nm and 10 nm, respectively, also occured during ST, although the amount of β' phase decreases with an increase in the ST time. The effect of solid solution hardening in the α, α_1, and α_2 phases is lower than that exerted by the precipitation hardening due to β' phases.

3.1.2. Hardening behavior of Ag–20Pd–12Au–14.5Cu alloy fabricated by liquid rapid solidification

An Ag–20Pd–14.5Cu–12Au alloy with a single α phase can be fabricated using a liquid rapid solidification (LRS) method that employs a melting mechanism, as shown schematically in Fig. 11 [12]. The critical temperature for the order–disorder transformation in the Cu–Pd binary phase diagram is below 1023 K, and hence, at 1023 K, the Cu-rich phase α_1 and Ag-rich phase α_2 decompose, as shown in the Ag–Cu binary phase diagram. Figure 12 shows TEM micrographs of an Ag–20Pd–14.5Cu–12Au alloy fabricated by the LRS method [13]. No precipitation is observed in the matrix.

As shown in Fig. 12 (b) and (c), the LRS alloy consists of a single α phase with face centered cubic structure (FCC). The tensile properties of the as-received Ag–20Pd–14.5Cu–12Au alloy (AS), AS subjected to ST at 1123 K for 3.6 ks in vacuum ($ST_{AS/3.6\,ks}$), LRS alloy (LRS), and LRS alloy subjected to ST at 1123 K for 3.6 ks in vacuum ($ST_{LRS/3.6\,ks}$) are shown in Fig. 13 [13]. The

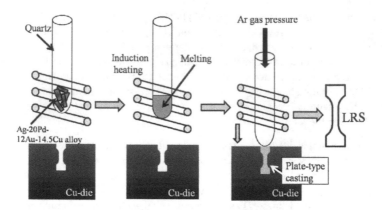

Figure 11. Schematic drawing of LRS method.

tensile strength and 0.2% proof stress of the AS alloy drastically increased after ST. The elongation of AS subjected to ST is smaller than that of the AS alloy. On the other hand, the tensile strength and 0.2% proof stress of the LRS alloy decrease after ST. The reduction in strain and the coarsening of the α phase during ST result in the decrease in the tensile strength and 0.2% proof stress and the increase in elongation. The tensile strength of the LRS alloy and solutionized LRS are relatively smaller than those of the AS alloy and the AS alloy subjected to the ST.

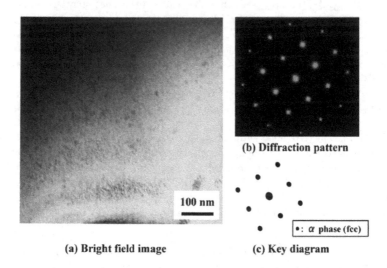

Figure 12. TEM micrographs of alloy fabricated by LRS: (a) bright field image, (b) diffraction pattern and (c) key diagram. Beam direction is parallel to [100].

Figure 14 shows the XRD profiles of the LRS alloy solutionized at 1173 K for 3.6 ks (1173WQ$_{LRS}$/3.6 ks) and the LRS alloy subjected to AT at 673 K for 1.8–28.8 ks following the ST (673WQ$_{LRS}$/1.8 ks-28.8 ks) [12]. A single α phase is identified in the solutionized LRS alloy, whereas, in the LRS alloy subjected to AT after the ST, α_2 and β phases are observed. The Vickers hardness of the solutionized LRS alloy and the LRS alloy subjected to AT are shown in Fig. 15. The hardness of the LRS alloy subjected to AT increases greatly as compared to that of the solutionized LRS alloy with a single α phase owing to the precipitation of β phase.

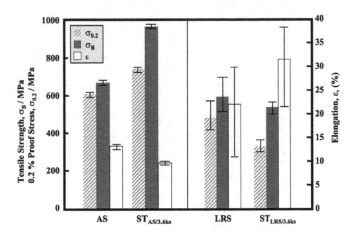

Figure 13. Tensile properties of AS, ST$_{AS/3.6ks}$, LRS, and ST$_{LRS/3.6ks}$.

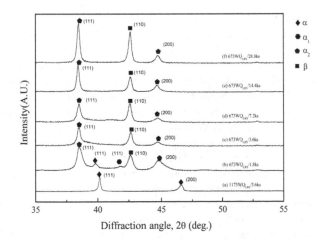

Figure 14. XRD profiles of (a) 1173WQ$_{LRS}$/3.6 ks, (b) 673WQ$_{LRS}$/1.8 ks, (c) 673WQ$_{LRS}$/3.6 ks, (d) 673WQ$_{LRS}$/7.2 ks, (e) 673WQ$_{LRS}$/14.4 ks, and (f) 673WQ$_{LRS}$/28.8 ks.

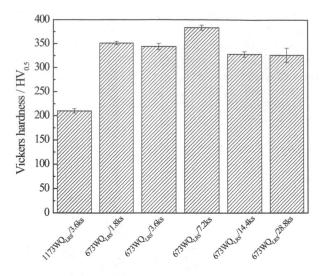

Figure 15. Vickers hardness of 1173WQ$_{LRS}$/3.6 ks, 673WQ$_{LRS}$/1.8 ks, 673WQ$_{LRS}$/3.6 ks, 673WQ$_{LRS}$/7.2 ks, 673WQ$_{LRS}$/14.4 ks, and 673WQ$_{LRS}$/28.8 ks.

3.2. Fatigue properties

Dental prosthetic products produced by dental casting method are subjected to cyclic stress, i.e., fatigue, because of mastication. Dental castings contain a number of casting defects such as microshrinkages, pores, and surface roughness. The effects of these casting defects on the fatigue properties of cast Ag–20Pd–14.5Cu–12Au alloy were investigated in comparison with the fatigue properties of a drawn Ag–20Pd–14.5Cu–12Au alloy. The tensile properties of the cast specimens and drawn specimens are shown in Fig. 16 [14]. The cast specimens were prepared using a lost wax method. The drawn alloy bars were solutionized at 1073K for 3.6 ks in vacuum and then cooled in air (D-1073AC (drawn)). The heat treatment produced a microstructure with a matrix similar to that in an as-cast alloy. For the mechanical testing, the following specimen dimension were used: gauge diameter 3 mm and gauge length 20 mm for cast specimens, gauge diameter 2 mm and gauge length 20 mm for drawn specimens. The surfaces of the cast specimens for tensile tests were sand blasted (non-polished). The tensile strength and 0.2% proof stress of the cast specimens were higher than those of the drawn specimens. The distribution of the elongation of the cast specimens was larger than that of the elongation of the drawn specimens. The amount of intermetallic β phase that leads to the high strength and low ductility is greater in the cast specimens than in the drawn specimens. The microstructure of the cast specimens may be coarser than that of the drawn specimens. The relationship between the volume fraction and the number of the microshrinkage as measured on the fracture surface of the non-polished cast specimen and the elongation is shown in Fig. 17 [14]. Although no correlation was obtained between the volume fractions of the micro-shrinkage and elongation, the elongation decreases with an increase in the number of the microshrinkage. The surfaces of some fatigue test specimens were finished by buff-polishing (polished). Drawn specimens with a gauge diameter of 5 mm and a gauge length of 20 mm were used for the fatigue tests. Fatigue tests were carried out in order to obtain an S–N curve for each specimen at a stress ratio, R, of 0.1 and a frequency of 10 Hz with a sine waveform in air at room temperature (295 K). As can be seen in Fig.18 [14], the fatigue strength of the non-polished specimen is similar to that of the polished specimen in both the low-cycle fatigue life region and the high-cycle fatigue life region. The distribution of the fatigue strength of both the cast specimens is greater than that of the fatigue strength of the drawn specimens. The fatigue strength of the non-polished cast specimens was 352–492 MPa ($\Delta\sigma_{max}$ (range of σ_{max}) = 140 MPa) at 10^5 cycles and 209–284 MPa ($\Delta\sigma_{max}$ = 75 MPa) at 10^6 cycles. The fatigue strength of the polished cast specimens was 347–565 MPa ($\Delta\sigma_{max}$ = 218 MPa) at 10^5 cycles and 233–251 MPa ($\Delta\sigma_{max}$ = 18 MPa) at 10^6 cycles. The fatigue strength of both cast specimens was lower than that of the drawn specimens, and is extremely low in the high-cycle fatigue life region, where N_f exceeds 10^5 cycles. The fatigue limits, which represent the fatigue strength for which the number of cycles to failure is over 10^7 cycles, are around 210 MPa. On the other hand, although the fatigue limit of the drawn specimen was not obtained, it is expected to be near 400 MPa. Figure 19 [14] shows SEM fractographs taken near the site at which fatigue crack initiated in the cast specimens and the drawn specimen, which then broke in the high-cycle fatigue life region. In the case of the drawn specimen, the fatigue crack initiates at the slip band on the specimen surface, but in the case of the cast specimens, the fatigue crack initiates from the microshrinkage near the specimen surface. In general, slip damage accumulates on the specimen surface, after which extrusion and intrusion take place. Next, the stress concentration occurs and a fatigue crack initiates along the slip plane. If there are polishing scars, defects, etc. on the specimen surface, stress concentration occurs, and the fatigue strength becomes lower. The sizes of the microshrinkage areas and pores whose size exceeds 10 μm were measured, because the microshrinkage areas and pores whose size is less than 10 μm were difficult to distinguish from dimples on the fracture surface in the measurement on the fractographs. The number and size of the microshrinkage, whose size exceeds 10 μm as measured on the fatigue fracture surface, are greater than those measured on the cross- section near the fatigue fracture surface. Therefore, the fatigue crack propagates by preferentially linking the areas of microshrinkage. The number and size of the pores measured on the fatigue fracture surface is nearly equal to those measured on the cross-section near the fatigue fracture surface. Therefore, the effect of the pores on the fatigue properties is much smaller than that of the microshrinkage.

In general, dental prosthetic materials sustain a stress of 20–230MPa during mastication. Moreover, they must be able to sustain such cyclic stress over 10,000,000 times (10^7 cycles), which is the calculated number of cycles that is equivalent to the number of times food will be chewed in a span of ten years. Therefore, the target value of the fatigue limit of the cast specimen is considered to be 230MPa, which is the greatest mastication stress. Since the fatigue strength of this cast specimen is strongly dependent on the size of the microshrinkage that acts as the fatigue crack initiation site, it is prudent to estimate the size of the microshrinkage. It is also beneficial to know the size that can be tolerated, in order to achieve reliability in casting that is subjected to fatigue fracture.

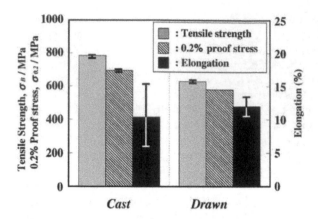

Figure 16. Tensile properties of non-polished cast specimens (Cast) and drawn specimens (Drawn: D-1073AC (drawn)).

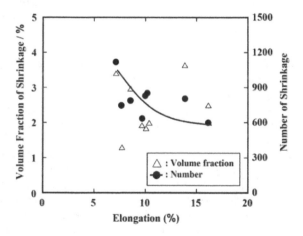

Figure 17. Relationships between volume fraction or number of shrinkage on fractograph and elongation of non-polished cast specimen.

3.3. Fretting–fatigue properties

Fretting–fatigue properties are also important for alloys that are used for dental applications, because during mastication, fretting occurs between the alloys and the teeth opposite them. Fig. 20 [15] shows the S–N curves of AS alloys subjected to ST at 1123 K for 3.6 ks followed by WQ and AT at 673 K for 1.8 ks followed by WQ that were obtained from plain fatigue and fretting–fatigue tests. The fretting–fatigue strength of the Ag–20Pd–14.5Cu–12Au alloy subjected to ST and AT decreases significantly as compared to the fatigue strength without fretting (plain–fatigue strength). The fretting–fatigue strength after the ST decreases by

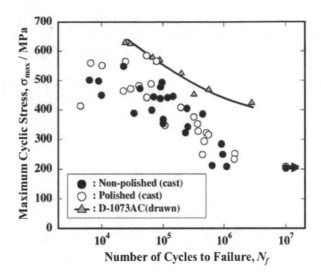

Figure 18. S-N$_f$ curves of non-polished cast specimen (Non-polished (cast)), polished cast specimen (Polished (cast)), and drawn specimen (D-1073AC(drawn)).

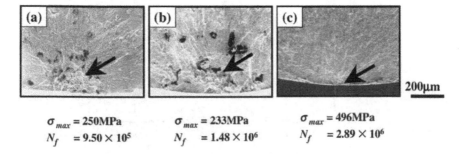

$\sigma_{max} = 250$MPa $\sigma_{max} = 233$MPa $\sigma_{max} = 496$MPa

$N_f = 9.50 \times 10^5$ $N_f = 1.48 \times 10^6$ $N_f = 2.89 \times 10^6$

Figure 19. SEM fractographs in high-cycle fatigue life region: (a) non-polished cast specimen, (b) polished cast specimen, and (c) drawn specimen. Arrows indicate crack initiation sites. σ_{max} and N$_f$ are the maximum cyclic stress and number of cycles to failure, respectively.

approximately 13% in the low-cycle fatigue life region and by approximately 40% in the high-cycle fatigue life region, as compared to the fatigue strength of the solutionized alloy. Moreover, the fretting–fatigue strength after the AT decreases by approximately 60% as compared to that after the ST, especially in the high-cycle fatigue life region. A schematic drawing of crack initiation from fretting damage region is shown in Fig.21 [15]. Although a slip between the specimen and a fretting pat does not occur in the stick region, a microslip between the specimen and the fretting pat occurs in the slip region during the deformation of the specimen. A significant stress concentration is generated by the damage to the specimen surface caused by the microslip. Fracture morphologies caused by crack initiation and propagation then appear. It can be observed that several traces of fretting wear are distributed in the slip region of both materials. These wear traces are generated by the accumulation of wear debris on the fretting pad or on the fretting–fatigue specimen. These traces of fretting wear are distributed more closely in the slip region of the material that was subjected to AT. Therefore, the fatigue life decreases significantly because the fretting–fatigue crack initiation life and the propagation life decrease in the material that was subjected to AT.

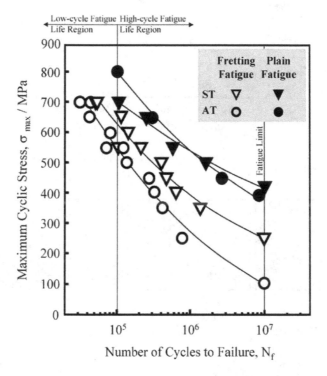

Figure 20. S–N curves of Ag–20Pd–14.5Cu–12Au alloy subjected to ST and AT obtained from plain fatigue and fretting fatigue tests.

3.4. Friction wear properties of Ag–20Pd–12Au–14.5Cu alloy in corrosive environments

Mastication also leads to friction wear in dental alloys and in teeth. As the friction wear progresses, this eventually causes problems with mastication. Therefore, the evaluation of the friction wear properties of dental alloys is quite important to the health of the teeth and oral cavity. The friction wear property of Ag–20Pd–14.5Cu–12Au alloy that was subjected to various heat treatments was evaluated in three corrosive environments: distilled water, 0.9% NaCl solution, and 3% NaCl solution. In the friction wear testing, the alloys were subjected to

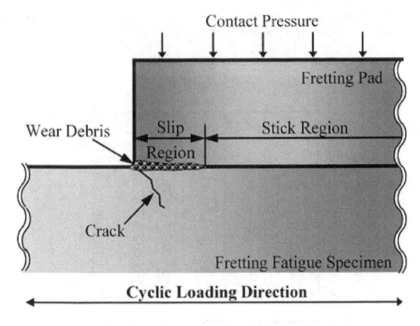

Figure 21. Schematic drawing of crack initiation from fretting damage region.

STs at 1073 and 1123 K subjected to WQ, AT at 673 K, and ST at 1073 K subjected to AC. It was found that the friction wear properties are influenced by the microstructures of this alloy as well as by the corrosive environments. The friction wear tests were performed using a pin-on-disk-type friction wear tester. The applied load, sliding diameter, sliding velocity, sliding distance, and test duration were 9.8 N, 3 mm, 31.4 mm/s (100 rpm), 4.71×10^5 mm, and 115 ks, respectively. The temperature of all the solutions was 310 K. The weight loss was calculated by subtracting the combined weight of a specimen and the mating material it after the friction wear test, from their combined weight before the test. Figure 22 [16] shows the total weight loss and wear surface roughness of specimens that were subjected to each heat treatment in each corrosive solution. The total weight loss (the sum of the weight losses of the specimen and the material opposite it) of the specimens was largest in distilled water, 0.9% NaCl and then 3% NaCl solution. A pin with a diameter of 1 mm, which was made from the as-received alloy, was used as the mating material. The weight losses of the specimens and the mating materials increased with a decrease in the kinematic viscosity of the solutions, due to the increase in the average friction coefficient during the friction wear tests. In every environment, the total weight loss of the specimen subjected to AT at 673 K, which gives a large amount of precipitated β phase, was small compared with that of the other heat-treated specimens, due to the higher degree of hardness near the contact surface, as also shown in Fig.4 [10]. The total weight loss increased with the surface roughness of the contact surface. The hardness near the contact surface changed the surface roughness of the contact surface. The mode of wear of these alloys in a corrosive environment is adhesive wear. No tarnish, which is corrosion caused by chloride ion and the production of silver chloride coatings were found on the wear marks or wear particles after the friction wear tests in each environment.

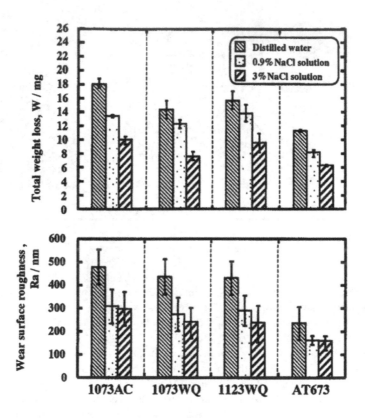

Figure 22. Total weight loss and wear surface roughness of specimen subjected to each heat treatment in each corrosive solution. 1073AC, 1073WQ, 1123WQ, and AT673 indicate specimens subjected to ST at 1073 K for 3.6 ks followed by AC or WQ, ST at 1123 K for 3.6 ks followed by WQ and AT at 673 K for 1.8 ks.

3.5. Corrosion properties

The study of the corrosion properties of dental alloys is very important due to their usage in severe oral environments. The formation of corrosion compounds on the surface causes the alloy to tarnish. The corrosion behaviors of commercial Ag-22.41Pd-15.64Cu-12.1Au alloys in various solutions were investigated by Ichinose [17]. The alloy was casted into a plate with 2 mm in thickness by heating at 973 K for 30 min. Table 2 [17] shows the rest-potential of the as-cast alloy in 1% NaCl solution, artificial saliva, human saliva, and 1% $C_3H_6O_3$ solution. The rest-potentials in 1% NaCl solution and 1% $C_3H_6O_3$ solution show obviously higher values than those for artificial and human saliva. The organic compounds in the artificial and human saliva inhibit the redox reaction by adsorbing on the surface of the alloy or by the formation of complexes with the metal. AgCl was formed on the surface of the alloy after anode polarization sweeping up to 1800 mV in 1% NaCl solution, artificial saliva, and human saliva, which contain Cl ion. 90% of the released ions of the as-cast alloy immersed in human saliva for 24 h were Cu ions (Fig.23 [17]). Cu contributes to the enhancement the hardness of the alloy. However, a large amount of Cu in the alloy decreases the corrosion resistance. The as-cast alloy was subjected to a softening treatment at 1073 K for 3 min followed by WQ (softened). An ingot of the commercial Ag-22.41Pd-15.64Cu-12.1Au alloy was subjected to ST at 1123 K for 2 h and then heated at 723 K for 1 h or 20 h (723 K 1h aged and 723 K 20 h aged, respectively). As shown in Fig. 24 [17], the amounts of released Cu and Ag ions depend on the heat treatment that the alloy is subjected to, because the corrosion behavior is influenced by the microstructure of the alloy. The amount of Cu ions released from the as-cast alloy is higher than that released from heat-treated alloys. Cavities formed by shrinkage during casting in the as-cast alloy are the reason for this phenomenon.

Solution	Rest–potential
1% NaCl solution	112.7 ± 22.4 mV
Artificial saliva	24.7 ± 17.2 mV
Human saliva	28.0 ± 20.4 V
1% $C_3H_6O_3$ solution	113.6 ± 37.7 mV

Table 2. Rest-potential of as-cast Ag-22.41Pd-15.64Cu-12.10Au alloy in various corrosive solutions.

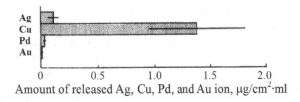

Amount of released Ag, Cu, Pd, and Au ion, $\mu g/cm^2 \cdot ml$

Figure 23. Amounts of ions released from as-cast Ag-22.41Pd-15.64Cu-12.10Au alloy immersed in human saliva for 24 h.

4. Summary

This chapter details the microstructure, the mechanical properties (hardness, fatigue, fretting-fatigue, and friction-wear), and the corrosion properties of the Ag–Pd–Cu–Au alloys, especially the Au-20Pd-14.5Cu-12Au alloy. Most studies on these alloys have been carried out in Japan and Korea. Although other dental materials such as high carat gold alloys, amalgam,

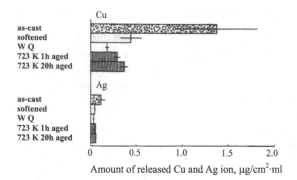

Figure 24. Cu and Ag release amounts from as-cast, softened, WQ, 723 K 1h aged, and 723 K 20 h aged Ag-22.41Pd-15.64Cu-12.10Au alloys immersed in human saliva for 24 h.

and non-precious alloys such as titanium and its alloys, cobalt-chromium alloys, and nickel–chromium alloys are also important, the authors intended to introduce present results of studies on the Ag–Pd–Cu–Au alloys to researchers who study dental materials all over the world through this chapter.

A variety of test results showed that the hardness of the alloy can be drastically increased through ST at a temperature over 1073 K subjected to WQ. The $L1_0$-type ordered phase (β' phase) precipitated during the quenching process leads to this unique hardening behavior. The hardness of the alloy increased with an increase in the cooling rate following ST, because the size of the β' phase decreased and the number of the β' phase increased with an increase in the cooling rate following ST.

It was also found that the fatigue strength of a cast alloy was considerably less than that of a drawn alloy. The fatigue crack of a cast alloy initiated preferentially at the shrinkage near the specimen surface. The deviation of the fatigue strength of the cast alloy became small by relating the fatigue life to the maximum stress intensity factor that was calculated, assuming that the shrinkage that begins as a fatigue crack initiation site becomes an initial crack. This means that the size of the shrinkage strongly affects the fatigue strength of this cast alloy. A tolerable shrinkage size that satisfies the target value of the fatigue limit (230 MPa) of this cast alloy was calculated to be below 80 μm, using a derived equation that describes the relationship between the maximum stress intensity factor and the number of the cycles to failure.

The fretting–fatigue strength of the Ag–20Pd–12Au–14.5Cu alloy subjected to ST and aging treatment decreased significantly as compared to the fatigue strength without fretting. The fretting–fatigue strength after the aging treatment decreased by approximately 60% as compared to that following the ST, especially in the high-cycle fatigue life region.

The total weight losses (the sum of the weight losses of a specimen and of the mating material) of specimens were largest in distilled water, subjected to 0.9% NaCl and then 3% NaCl solution. In every environment, the total weight loss of a specimen subjected to aging treatment at 673

K, which gives a large amount of precipitated β phase, was small compared with that of the other heat treated specimens, due to the higher degree of hardness near the contact surface.

The Ag-Pd-Cu-Au alloys have excellent mechanical and corrosion properties, but the relatively high cost and supplied amounts of these alloys are issues to be used widely. The authors hope that the Ag-Pd-Cu-Au alloys is further investigated by many researchers for its wide usage.

Acknowledgements

This study was supported in part by ISHIFUKU Metal Industry Co., Ltd. for their support during this study. This study was financially supported in part by a Grant-in-aid for Scientific Research from the Japan Society for the Promotion of Science (Grant Number 21360332), the Global COE program "Materials Integration International Center of Education and Research, Tohoku University," Ministry of Education, Culture, Sports, Science and Technology (MEXT) of Japan, and Tohoku Leading Women's Jump Up Project, Tohoku University. The authors are very grateful to Dr. YH. Kim (Institute for Materials Research, Tohoku University) and Prof. H. Fukui (Aichi-Gakuin University) for their experimental work and fruitful discussion.

Author details

Junko Hieda, Mitsuo Niinomi, Masaaki Nakai and Ken Cho

Department of Biomaterials Science, Institute for Materials Research, Tohoku University, Katahira, Aoba-ku, Sendai, Japan

References

[1] Ohta M, Shiraishi T, Yamane M. Phase transformation and age-hardening of Au-Cu-Pd ternary alloys. Journal of Materials Science 1986;21(2) 529-535.

[2] Winn H, Tanaka Y, Shiraishi T, Udoh K, Miura E, Hernandez RI, Takuma Y, Hisatsune K. Two types of checkerboard-like microstructures in Au–Cu–Pd ternary alloys. Journal of Alloys and Compounds 2000;306(1-2) 262-269.

[3] Seol HJ, Son KH, Yu CH, Kwon YH, Kim HI. Precipitation hardening of a Cu-free Au–Ag–Pd–In dental alloy. Journal of Alloys and Compounds 2005;402(1-2) 130-135.

[4] Seol HJ, Shiraishi T, Tanaka Y, Miura E, Hisatsune K, Kim HI. Ordering behaviors and age-hardening in experimental AuCu–Zn pseudobinary alloys for dental applications Biomaterials 2002;23(24) 4873-4879.

[5] Hisatsune K, Sakrana A, Hamasaki K, Hernandez R, Salonga JP. Phase transforma-
     tion in a dental gold alloy for soldering. Journal of Alloys and Compounds
     1997;261(1-2) 308-312.

[6] Lee JH, Yi SJ, Seol HJ, Kwon YH, Lee JB, Kim HI. Age-hardening by metastable phas-
     es in an experimental Au–Ag–Cu–Pd alloy. Journal of Alloys and Compounds
     2006;425(1-2) 210-215.

[7] Santos ML, Acciari HA, Vercik LCO, Guastaldi AC. Laser weld: microstructure and
     corrosion study of Ag–Pd–Au–Cu alloy of the dental application. Materials Letters
     2003;57(13-14) 1888-1893.

[8] Seol HJ, Kim GC, Son KH, Kwon YH, Kim HI. Hardening mechanism of an Ag–Pd–
     Cu–Au dental casting alloy, Journal of Alloys and Compounds 2005;387(1-2) 139-146.

[9] Fukui H, Shinoda S, Mukai M, Yasue K, Hasegawa J. Effect of heat treatment on me-
     chanical properties of type IV gold and 12wt% Au-Pd-Ag alloys. The Japanese Soci-
     ety for Dental Materials and Devices 1992;11(1) 141-148.

[10] Fukui H, Mukai M, Shinoda S, Hasegawa J. Strengthening mechanism of Au-Pd-Ag-
     Cu system. The Japanese Society for Dental Materials and Devices 1993;12(6) 685-690.

[11] Kim YH, Niinomi M, Hieda J, Nakai M, Fukui H. Formation of L10-type ordered β′
     phase in as-solutionized dental Ag–Pd–Au–Cu alloys and hardening behavior. Mate-
     rials Science and Engineering: C 2012;32(3) 503–509.

[12] Kim YH, Niinomi M, Nakai M, Akahori T, Kanno T, Fukui H. Mechanism of unique
     hardening of dental Ag–Pd–Au–Cu alloys in relation with constitutional phases.
     Journal of Alloys and Compounds 2012;519 15–24.

[13] Akahori T, Niinomi M, Nakai M, Tsutsumi H, Kanno T, Kim YH, Fukui H. Relation-
     ship between unique hardening behavior and microstructure of dental silver alloy
     subjected to solution treatment. Journal of the Japan Institute of Metals 2010;74(6)
     337-344.

[14] Mizumoto T, Niinomi M, Nakano Y, Akahori T, Fukui H. Fatigue properties of cast
     Ag-Pd-Cu-Au-Zn alloy for dental applications in the relation with casting defects.
     Materials Transactions 2002;43(12) 3160-3166.

[15] Akahori T, Niinomi M, Nakai M, Kawagishi W, Fukui H, Fretting-fatigue properties
     and fracture mechanism of semi-precious alloy for dental applications. Journal of
     The Japan Institute of Metals 2008;72(1) 63-71.

[16] Mizumoto T, Niinomi M, Akahori T, Katou K, Fukui H. Friction wear properties of
     dental Ag-Pd-Cu-Au alloy in corrosive environments. The Japanese Society for Den-
     tal Materials and Devices 2003; 22(6) 459-468.

[17] Ichinose S. Corrosion behavior of dental Au-Pd-Cu-Au alloy in various solutions.
     The Japanese Society for Dental Materials and Devices 1992;11(1) 149-168.

[18] Seol HJ, Lee DH, Lee HK, Takada Y, Okuno O, Kwon YH, Kim HI. Age-hardening and related phase transformation in an experimental Ag–Cu–Pd–Au alloy. Journal of Alloys and Compounds 2006;407(1-2) 182-187.

[19] Yu CH, Park MG, Kwon YH, Seol HJ, Kim HI. Phase transformation and microstructural changes during ageing process of an Ag-Pd-Cu-Au Alloy. Journal of Alloys and Compounds 2008;460(1-2) 331-336.

[20] Kanzawa Y, Uzuka T, Kondo, Shoji M. Study on the Ag-Pd alloy. Journal of the Japan Society for Dental Apparatus and Materials 1963;4 157-160.

[21] Yasuda K. Study on the age-hardeability of dental precious metal alloys. Journal of the Japan Society for Dental Apparatus and Materials 1969;10 156-166.

[22] Ohta M, Hisatsune K, Yamane M. Study on the age-hardenable silver alloy. Journal of the Japan Society for Dental Apparatus and Materials 1975;16 144-149.

[23] Ohta M, Hisatsune K, Yamane M. Age Hardening of Ag-Pd-Cu dental alloy. Journal of the Less-Common Metals 1979;65(1) 11-21.

[24] Ohta M, Shiraishi T, Hisatsune K, Yamane M. Age-hardening of dental Ag-Pd-Cu-Au alloys. Journal of Dental Research 1980;59(11) 1966-1971.

[25] Tanaka Y, Miura E, Shiraishi T, Hisatsune K. Nano-precipitates generated in the dental silver–palladium–gold alloy. Materia Japan 2004;12 1036.

[26] Tanaka Y, Seol HJ, Ogata T, Miura E, Shiraishi T, Hisatsune K. Hardening mechanism of dental casting gold-silver-palladium alloy by higher-temperature heat-treatment. The Japanese Society for Dental Materials and Devices 2003;22 (2) 69.

Chapter 10

Hydroxylapatite (HA) Powder for Autovaccination Against Canine Non Hodgkin's Lymphoma

Michel Simonet, Nicole Rouquet and
Patrick Frayssinet

Additional information is available at the end of the chapter

1. Introduction

Lymphoma is the most common neoplasm of the canine hemolymphatic system. It represents about 15% of all malignant neoplasms. It has a very poor prognosis, the mean survival with high grade non Hodgkin's lymphomas being two months without treatment [1]. Incidence is increasing.

Lymphomas in dogs, as in humans, can be divided into numerous types depending on the cell line involved and their immunophenotype [2]. T lymphomas have a worse prognosis than B lymphomas and late clinical stages obviously have a very short survival period.

Lymphomas are known in human medicine to respond to chemotherapy, and some of them can even be cured by complex chemotherapy protocols, although severe side effects are noted.

Chemotherapy protocols have also been developed for dogs in the last 40 years. They have proved to be effective for the overall survival of the treated animal. Although the order of drug administration and duration of the maintenance part of the protocol vary considerably, most oncologists agree that a doxorubicin-based (eg CHOP) combination chemotherapy protocol provides the longest period of disease control and overall survival [3].

Even with chemotherapy, survival is relatively short and adjuvant therapies have been developed to improve prognosis. Immunotherapy protocols are of particular interest for this purpose as they may arm immune system cells against the abnormal proteins synthesized by cancer cells [4]. It is a selective way of destroying cancer cells and a treatment with much fewer side effects than chemo- or radiotherapy.

The immune system can destroy cancer cells by different methods:

- Synthesis of TNF-α (tumor necrosis factor alpha) and an oxygen intermediate such as nitric oxide by macrophages activated by IFN-γ (interferon gamma)

- Activation of NK (natural killer) cells by IL-2 (interleukin 2)

- Adsorption of an antibody against tumor cell antigens targeting macrophages and cytotoxic T lymphocytes.

- Activation of CD8+ T lymphocytes by an MHC(major histocompatibility complex) - mediated cell contact mechanism between antigen-presenting cells (APCs) and CD8 cells

Several kinds of immunotherapy protocol are available both in human and veterinary medicine [4, 5, 6, 7]. Heat shock proteins (HSPs) such as gp96 or HSPs70 which are synthesized by the cells submitted to stress are advantageous vaccination adjuvants due to their chaperone properties and their role in antigen presentation [8]. As chaperone molecules, almost all the cell peptides are associated with these proteins and HSP purification provides a fingerprint of the cell's protein synthesis [9]. This is particularly useful for cancer cells which synthesize numerous abnormal proteins during their natural progress [10]. These cells being genetically unstable, their abnormal protein synthesis differs from patient to patient and during the course of the disease. The HSPs and their associated peptides (AAPs) have special receptors (CD91) on dendritic cells which allow the internalization of the AAPs and their modification in order to be expressed at the surface of class I HLA proteins on the cell membrane, triggering activation of the CD8 T cells if they are abnormal [11].

Cancer cells are stressed by the mechanical and metabolic characteristics of the tumour. They synthesize many HSPs [12]. We thus isolated these proteins in order to make an autologous vaccine against the tumour. The HSPs were purified using a hydroxylapatite powder (HA) column. The powder carrying the HSPs was then injected subcutaneously to stimulate the immune system's response to the tumour.

Purification of HSPs using classical way is long and tedious. The use of hydroxylapatite powder allows a much faster purification process. Hydroxylapatite chromatography has been described by Tiselius in the early seventies. Hydroxylapatite chromatography is an adsorption chromatography. The adsorption mechanism is very poorly understood. The surface of the material is occupied bu Ca^{++} and PO_4^-. These ions are supposed to interact with the chemical groups of the proteins. However, post synthesis treatment such as sintering or spray- drying process modify the physico-chemical properties of the material surface. Furthermore, the interaction of the material surface with biological fluids triggers epitaxial growth of carbonated apatite at the surface of the material [13].

It was decided that the proteins purified will be injected carried by the particles for several reasons: the hydroxylapatite particles have been described as vaccine adjuvant, they are phagocytosed by the APCs and can deliver the proteins directly in the APCs, they trigger an afflux of APCs at the injection site [14]. Most of the adjuvants used in antiinfectious vaccines are nano or microparticular.

The aims of this study was to check the feasibility of this protocol using HA-particles with dogs suffering of high grade lymphoma and to know if secondary effects were detected.

2. Materials and methods

2.1. Dogs to be treated

Two dogs (Poodle, 6 years, Jagdterrier, 8 years) suffered from polyadenopathy without any sign of immune deficiency. One dog (mixed breed, 10 years) had a liver metastasis. The last one had a cutaneous form. Their general condition remained reasonable, with no real weight loss or fever. One dog (Poodle) had a splenomegaly. The blood numeration revealed that the white cells and calcaemia for both dogs were in the normal range. Node biopsies were performed. One was sent to the pathologist and the other was frozen (-20°C) and used to manufacture the vaccine. Disease staging was performed using the WHO-staging criteria for canine lymphoma.

A chemotherapy treatment was proposed by the physician but rejected by the dog's owners due to side effects and an informed consent was signed.

After vaccination, the dogs were subjected to a clinical examination whenever they came for the following injection and side effects noted. The volume of a control node was externally measured.

2.2. Toxicity and response assessment

The side effects were graded every week for the first month and every month for the next five months according to the National Cancer Institute's common Toxicity Criteria (version 2.0).

The dogs were also submitted to a physical examination at the same frequency to assess their clinical response. A complete response (CR) was defined as the disappearance of all the nodes and metastasis for at least 4 weeks. A partial response (PR) was defined as a decrease by at least 50% of the product of the 2 longest lengths of all the nodes without the appearance of new lesions for at least 4 weeks. A minor response (MR) was defined as a decrease by less than 50% using the same criteria. Stable disease (SD) was defined as the same criteria unchanged for at least 4 weeks. Progressive disease (PD) was defined as an increase by >25% of the product of the 2 longest lengths of all the nodes for at least 4 weeks or when new lesions appeared.

2.3. Hydroxylapatite powder characteristics

Hydroxylapatite powders (Fig. 1) can be used for adsorption chromatography under atmospheric or high pressure. In order that the protein solution did not fill in the column and to avoid the compaction, the powder was spray-dried then sintered at 1000°C.

The HA was transformed into a ceramic powder according to the following protocol. The synthesized calcium phosphate was suspended in a slurry which is liquid, spray-dried, then sintered. The spray-dried material was heated almost to fusion temperature which favors the migration of matter between the grains and the formation of bridges. As the surface energy was smaller for large than for small grains, their size increased and the distance between the grain centers and the particle surface area decreased.

Powder characteristics	
Nature of the charged groups	PO_4^{3-}, OH^-, Ca^{2+}
Electrocinetical potential (mV)	-35
Hydrophobicity	+
Surface pH	7,8
Granulometry (μm)	0-25
Surface area (m²/gr)	4
Shape	spherical

Table 1. Characteristics of the powder

The sintering considerably reduced the surface area making the amount of proteins adsorbed on the powder lower. It also stabilized the powder structure. The powder was submitted to dissolution/ precipitation processes when soaked inside a saline solution [13]. The modification occurring at the powder surface affected the adsorption properties of the powder. The reduced surface area decreased the interactions with the saline solution containing the proteins. There was a microporosity between the ceramic grains inside the same particle allowing the protein solution to diffuse inside the particles. The characteristics of the powder used in this experiment was given in table 1

As the chromatography was carried out under atmosphere, the granulometry of the powder was an important factor in order to avoid any plugging of the column. The HSPs could be eluted from the powder by 200-300 mM NaCl solutions. The powder solution in NaCl was not stable enough to be injected as it decanted too fast in the syringe. Thus to improve the injectability the powder was put in suspension in a 2% solution of carboxymethylcellulose in 20 mM NaCl.

2.4. Vaccine manufacturing protocol

The tumor tissue and all the materials used to prepare the vaccine were handled in sterile conditions under a laminar flow. The frozen tumor (200 mgr) tissue was homogenized using a bead tissue homogenizer. 1 ml of $NaHCO_3$ (30 mM, pH 7) was added for 1 ml of homogenate. The resulting homogenate was then centrifuged at 1000 g for 15 mn at 4°C to remove all cell fragments.

The supernatant containing the cytoplasmic proteins was used for protein purification by HA column chromatography as follows: a) two precipitations with ammonium sulphate (first at 50% and then at 70%) recovering the pellets. The last pellet was resuspended in 1 ml phosphate buffer (20 mM, pH 7). The column was filled (chromatography columns, Poly-prep, Cat. 731-1550, Bio Rad) with 0.2 gr of HA (0-25 μm), equilibrated with 10 volumes of phosphate buffer (20 mM pH7). The resuspended pellet was then added. The column was then washed with 3 ml of a 100 mM NaCl solution (fig.2).

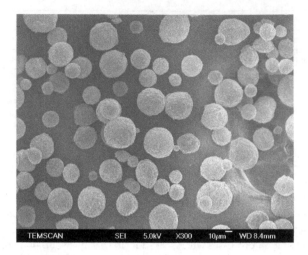

Figure 1. SEM of the HA-powder used for the vaccine.

The powder was then suspended in 5 ml carboxymethylcellulose (CMC) solution (2% in 20mM NaCl). 0.5 ml of this solution was used for each vaccine shot.

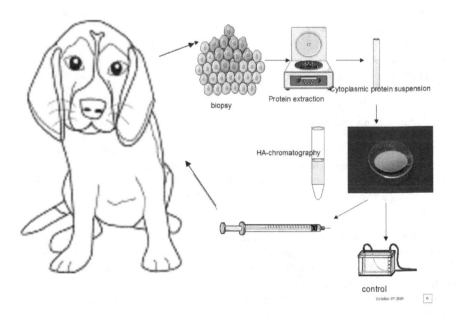

Figure 2. Autovaccine manufacturing scheme

0.2 ml of the previous solution was used to make electrophoretic control. The solution was centrifuged at 1000g 30 for seconds. The supernatant was discarded and the powder in the pellet washed with 0.1 ml of a 0.5 M NaCl solution. The solution was again centrifuged and the supernatant was used for a SDS-Page and for protein quantification using UV spectrometer. 10 μl of the solution was also used for dot blot with anti HSP70 and anti gp90 antibodies on a nitrocellulose membrane. The antibody labelling was evidenced using a westernbreeze™ (invitrogen) kit according to the manufacturer instructions.

2.5. Vaccination protocol

The dogs were injected with 0.5 ml (about 40 μg of proteins) of the vaccine subcutaneously on day 0. The dose schema consisted of 0.5 ml/dose every week for one month, followed by one dose every month for four months.

2.6. activation of TLR2 and 4

Some HSPs are TLR (Toll like receptor) agonist and the TLR activation was checked using two cell lines secreting an embryonic phosphatase alkaline when the TLR 2 or 4 are stimulated.

Two cell lines were used for TLR receptor stimulation. HEK-Blue™-hTLR2 and HEK-Blue™-hTLR4 cells (invivogen –France) were grown in DMEM supplemented with 10% fetal calf serum and 0,5% normocin (invivogen-France) to avoid mycoplasma contamination. 20000 cells were introduced in wells of 96-well plate, 4 hours later 20 μl of different concentrations of the vaccine was added and incubated at 37°C for 20 hours. Then the medium was removed and replaced by 180 μl of resuspended QUANTI- blueTM (Invivogen) and incubated for 1 hour and the positivity evaluated. The negative control was the HA- powder without any protein immobilized on its surface. The minimal concentration turning blue the medium was noted. It was estimated that the vaccine was functional when the minimal active concentration was less than the vaccine concentration.

3. Results

All the vaccine dilutions stimulated the TLR 4 but not the TLR2. The negative control (HA powder) did not stimulate any TLR. The SDS PAGE revealed two bands in the 95 kDa region which were previously demonstrated to be HSPs rich bands (fig. 3) The dot blots revealed that all the vaccine contained gp96 and HSP70 but the amount was different (fig.3 and 4).

Neither dog showed side effects after the injections, whether systemic or local. Two showed a decrease in nodule volume of less than 50% following the first month of injections and were rated MR. The other were rated SD. All dogs were rated PD about one month before they died.

No sign of infection such as fever was observed during the first month of vaccination. The Jagdterrier was diagnosed with an abscess of the collar by the fourth month, which was cured surgically. The lung radiographs did not reveal any lung metastases. The blood count did not show any anomaly in the white cell count up to the last month of survival.

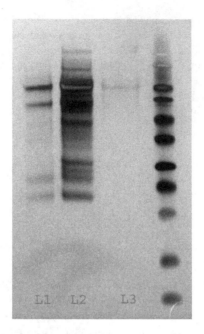

Figure 3. L1 was obtained after washing the powder with 0.3M NaCl, L2 was obtained after washing at 0.02M, L3 was obtained with 0.5M. At 0.02M almost all the contaminant proteins are eluted from the powder. At 0.3 M, the remaining proteins after the 0.02M elution are located in the 95 and 70 kDa zone. The 0.5 M column shows that after after 0.3 M there is almost no proteins remaining on the powder.

The poodle was euthanazised 11 months, and the Jagdterrier 6 months, after the disease was discovered. During their survival period, both dogs had a normal activity. The Jagdterrier was still hunting two weeks before to be euthanazied. The two other dogs were euthanazied at 155 and 173 days (table 2). The mean overall survival time is 210 days.

Dog number	Breed	Histology	Stage	OS	Immunophenotype
1	Jagd terrier	Centoblastic polymorphic	IIIb	330	B cell
2	Poodle	Centroblastic polymorphic	IIIb	180	B cell
3	mixed	Centroblastic polymorphic	IVb	173	B cell
4	cocker	cutaneous	IVb	155	T cell

Table 2. Characteristics of the dogs treated by the vaccination protocol and overall survival time (OS) in days.

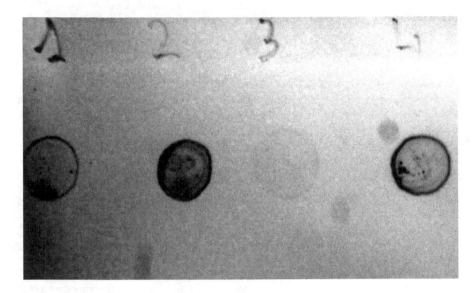

Figure 4. Dot blot after anti gp90 labelling

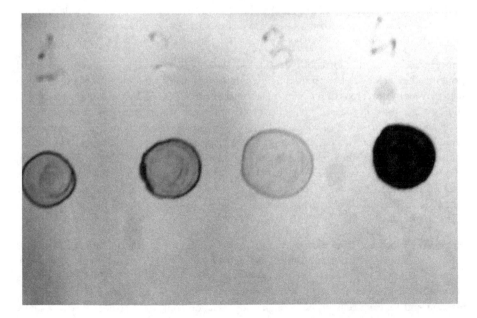

Figure 5. Dot blot after anti HSP70 labelling

4. Discussion

This experiment showed the feasibility of this protocol as an autologous vaccine for cancer in dogs in veterinary practice. We have also developed an *in vitro* test to assess the functionality of purified heat shock proteins. This test checks in a few minutes the vaccine's ability to stimulate antigen-presenting cells (APCs) through toll-like receptor (TLR) activation. Even if the sample size is small, the dogs' overall survival (210 days) was much higher than expected, as the average OS for this type of pathology is two months. In larger series of stage Vb lymphomas associating chemotherapy and the same vaccine protocol, we could demonstrate that after vaccination the dogs showed a delayed cutaneous hypersensibility after their own tumor antigen injection in the derm (Marconato, unpublished results).

High grade lymphomas in dogs are an interesting model for cancer vaccines because survival is very short, so the effect on OS is very easy to measure. The clinical efficiency of vaccine is not always related to the vaccine's effect on biological parameters. Models with a short life expectancy are thus of interest. Furthermore vaccination without the use of other drugs is of particular interest.

The amount of proteins used in this vaccine was justified by the different experiments published about autovaccines using HSPs in animals and humans. Furthermore we checked that the amount of proteins could activate 20000 APCs *in vitro*. The presence of the tumor proteins at the surface of the HA-particles allows the activation of the TLRs. It indicates that the proteins are immobilized at the surface of the particles and their adsorption does not denaturize these proteins.

Cancer vaccines are the focus of great interest. Although cancer cells synthesise abnormal proteins, they are are not recognised by the immune system. Different immunosuppression mechanisms by cancerous tumours have been described [15]. The use of multiantigen vaccines could reduce the cancer cell's "invisibility" to the immune system compared to monoproteic vaccines. Different kinds of immune therapy are under investigation. Cell engineering immunotherapy protocols have been tested, including activation of dendritic cells *in vitro* by tumour antigens before being reinjected into the patient [16]. Other trials concern amplification of the intratumoural lymphocytes (TILs) *in vitro* [17] before being reinjected into the donor. Recently, different types of antibodies were approved for the oncology field, in particular antibodies against VEGF (Vascular endothelial growth factor) to inhibit tumour vascularization [18, 19].

Heat Shock Proteins (HSPs) have proved to be of therapeutic interest in human medicine for some applications. In order to be useful as a cancer vaccination, these HSPs must be made available to APCs. HA-powder is a good material for use as a vector of HSPs to APCs. It has been shown that when injected in the dermis or subcutaneous tissue, it triggers a foreign body reaction and that the cells of this foreign body reaction could be transfected with a DNA molecule carried by the particles [20]. It suggests that, further to DNA vectorisation, the particles could help in the transfection of HSPs and their associated peptides in APCs.

Although gp96 has been described as able to stimulate TLR4, it is not sure that these proteins are the only proteins responsible for TLRs stimulation in this case. There are contaminating proteins in various bands of the SDS which could interfere with the TLRs. The non stimulation of the TLR2 indicates that the TLR4 is not activated by contaminating endotoxins.

Hydroxyapatite has been used as an adjuvant for various infectious vaccines such as diphtheria and tetanus [21]. The Hydroxyapatite lattice is a hexagonal structure which allows numerous substitutions. Ions and small amino acids can thus be trapped in the HA lattice. Consequently, HA powder has been used to purify DNA, proteins or even viruses from biological solutions [22]. In this case, the surface properties of the particles allowed both the purification of HSPs and their use as a vector to APCs and as an adjuvant.

The HA-powder characteristics seems well suited for its role of cancer vaccine adjuvant. The granulometry range allows the phagocytosis by the APCs as it was demonstrated previously [14]. Furthermore, the grain boundaries in each particle is degraded by the cells making the particles fragmented and thus decreasing the real granulometry a few days after injection. It was also demonstrated that the phagocytosis of these particles by the APCs induced the synthesis of various cytokines and lymphokines necessary for the cross-priming of the CD8. The HA-adjuvant effect does not seem to be due to TLR activation as HA-particles alone do not trigger TLR2 and 4 activation. Other mineral adjuvants such as aluminum oxide have been demonstrated to activate the inflamasome. The inflamasome is a multi-protein complex involved in the production of mature IL-1β. The alumn-induced release of IL-1β in macro-phages is done under activation of the NLRP3 [23]. It is suggested from unpublished results that the adjuvancy effect of the HA-particles is also due to the inflamasome activation.

Tumor associated antigens show a very poor antigenicity. Thus the presence of an adjuvant like calcium phosphate particles is essential in order to increase the visibility of these antigens by the patient immune system.

This method was used in a short pilot study in humans and proved to be very safe, as only local effects (erythema) were reported in some patients (24). Although it was not the goal of the pilot study, some remission in the extent of the tumour was observed and constituted a good proof of concept. Gp96 has already been used in human medicine to treat a series of patients with indolent non Hodgkin's lymphoma [23]. The results are difficult to compare, as the patients could have been treated by chemo- or radiotherapy more than six weeks before the vaccination protocol. However, at three months most of the patients were rated SD, including those who were resistant to previous therapy. No patients suffered side effects.

5. Conclusions

The HA-particles are essential in this protocol both for their adsorption properties for proteins of interest and their adjuvant properties. They constitute a tool which allows to purify tumor associated antigens in a fast and reproducible way.

The overall survival of the four dogs was much better than expected. These preliminary results nonetheless show that the technique is feasible in private veterinary medicine. They are consistant with other results obtained with canine osteosarcomas or with a series of stage Vb lymphomas treated by chemotherapy and this protocol.

The association of the HA-particles to tumor associated antigens and HSPs did not trigger any adverse effects, confirming the safe results obtained for other applications in human medicine.

This technique could also be combined with conventional chemo- or radiotherapy to increase the animal's overall survival.

Author details

Michel Simonet[1], Nicole Rouquet[2] and Patrick Frayssinet[2*]

1 Veterinary hospital, Nuit Saint Georges, France

2 Urodelia, St Lys, France

References

[1] C. Fournel-Fleury, F. Ponce, P., Felman, A. Blavier, C. Bonnefont, L. Chabanne, T. Marchal, J.L. Cadore, I. Goy-Thollot, D. Ledieu, I. Ghernathi, J.P. Magnol, Canine T-cell lymphomas: a morphological, immunological, and clinical study of 46 new cases. Vet Pathol 39: 92-109 (2002).

[2] R. Chun, Lymphoma: which chemotherapy protocol and why? Top Companion Anim Med.;24: 157-62 (2007)

[3] L. Marconato, The staging and treatment of multicentric high-garde lymphoma in dogs: A review of recent developments and future prospects. The Veterinary Journal, 188: 34-38 (2011).

[4] T., F., Greten, E.M., Jaffee, Cancer vaccines, Journal of clinical oncology, 17: 1047-1060 (1999).

[5] C. J. Wheeler, K. L. Black, G. Liu, M. Mazer, X.-X. Zhang, S. Pepkowitz, D. Goldfinger, H. Ng, D. Irvin, and J. S. Yu. Vaccination elicits correlated immune and clinical responses in glioblastoma multiforme patients. Cancer Research 68 : 5955-5964, (2008).

[6] B. Klein, K. Tarte, A. M. Conge, L. Zhao-Yang, and J. F. Rossi. Stratégie de vaccination antitumorale. Biotech Médecine 23, (2002).

[7] Y. Akiyama, R. Tanosaki, N. Inoue, M. Shimada, Y. Hotate, A. Yamamoto, N. Yamazaki, I. Kawashima, I. Nukaya, K. Takesako, K. Maruyama, Y. Takaue, and K. Yama-

gushi. Clinical response in japanese metastatic melanoma patients treatted with peptide cocktail-pulsed dendritic cells. Journail of Translational Medicine 3: 4-14, (2005).

[8]   A. Murshid, J. Gong, and S. K. Calderwood. Heat-shock proteins in cancer vaccines: agents of antigen cross presentation. Expert Rev Vaccines 7: 1019-1030, (2008).

[9]   D. R. Ciocca and S. K. Calderwood. Heat shock proteins in cancer: diagnostic, prognostic, predictive, and treatment implications. Cell Stress & Chaperones 10: 263-270, (2005)

[10] J. Kaiser. A detailed genetic portrait of the deadliest human cancers. Science 321: 1280-1281, (2008).

[11] C. V. Nicchitta, D. M. Carrick, and J. C. Baker-LePain. The messenger and the message: gp96 (grp94)-peptide interactions in cellular immunity. Cell Stress & Chaperones 9 : 325-331, (2004).

[12] M. Romanucci, A. Marinelli, S. Giuseppe, and L. Della Salda. Heat shock protein expression in canine malignant mammary tumours. BMC Cancer 6: 171-183, (2006).

[13] M. Heughebaert, R.Z. LeGeros, M. Gineste ,A. Guilhem, G. Bonel, Physico chemical characterization of deposits associated with HA-ceramics implanted in osseous sites. J Biomed Mater Res. 22(3 Suppl): 257-68 (1988)

[14] P. Frayssinet, A. Guilhem, Cell transfection using HA-ceramics. Bioprocessing Journal, 3, 4 (2004)

[15] W. Zou. Immunosuppressive networks in the tumour environment and their therapeutic relevance. Nature Reviews 5: 263-274, (2005).

[16] L. M. Liau, R. M. Prins, S. M. Kiertscher, S. K. Odesa, T. J. Kremen, A. J. Giovannone, J.-W. Li, D. J. Chute, P. S. Mischel, T. F. Cloughesy, and M. D. Roth. Dendritic cell vaccination in glioblastoma patients induces systemic and intracranial T-cell responses modulated by the local central nervous system tumor microenvironment. Clinical Cancer Research 11: 5515-5525, (2005).

[17] G. P. Dunn, I. F. Dunn, and T. W. Curry. Focus on TILs: prognostic significance of tumor infiltrating lymphocytes in human glioma. Cancer Immunity 7: 12-27, (2007).

[18] K. Miller, M. Wang , J. Gralow, M. Dickler, M. Cobleigh, E.A. Perez, T. Shenkier, D. Cella, N.E. Davidson: Paclitaxel plus bevacizumab versus paclitaxel alone for metastatic breast cancer. N Engl J Med , 357: 2666-2676, (2007).

[19] N. Ferrara, K. J. Hillan, H.-P. Gerber, W. Novotny. Discovery and development of bevacizumab, an anti-VEGF antibody for treating cancer. Nature Reviews Drug Discovery, 3: 391-400, (2004)

[20] P. Frayssinet, N. Rouquet, M. Bausero, and P.O. Vidalain, Calcium Phosphates for Cell Transfection. In: P. Ducheyne, K.E. Healy, D.W. Hutmacher, D.W. Grainger, C.J. Kirkpatrick (eds.) Comprehensive Biomaterials, vol. 1, pp. 259-265 Elsevier (2011).

[21] Q. He, A.R. Mitchell, S.L. Johnson, C. Wagner-Bartak, T. Morcol, S. J. D., Bell, Calcium Phosphate Nanoparticle Adjuvant, Clinical and diagnostic laboratory immunology, 899–903 (2000)

[22] P. Gagnon, P., Ng,J., Zhen, C. Aberin, J. He, H. Mekosh, L. Cummings, , S. Zaidi, R. Richieri, A ceramic hydroxyapatite-based purification platform. Simultaneous removal of leached protein A, aggregates, DNA, and endotoxins from Mabs. Bioprocess International, 50-60 (2006).

[23] V. Hornung, F. Bauernfeind, A. Halle, E. Samstad, H. Kono, K.L. Rock, K. A. Fitzgerald, E. Latz, Silica crystals and aluminum salts mediate NALP-3 inflammasome activation via phagosomal destabilization. Nat Immunol.; 9(8): 847–856 (2008)

[24] D.R. Ciocca, P. Frayssinet, F.D. Cuello-Carion, A pilot study with a therapeutic vaccine based on hydroxyapatite ceramic particles and self-antigens in cancer patients. Cell Stress &Chaperones; 12: 33-43, 2007

[25] Y. Oki, P. McLaughlin, L. E. Fayad, B. Pro, P. F. Mansfield, G. L. Clayman, L. J. Medeiros, L. W. Kwak, P. K. Srivastava, and A. Younes. Experience with Heat shock protein-peptide complex 96 vaccine therapy in patients with indolent non-hodgkin lymphoma. Cancer 109: 77-83, (2007).

Chapter 11

Ceramic-On-Ceramic Joints: A Suitable Alternative Material Combination?

Susan C. Scholes and Thomas J. Joyce

Additional information is available at the end of the chapter

1. Introduction

Total hip replacement (THR) surgery has been available for several decades and is now a relatively common procedure. Since the introduction of the Charnley metal-on-ultra-high molecular weight polyethylene (UHMWPE) hip prosthesis, THR is seen as one of the most successful orthopaedic operations available today. There are currently over 80,000 hip replacement procedures carried out in England and Wales [1] each year and THR has now become more popular with the younger, more active patient. This is shown in the statistics reported in the National Joint Registry; 12% of the patients who undergo THR are under the age of 55 and 85% of these are recorded as being either fit and healthy (16%) or with mild disease that is not incapacitating (69%) [1]. However, failure of these artificial joints does occur, leading to the need for revision surgery; approximately 10% of the THR procedures reported are revision operations [1].

Failure, in many cases, is due to aseptic loosening [1, 2]. With the conventional metal-on-UHMWPE joint this has been shown to be due to wear particle induced osteolyisis [3]. Although 90% of these joints are operating well 15 years after implantation [2] this wear particle induced osteolysis may lead to repetitive revision requirements for the younger, more active patient.

An alternative to the conventional metal-on-UHMWPE type of hip joint is to use ceramic-on-ceramic joints. Ceramic-on-ceramic joints were first introduced in the early 1970s but often resulted in poor performance due to fixation problems, poor quality alumina as a result of inadequately controlled grain size and other material properties (leading to catastrophic wear), and sub optimal design parameters such as too large a clearance. The work of many people over the years, including material scientists and engineers, has improved the quality of these ceramics. Therefore, since the introduction of the standard for ceramic production

(ISO 6474:1981 (second-generation ceramics), which was replaced with ISO 6474:1994 (third-generation ceramics) and has now been replaced by ISO 6474-1:2010 (fourth-generation ceramics)) the performance of these all ceramic bearings has been greatly improved [4, 5]. The third and fourth-generation alumina ceramics are manufactured using hot isostatic pressing. This produces a material that is highly pure with a small grain size ($\leq$ 2.5 µm and many manufacturers produce ceramics with even smaller grain sizes) that provides material strength and minimises the risk of fracture. The majority of the ceramic-on-ceramic joints discussed in this chapter were produced using third-generation ceramics.

Ceramic-on-ceramic hip prosthesis performance will be reviewed in this chapter (*in vitro* and *in vivo*) along with a discussion of the concerns with ceramic-on-ceramic joints that happen in a minority of cases such as joint "squeaking" and component fracture. The majority of articles reviewed discuss the performance of alumina-on-alumina joints. There are, however, other ceramic materials available on the market today for use in orthopaedic surgery, for example BIOLOX® delta (an alumina matrix composite containing 72.5% alumina, 25.5% zirconia, and 2% mixed oxides). The reader will be made aware when joints made from this material are discussed.

2. Ceramic-on-ceramic hip prosthesis performance

The performance of ceramic-on-ceramic hip joints has been evaluated using data obtained from joints operating well within the body, prostheses retrieved due to joint failure and also tests performed within the laboratory. Firstly, the *in vitro* laboratory tests results will be discussed, then the *in vivo* data will be given. In addition to this, "squeaking", one of the most common concerns relating to ceramic-on-ceramic joints will be discussed.

2.1. *In vitro*

The majority of recent papers discussing the tribology (lubrication, friction and wear) of ceramic-on-ceramic hip joints detail tests done under 'severe' conditions such as malpositioning, edge-loading or microseparation. There are, however, some earlier studies that describe how these joints operate under 'standard' conditions.

A well positioned ceramic-on-ceramic hip, tested under the loads and motions expected during the standard walking cycle, performs exceptionally well in terms of friction, lubrication and wear [6-24]. Friction tests using different viscosities of carboxy-methyl cellulose (CMC) solution show that these joints operate close to full-fluid film lubrication with very low friction factors (0.002 at physiological viscosities) [6, 12]. These ceramic-on-ceramic joints have been shown to have very low surface roughness values that play a part in this low friction [6]. Tests were also performed using different viscosities of bovine serum [6, 12]. Bovine serum is often used in the laboratory as a replacement for the body's natural lubricating fluid, synovial fluid, as it contains proteins that act in a similar manner to those present in synovial fluid and although CMC fluids replicate the shear-thinning behaviour of synovial fluid, they do not contain any proteins. The introduction of these proteins into the lubricating fluid resulted in higher friction (0.03 at physiological viscosities) and mixed lubrication. These results are shown as Stribeck plots in Figure 1. A Stribeck plot shows the measured friction factor plotted against Sommerfeld number (a dimensionless parameter dependent on the lubricant viscosity, the entraining velocity of the bearing surfaces, the joint radius and the load applied). A rising trend of friction factor with increasing Sommerfeld number is indicative of a full-fluid film lubrication regime, whereas a falling trend is normally indicative of mixed lubrication. In full-fluid film lubrication, the surfaces are completely separated by the lubricant and the friction generated is due solely to the shearing of the lubricant film. In mixed lubrication, the load is carried in part by the contact between the asperities of the bearing surfaces and also by the pressure generated within the lubricant. Although the bovine serum tests suggested that these ceramic-on-ceramic joints were operating in mixed lubrication with some asperity contact, there was no surface damage evident on the joints after testing. It was speculated that the proteins that adhere to the ceramic surfaces when using protein-based lubricants produce a sufficiently thick layer to penetrate the fluid film and result in protein-to-protein contact and shearing. It is likely that the subsequent friction developed by the protein-to-protein contact is greater than that due to the shearing of the lubricant film alone. Therefore, although higher friction and mixed lubrication is encountered when testing under more physiological lubricating conditions, there is still little asperity contact during the normal walking cycle [12].

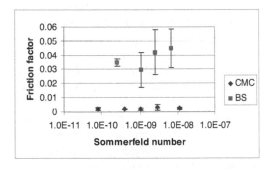

Figure 1. Stribeck plot for ceramic-on-ceramic joints (Scholes *et al* (2006) [12]). CMC: CMC fluids; BS: bovine serum.

With this good lubrication and low surface roughness the wear volumes produced under 'standard' conditions in the laboratory have, inevitably, been shown to be very low (less than 0.4 mg/million cycles cf. approximately 35 mg/million cycles for conventional metal or ceramic-on-UHMWPE joints, see Table 1), and sometimes almost immeasurable. As these ceramic-on-ceramic joints are working close to full-fluid film lubrication there is little or no contacting of the asperities on the joint surfaces leading to this low wear and friction [6, 12]. Also, laboratory studies have shown that cup malpositioning and elevated swing phase load testing have not significantly affected the wear of these joints [21, 22, 25, 26], see Table 2. This combination should, therefore, lead to a very successful artificial joint.

Reference	Material combination	Components	Wear rate (mg/million cycles)
[27]	Metal-on-UHMWPE	UHMWPE cup	47.4
[27]	Ceramic (zirconia)-on-UHMWPE	UHMWPE cup	37.9
[28]	Metal-on-UHMWPE	UHMWPE cup	~33.7
[28]	Ceramic (zirconia)-on-UHMWPE	UHMWPE cup	~29.0
[29]	Metal-on-UHMWPE	UHMWPE cup	~40.9
[29]	Ceramic (zirconia)-on-UHMWPE	UHMWPE cup	~29.5
[13]	Ceramic-on-ceramic	Head and cup	~0.25
[16]	Ceramic-on-ceramic	Head and cup	~0.16
[17]	Ceramic-on-ceramic	Head and cup	< 0.04
[18]	Ceramic-on-ceramic	Head and cup	0.09
[24]	Ceramic-on-ceramic	Head and cup	~0.20

Table 1. Wear rates found for well-positioned conventional metal or ceramic-on-UHMWPE and ceramic-on-ceramic joints under standard testing conditions

More severe loading conditions have, however, given slightly different results. Microseparation was first introduced during the swing phase of the walking cycle on the Leeds hip wear simulator [30] to replicate the stripe wear sometimes seen on retrieved ceramic-on-ceramic joints. Microseparation was incorporated in the simulator studies at Leeds because a year earlier, it was suggested by Mallory *et al* (1999) [31] that this separation of the femoral head and acetabular cup can occur in conventional metal-on-UHMWPE joints. Nevelos *et al* (2000) [30] hypothesised that a similar mechanism may take place in ceramic-on-ceramic joints resulting in the visible stripe wear found on some retrievals. Microseparation was, therefore, set up in the simulator and involved separation of the femoral head and acetabular cup during the swing phase of walking leading to relocation (with rim contact and edge-loading) during heel strike before the head then relocated in the cup in the stance phase (see Figure 2). The surface damage caused by this rim contact resulted in what is known as stripe wear.

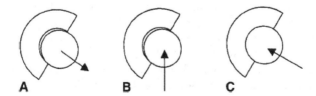

A   B   C

Figure 2. Microseparation as applied in the Leeds simulator by Nevelos *et al* (2000) [30]. (A) Swing phase: microseparation. (B) Heel-strike: rim contact. (C) Stance phase: relocation.

Using this microseparation technique, Nevelos *et al* (2000) [30] found slightly higher wear rates with ceramic-on-ceramic joints than found under 'standard' conditions (see Table 2). This study, however, was relatively short-term (800,000 cycles). Longer-term tests performed by Stewart *et al* (2001) [32] on the same simulator gave similar results to those found by Nevelos *et al* (2000) [30]. Other workers have also found an increase in wear rate with microseparation [33]. More recent work performed by Al-Hajjar *et al* (2010) [25] studied BI-OLOX® delta couplings. These joints gave lower wear than that found for alumina-on-alumina joints. Microseparation of the BIOLOX® delta joint surfaces, again, resulted in higher wear. The wear rates found using microseparation are, however, still extremely low in comparison with conventional joints (see Tables 1 and 2).

Reference	Wear conditions	Components	Average wear rate (mg/million cycles)
[11]	Standard	Cup only	< 0.02
[13]	Standard	Not stated	~0.25
[16]	Standard	Head and cup	~0.16
[17]	Standard	Head and cup	< 0.04
[18]	Standard	Head and cup	0.09
[19]	Standard	Cup only	~0.40
[21]	Standard	Not stated	~0.24
[22]	Standard	Cup only	~0.32
[24]	Standard	Head and cup	~0.20
[21]	Elevated cup angle	Not stated	~0.20
[25]	Elevated cup angle	Not stated	0.20
[22]	Elevated swing phase load	Cup only	0.36
[25]	Microseparation	Not stated	0.52
[30]	Microseparation	Not stated	4.78 (after 800,000 cycles)
[32]	Microseparation	Not stated	(mild) ~0.40 (severe) ~5.17
[33]	Microseparation	Head and cup	1.55

Table 2. Wear rates found for alumina-on-alumina joints under standard testing conditions and microseparation

It is still unknown if it is this microseparation that causes the stripe wear that is observed on some retrievals or whether this type of wear is due simply to edge-loading of the head on the cup through a different mechanism. Higher rates of wear including the appearance of stripe wear may also be due to a steep acetabular cup implantation angle or repeated dislocations [34]. Microseparation, or edge-loading, may occur during various different physical activities such as stair climbing, standing from squat position and deep flexion. It may, however, also occur during walking. These simulator studies incorporating microseparation of the head and cup into the walking cycle are therefore a severe testing method. The resulting rim contact and stripe wear does, however, replicate the more severe conditions that these joints may encounter thus producing the same effect that is seen on some retrievals but not necessarily through the correct corresponding actions.

If, and when, wear of these ceramic components occurs it is important to understand how the body is likely to react to these wear particles. It is well known that wear particle induced osteolysis is a major concern for conventional metal-on-UHMWPE joints [3] but is this the case for ceramic-on-ceramic prostheses? Promisingly, several workers have shown that the cellular response to ceramic particles is less severe than that due to polyethylene particles [35, 15]. An important point to note with the laboratory tests discussed above is that, even under extreme loading and motion conditions, these joints provide low wear with a minimal adverse tissue reaction to these wear particles. As stated by Fisher *et al* (2006) [15], the combination of low wear and low reactivity means that '...ceramic-on-ceramic bearings address the tribological lifetime demand of highly active patients.'.

2.2. *In vivo*

As shown above, the laboratory test results for ceramic-on-ceramic joints are very promising. Is this mirrored by the *in vivo* performance? There are many publications detailing the performance of ceramic-on-ceramic hip joints in the body. A selection of these papers is discussed below to give a general overview of joint performance using this material combination.

The short-term (mean follow-up of 50.4 months) performance of ceramic-on-ceramic joints was compared to that of metal-on-highly cross linked polyethylene (XLPE) joints in a study reported by Bascarevic *et al* (2010) [36]. Seventy-five metal-on-highly XLPE hips (72 patients) and 82 ceramic-on-ceramic hips (78 patients) were assessed. Both were found to work well with no revisions performed on the ceramic-on-ceramic joints compared with 2 revisions necessary for the metal-on-highly XLPE group. The authors commented that ceramic-on-ceramic components manufactured using third-generation ceramics were "especially suited for hip arthroplasty in young and active persons".

A comparative study was also performed by Amanatullah *et al* (2011) [37]. The short-term performance (60 months) of 125 ceramic-on-ceramic hip joints was assessed against 95 ceramic-on-UHMWPE prostheses. In this study both the material combinations preformed well and no statistically significant difference was found between the clinical outcome scores for the two types of prosthesis, however, one important point to note is that audible noise such as "squeaking" did occur in 3.1%. of the ceramic-on-ceramic hips. "Squeaking" is a phenomenon reported by others and this will be discussed later. It was noted that this is a short-term study (five years) and, as the metal-on-UHMWPE hips did not produce as low wear rates in the radiographic analysis, osteolysis may occur at a later stage.

Another short-term study comparing the results of 525 hips (421 ceramic-on-ceramic and 104 metal-on-UHMWPE) was reported by Johansson *et al* (2011) [38]. These joints had been implanted for an average of 59 months. The survival rates were 98% and 92% for the ceramic-on-ceramic and metal-on-UHMWPE hip joints respectively.

A short-term study (60 month follow-up) reported by Nikolaou *et al* (2012) [39] assessed and compared the performance of 36 metal-on-UHMWPE, 32 metal-on-highly XLPE and 34 third-generation ceramic-on-ceramic hip joints. The apparent wear of the bearing surfaces was assessed radiologically. The ceramic-on-ceramic joints showed the lowest wear (mean linear wear 0.035 mm) and the metal-on-highly XLPE gave nearly 3 times lower wear than the metal-on-UHMWPE joints (0.329 mm cf. 0.869 mm). At 60 months, no difference in clinical outcome was found for these three different material combinations. "Squeaking" was observed in 3 (8.8%) of the ceramic-on-ceramic joints; no revision procedures were necessary as a results of this squeaking though.

Early to mid-term results were also reported by Stafford *et al* (2012) [40]. At a mean follow-up of 59 months six of these 250 ceramic-on-ceramic hips were revised. Two were revised for recurrent dislocation secondary to impingement, two for deep infection, one for recurrent dislocation and one due to fracture of the femoral head. Although no patients experienced "squeaking", six described a grinding or crunching noise that was experienced mainly during deep flexion. One of these "squeaking joints" was a BIOLOX® delta ceramic prosthesis. Again, no revision surgery was performed on these noisy joints.

Mesko *et al* (2011) [41] assessed the outcome of 930 ceramic-on-ceramic hips over 10 years that were implanted by nine different surgeons. The survivorship at 10 years (96.8%) was referred to as 'excellent' with 0.9% fracture, 2.3% dislocation and 2.5% reported incidents of noise such as clicking, squeaking, popping, or creaking.

Another 10 year follow-up was reported by Yeung *et al* (2012) [42]. The clinical information was available for 244 hips (227 patients) and the radiographic information was available for 184 hips (172 patients). The success of these joints led to an overall survival rate of 98% (again, with revision for any reason as the end point).

In a multicentre study performed by Capello *et al* (2008) [43], 452 patients (475 hips) were assessed. The majority of the hips implanted were ceramic-on-ceramic (380) whilst the remainder (95) were conventional metal-on-UHMWPE and used as a comparison. The average patient age was 53 years and there was an average 8 year follow-up period. The authors found the clinical results to be excellent. The ten-year Kaplan-Meier survivorship (with revision of either component for any reason given as the end-point) was stated as 95.9% for the ceramic-on-ceramic hip joints and 91.3% for metal-on-UHMWPE. The ceramic joints, therefore, performed better than the conventional joints and because one of the major causes of failure for conventional metal-on-UHMWPE joints is late aseptic loosening due to osteolysis, a longer term study is likely to give a greater difference in survivorship ratings. Of the ceramic-on-ceramic failures requiring revision, only 2/380 (0.5%) were due to ceramic fractures. Therefore, overall it was concluded that the third-generation ceramic-on-ceramic hip joints performed well clinically and radiographically in this young patient group. Although these joints performed relatively well "squeaking" was reported in 3/380 (0.8%) cases for the ceramic-on-ceramic joints.

In the study reported by Lee *et al* (2010) [44], the ten year survival rate of 88 ceramic-on-ceramic hip joints, with revision of either the head or the cup for any reason being as the end point, was 99.0%. These results were taken after a minimum of 10 years postoperatively and are, indeed, very promising.

A long-term study on earlier generation ceramic joints was performed by Hernigou *et al* (2009) [45]. This was a comparative study which investigated the wear and osteolysis of 28 bilateral arthroplasties (one ceramic-on-ceramic and the contralateral ceramic-on-UHMWPE). All of these joints (ceramic-on-ceramic and ceramic-on-UHMWPE) had lasted 20 years without the need for revision surgery. Computer tomography (CT scan) was used to assess the number and volume of osteolytic lesions present. Fewer osteolytic lesions were found on the side with the ceramic-on-ceramic joint; there were 13 cases of pelvic osteolysis found and 15 joints showed evidence of femoral osteolysis (cf. 24 joints with pelvic osteolysis and 23 with femoral osteolysis for the ceramic-on-UHMWPE joints). Also, in each patient, the diameter, surface and volume of osteolysis was substantially lower on the side with the ceramic-on-ceramic hip implant than the ceramic-on-UHMWPE joint. It must also be remembered that these joints were manufactured using first-generation ceramics and the ceramics produced to the standard expected for third and fourth-generation ceramics are expected to perform even better.

Another longer-term study (mean 20.8 years), again with earlier generation ceramics, performed by Petsatodis *et al* (2010) [46] also showed good results. There were 100 patients in this study, all with at least one ceramic-on-ceramic hip joint (109 hips) and, again, a young patient population (average age 46 years). The cumulative rate of survival was quoted as being 84.4% at 20.8 years.

Although these results are promising, in the majority of cases, the follow-up period particularly for the third generation ceramics, was only short-term. It will, therefore be very interesting to evaluate the performance of these third and fourth-generation ceramic-on-ceramic joints, along with the metal and ceramic-on-highly XLPE, on a longer-term basis. These results are eagerly anticipated.

The papers discussed so far have shown exceptional performance of ceramic-on-ceramic joints and suggests that these joints may perform better than metal or ceramic-on UHMWPE. This, however, is not reflected in the data described in the National Joint Registry (NJR) of England and Wales (2011) [1]. Promisingly though, the NJR states that there is 'little substantive difference' in the risk of revision for ceramic-on-ceramic, ceramic-on-polyethylene or metal-on-polyethylene joints. It is, however, not stated whether this polyethylene is UHMWPE or XLPE and the differences in performance between these two materials is not listed.

Although, as discussed above, many of these ceramic-on-ceramic hip joints perform exceptionally well, early dislocation is seen as a possible concern due to limited modular neck length and other factors. In the majority of the published literature referred to in this text [47, 36, 48, 43, 49, 50, 46, 51-57, 41, 40], the occurrence of dislocation is 0% - 2.3%. The number of dislocations was higher (6%) in a study reported by Chevillotte *et al* (2011) [58], however, no reoperation was required for any of these cases. Colwell *et al* (2007) [53] summarised other published literature detailing the number of dislocations in ceramic-on-ceramic hip joints in comparison with metal-on-polyethylene and found no difference between the two material combinations. In addition to this Amanatulla et al (2011) [37] and Bascarevic et al (2010) [36] showed no difference in the number of dislocations for ceramic-on-ceramic and ceramic-on-UHMWPE or metal-on-highly XLPE hip prostheses. Often there is no need for revision surgery after dislocation, unless it is recurrent dislocation.

Component fracture in ceramic-on-ceramic hips is another cause for concern for many surgeons and patients. The fracture rates of ceramic joints have been dramatically reduced since the introduction of third and fourth-generation ceramics with the new material processing methods. Ceramic-on-ceramic joints have strict regulations that must be abided by with regard to material properties such as burst strength; as discussed in work reported by Salih et al (2009) [59]. However, fracture of these components does still occur, leading to catastrophic joint failure and revision surgery. In the majority of cases though, this fracture rate is extremely low (0% - 0.5%) [60, 61, 43, 49, 45, 50, 46, 51, 48, 55, 57, 40]. Some reports do, however, give a higher rate of post-operative fracture (1-2.3%) [62, 44, 37, 42, 47, 39]. Fracture is often associated with trauma, however a multicentre review reported by Park et al (2006) [63] discussed the performance of 357 third-generation ceramic-on-ceramic THRs and fracture occurred under normal activities in six of these hips (1.7%). This design used a polyethylene-ceramic composite liner within a titanium alloy shell and the high rate of fracture led to the authors discontinuing its use. It must be recognised though that, in general, the rate of fracture for ceramic-on-ceramic hip joints is very low. In fact, an article describing the fracture of ceramic joints (Hannouche et al (2003) [64]) stated that during a 25 year period (1977 – 2001) 11 (less than 0.004%) of the 3300 ceramic-on-ceramic joints reported on failed due to fracture. This low rate of fracture is from ceramics produced using earlier versions of the ISO standard and, so, this is expected to reduce even further and many studies using third-generation ceramics have reported no failures due to fracture [51, 36, 65, 66], Fracture must, however, still be recognised as a risk (albeit very low) with ceramic-on-ceramic joints.

For what other reasons does failure occur? Savarino et al (2009) [67] analysed the clinical, radiographic, laboratory and microbiological data from 30 retrieved ceramic-on-ceramic hip components. They concluded that failure was due to malpositioning of the joint during surgery leading to mechanical instability, or trauma or infection. Loosening in this selection of joints was not due to wear debris induced osteolysis. They indicated that the wear debris produced by these joints and the osteolysis present were the effect of the loosening, rather than the cause. It is stated that correct positioning of the implant is crucial. This has also been stated by other workers [54].

A case study was reported by Nam et al (2007) [68] discussing a failed ceramic-on-ceramic hip joint where failure was stated as being caused by alumina debris-induced osteolysis. A sixty-three year old woman underwent bilateral THR in 1998. Eight years later the patient returned to the clinic for routine follow-up and was experiencing no discomfort or worrying symptoms. However, the radiographs taken showed expansive osteolytic lesions. After revision surgery a histologic analysis of the retrieved tissues showed alumina particles within the cytoplasm of macrophages and in intercellular tissue suggesting wear particle induced osteolysis. Alumina wear particle-induced osteolysis is, however, a very rare phenomenon.

Chang *et al* (2009) [69] reported on the clinical and radiographic outcomes when using third-generation ceramic-on-ceramic joints in revision THR of 42 failed metal-on-UHMWPE hips. This was an interesting study as most published literature discuss the choice of bearing material for primary surgery and, as stated by the authors, '...few studies have focussed on the choice of bearing surface in revision...'. This was a young patient group (mean age: 48.8 years, range: 32 – 59 years) and the mean length of time between primary and revision surgery was 9.5 years (range: 3.3 – 16.1 years). The mean duration of follow-up after this revision surgery was 64 months (range: 38 – 96 months). At the time of publication of this article, no hips needed additional revision surgery and no hips showed radiolucent lines, acetabular cup migration or osteolysis. This study gives very favourable results for the use of ceramic-on-ceramic hip joints in revision surgery, especially for the younger patient as the likelihood of the need for further revision is greater.

3. The "squeaking" hip

Another concern with hard-on-hard bearing couples such as ceramic-on-ceramic and metal-on-metal is the incidence of noise or "squeaking" in these joints. Audible sounds such as squeaking, clicking, snapping, cracking, grinding, rustling, crunching and tinkling are all referred to in this text as "squeaking". "Squeaking" can be present during different kinds of activity including stair climbing, bending forward, squatting, standing from a chair and walking. The occurrence of this "squeaking" has been reported by many workers to different degrees.

Jarrett *et al* (2009) [52] described a group of 131 patients from which 14 (10.7%) suffered an audible "squeak" during normal activities (however, only 4 of these patients were able to reproduce the "squeak" during the clinical review session). They stated that none of the patients had undergone revision surgery specifically because of "squeaking", however, longer-term follow-up was needed to monitor this noise.

Mai *et al* (2010) [70] reported noise or "squeaking" in 17% of 320 ceramic-on-ceramic hips and Keurentjes *et al* (2008) [71] found "squeaking" in 20.9% of cases. From their study they concluded that short neck length of the femoral component was a potential risk factor for "squeaking".

A study performed by Cogan *et al* (2010) [72] reported on the occurrence of "squeaking" in a patient population with at least one ceramic-on-ceramic hip; 10.6% of 265 hips demonstrated "squeaking". Two other published studies report on "squeaking" in 15% and 8.8% of the patient population [44, 39]. Other published literature suggests that "squeaking" occurs in 0% - 6% of patients [73-75, 40, 65, 50, 61, 56, 76, 43, 49, 51, 37, 58, 41, 77]. The "squeaking" phenomenon tends to appear at an average of 28.8 months (range of averages 5.7 - 66 months) post-operatively.

After 10 years of follow-up Chevillotte *et al* (2012) [73] discussed the performance of 100, third-generation ceramic-on-ceramic joints. By use of a questionnaire, 5% of these patients reported the occurrence of "squeaking". All of these patients were active, sporty and heavy men. "Squeaking" was not related to any malpositioning, wear or loosening of the joint and none of the 100 patient group suffered from any component fracture. In this paper it was stated that "squeaking" noise seems to be an isolated phenomenon with no consequences for the patient regarding functional results and on the implant longevity at 10 years of follow-up'.

The largest study to date (Sexton *et al* (2011)) [75] reported on the occurrence of "squeaking" and the role of patient factors and implant positioning in 2406 ceramic-on-ceramic hips at a mean follow-up of 10.6 years. Seventy-four hips (73 patients, 3.1%) made "squeaking" sounds at a mean time post-operatively of 40 months. Taller, heavier and younger patients with higher activity levels were found to be more at risk of developing a "squeaking" hip. However, there was no relationship between BMI and the prevalence of "squeaking". Interestingly, it was found that at a mean follow-up of 9.5 years, 11 of these hips (15%) had stopped "squeaking". Therefore, "squeaking" is not necessarily a permanent complication.

There is great debate over the cause of "squeaking" in ceramic-on-ceramic THRs. Several possible causes of "squeaking" are edge-loading [78], component malpositioning [78-80] or component or stem design [74, 81, 70, 77]. Other workers have also related "squeaking" to patient weight, height or age [70, 78, 79]. It is possible that a number of factors need to be present to initiate the "squeaking" phenomenon. The occurrence of "squeaking" has not been found to compromise the results of ceramic-on-ceramic hip joints; however, some patients do request revision surgery in order to solve the "squeaking" issue [82].

Recently, laboratory studies have been performed in an attempt to re-create the conditions required to generate this "squeaking". Some authors have observed "squeaking" with ceramic-on-ceramic hip joints lubricated under dry conditions [83, 84, 73]. However, such an extreme lubrication regime is not expected to occur *in vivo* [85]. Work performed by Currie *et al* (2010) [86] suggested that the rolling/sliding mechanism of the bearing surfaces can induce vibration, of an audible frequency, resulting in "squeaking". Under lubricated conditions, Sanders *et al* (2012) [85] were able to reproduce the "squeak" using edge-loading during short-term wear tests. The "squeaking" was found to occur with a high contact force centred above or near the margin of the wear patch on a previously edge-worn femoral head. The authors state 'the results reveal key conditions that yield recurrent squeaking *in vitro* in various scenarios without resorting to implausible dry conditions'. In support of this, Walter *et al* (2011) [87] analysed 12 ceramic-on-ceramic components retrieved from "squeaking" joints and compared these with 33 'silent' ceramic-on-ceramic hip retrievals. All 12 "squeaking" hips showed evidence of edge-loading with up to 45 times greater wear than that reported for then the 33 'silent' hips [54]. The authors suggested that although the causes of "squeaking" are unknown, the high contact pressures experienced during edge-loading may result in a breakdown of the fluid film lubrication leading to some asperity contact and an increase in friction. Also, any surface damage, which may have been caused by the edge-loading, will result in an increased roughness of the bearing surfaces thus leading to possible destruction of the fluid film leading to asperity contact.

Although there are a few reports on poor ceramic-on-ceramic hip prosthesis performance, the majority of authors give good and optimistic results. There have been little or no fractures, dislocation, infection or osteolysis. Also, the few patients suffering from "squeaking" hips have, in the majority of cases, had no need for revision surgery. These are, therefore, excellent results, but Lee *et al* (2010) [44] did suggest that these small risks should be a concern to surgeons and that patients should also be made aware of these before surgery. In addition to this, they mentioned that longer-term follow-up is needed to assess the effects of these small risks on the prosthesis performance.

4. The younger patient

As these artificial hip joints have been found to perform well in the younger patient (45 to 55 years), some surgeons have chosen to replace the diseased joints of even younger patients with this material combination.

A case study was reported by Capello and Feinberg (2009) [88] where ceramic-on-ceramic joints were implanted in a 13 year-old child with bilateral end-stage arthritis of the hip. Seven and eight years post-operatively the patient had no pain, no limp, and was able to walk long distances. The radiographs showed no implant loosening, osteolysis or wear. This is a very encouraging result, however, it was stated that the patient is still very young (20 years of age at the time of report) and, therefore, the need for revision surgery will be more than likely.

Other studies on younger patients have not had as good results as those reported by Capello though. Nizard *et al* (2008) [89] reported on ceramic-on-ceramic hips that had been implanted in a group of 101 patients (132 hips) younger than 30 years old (mean age: 23.4 years, range: 13 – 30 years). These joints were implanted from 1977 to 2004 and, because of this, different implant designs and modes of fixation were used. Of these 132 joints, 17 were revised for aseptic loosening leading to a survivorship of 82.1% at 10 years and 72.4% at 15 years. These survivorship rates are quite low and may create cause for concern. It was, however, found that the higher rate of failures of joints replaced for treatment of slipped capital epiphysis or trauma influenced the survivorships greatly. Also, these artificial hip joints were implanted over a period of 26.5 years, during which time the ceramic materials have been improved and the fixation methods have changed. It is hoped that ceramic of the new generation with improved prosthesis design and mode of fixation will perform better and provide improved longer-term results.

5. Overview

From the results reported here it is clear that ceramic-on-ceramic hip joints have good tribological results: low friction, good lubrication and very low wear *in vitro* and *in vivo*. In addition to this, ceramic particles are biologically inert. Also, the fracture risk is relatively low. With good implant positioning these joints have the potential to perform incredibly well. These bearings, therefore, deserve to be high on the list for both primary and revision implants, especially for the younger, more active patient. However, for the best results, the choice of bearing combination/design should be patient-specific; as one design does not suit all.

Author details

Susan C. Scholes and Thomas J. Joyce

*Address all correspondence to: susan.scholes@newcastle.ac.uk

School of Mechanical and Systems Engineering, Newcastle University, Newcastle-upon-Tyne, UK

References

[1] National Joint Registry for England and Wales. 8th Annual Report. 2011.

[2] The Swedish Hip Arthroplasty Register. Annual Report 2008. 2008.

[3] Harris WH. The Problem Is Osteolysis. Clin Orthop Rel Res. 1995(311):46-53.

[4] Sedel L, Kerboull L, Christel P, Meunier A, Witvoet J. Alumina-on-Alumina Hip-Replacement - Results and Survivorship in Young-Patients. J Bone Joint Surg-Br Vol. 1990;72(4):658-63.

[5] Walter A. On the Material and the Tribology of Alumina Alumina Couplings for Hip-Joint Prostheses. Clin Orthop Rel Res. 1992(282):31-46.

[6] Scholes SC, Unsworth A. Comparison of friction and lubrication of different hip prostheses. Proc Inst Mech Eng Part H-J Eng Med. 2000;214(H1):49-57.

[7] Scholes SC, Unsworth A, Hall RM, Scott R. The effects of material combination and lubricant on the friction of total hip prostheses. Wear. 2000;241(2):209-13.

[8] Scholes SC, Unsworth A, Goldsmith AAJ. A frictional study of total hip joint replacements. Phys Med Biol. 2000;45(12):3721-35.

[9] Vassiliou K, Scholes SC, Unsworth A. Laboratory studies on the tribology of hard bearing hip prostheses: ceramic on ceramic and metal on metal. Proc Inst Mech Eng Part H-J Eng Med. 2007;221(H1 Special Issue):11-20.

[10] Scholes SC, Green SM, Unsworth A. The friction and lubrication of alumina-on-alumina total hip prostheses - The effect of radial clearance and wear testing. Bioceramics 14. Key Engineering Materials, 2002. p. 535-9.

[11] Scholes SC, Green SM, Unsworth A. Nanotribological characterisation of alumina femoral heads using an atomic force microscope. Bioceramics 14. Key Engineering Materials, 2002. p. 543-7.

[12] Scholes SC, Unsworth A. The effect of proteins on the friction and lubrication of arti-
      ficial joints. Proc Inst Mech Eng Part H-J Eng Med. 2006;220(H6):687-93.

[13] Spinelli M, Affatat S, Corvil A, Viceconti M. Ceramic-on-ceramic vs. metal-on-metal
      in total hip arthroplasty (THA): do 36-mm diameters exhibit comparable wear per-
      formance? Materialwissenschaft Und Werkstofftechnik. 2009;40(1-2):94-7. doi:
      10.1002/mawe.200800381.

[14] Brockett C, Williams S, Jin Z-M, Isaac G, Fisher J. Friction of total hip replacements
      with different bearings and loading conditions. Journal of Biomedical Materials Re-
      search Part B-Applied Biomaterials. 2007;81B:508-15.

[15] Fisher J, Jin ZM, Tipper J, Stone M, Ingham E. Presidential guest lecture - Tribology
      of alternative beatings. Clin Orthop Rel Res. 2006(453):25-34. doi:10.1097/01.blo.
      0000238871.07604.49.

[16] Essner A, Sutton K, Wang A. Hip simulator wear comparison of metal-on-metal, ce-
      ramic-on-ceramic and crosslinked UHMWPE bearings. Wear. 2005;259:992-5. doi:
      10.1016/j.wear.2005.02.104.

[17] Richardson HA, Clarke IC, Williams P, Donaldson T, Oonishi H. Precision and accu-
      racy in ceramic-on-ceramic wear analyses: influence of simulator test duration. Pro-
      ceedings of the Institution of Mechanical Engineers Part H-Journal of Engineering in
      Medicine. 2005;219(H6):401-5. doi:10.1243/095441105x34428.

[18] Oonishi H, Clarke IC, Good V, Amino H, Ueno M. Alumina hip joints characterized
      by run-in wear and steady-state wear to 14 million cycles in hip-simulator model.
      Journal of Biomedical Materials Research Part A. 2004;70A(4):523-32. doi:10.1002/
      jbm.a.30021.

[19] Smith SL, Unsworth A. An in vitro wear study of alumina-alumina total hip prosthe-
      ses. Proceedings of the Institution of Mechanical Engineers Part H-Journal of Engi-
      neering in Medicine. 2001;215(H5):443-6.

[20] Clarke IC, Good V, Williams P, Schroeder D, Anissian L, Stark A et al. Ultra-low
      wear rates for rigid-on-rigid bearings in total hip replacements. Proc Inst Mech Eng
      Part H-J Eng Med. 2000;214(H4):331-47.

[21] Nevelos JE, Ingham E, Doyle C, Nevelos AB, Fisher J. The influence of acetabular cup
      angle on the wear of "BIOLOX Forte" alumina ceramic bearing couples in a hip joint
      simulator. J Mater Sci-Mater Med. 2001;12(2):141-4.

[22] Nevelos JE, Ingham E, Doyle C, Nevelos AB, Fisher J. Wear of HIPed and non-HIPed
      alumina-alumina hip joints under standard and severe simulator testing conditions.
      Biomaterials. 2001;22(16):2191-7.

[23] Shishido T, Clarke IC, Williams P, Boehler M, Asano T, Shoji H et al. Clinical and
      simulator wear study of alumina ceramic THR to 17 years and beyond. Journal of Bi-
      omedical Materials Research Part B-Applied Biomaterials. 2003;67B(1):638-47. doi:
      10.1002/jbm.b.10048.

[24] Tipper JL, Firkins PJ, Besong AA, Barbour PSM, Nevelos J, Stone MH et al. Characterisation of wear debris from UHMWPE on zirconia ceramic, metal-on-metal and alumina ceramic-on-ceramic hip prostheses generated in a physiological anatomical hip joint simulator. Wear. 2001;250:120-8.

[25] Al-Hajjar M, Leslie IJ, Tipper J, Williams S, Fisher J, Jennings LM. Effect of cup inclination angle during microseparation and rim loading on the wear of BIOLOX (R) delta ceramic-on-ceramic total hip replacement. Journal of Biomedical Materials Research Part B-Applied Biomaterials. 2010;95B(2):263-8. doi:10.1002/jbm.b.31708.

[26] Affatato S, Traina F, Toni A. Microseparation and stripe wear in alumina-on-alumina hip implants. International Journal of Artificial Organs. 2011;34(6):506-12. doi: 10.5301/ijao.2011.8457.

[27] Smith SL, Unsworth A. A comparison between gravimetric and volumetric techniques of wear measurement of UHMWPE acetabular cups against zirconia and cobalt-chromium-molybdenum femoral heads in a hip simulator. Proc Inst Mech Eng Part H-J Eng Med. 1999;213(H6):475-83.

[28] Bigsby RJA, Hardaker CS, Fisher J. Wear of ultra-high molecular weight polyethylene acetabular cups in a physiological hip joint simulator in the anatomical position using bovine serum as a lubricant. Proc Inst Mech Eng Part H-J Eng Med. 1997;211(3):265-9.

[29] Barbour PSM, Stone MH, Fisher J. A hip joint simulator study using simplified loading and motion cycles generating physiological wear paths and rates. Proc Inst Mech Eng Part H-J Eng Med. 1999;213(H6):455-67.

[30] Nevelos J, Ingham E, Doyle C, Streicher R, Nevelos A, Walter W et al. Microseparation of the centers of alumina-alumina artificial hip joints during simulator testing produces clinically relevant wear rates and patterns. J Arthroplast. 2000;15(6):793-5.

[31] Mallory TH, Lombardi AV, Dennis DA, Komistek RD, Fada RA, Northcut E, editors. Do total hip arthroplasties piston during leg lift manoeuvres and gait. An in vivo determination of total hip arthroplasty during abduction/adduction leg lift and gait. 66th Annual Meeting of the American Academy of Orthopaedic Surgeons; 1999; Anaheim, California.

[32] Stewart T, Tipper J, Streicher R, Ingham E, Fisher J. Long-term wear of HIPed alumina on alumina bearings for THR under microseparation conditions. J Mater Sci-Mater Med. 2001;12(10-12):1053-6.

[33] Manaka M, Clarke IC, Yamamoto K, Shishido T, Gustafson A, Imakiire A. Stripe wear rates in alumina THR - Comparison of microseparation simulator study with retrieved implants. Journal of Biomedical Materials Research Part B-Applied Biomaterials. 2004;69B(2):149-57. doi:10.1002/jbm.b.20033.

[34] Nevelos JE, Ingham E, Doyle C, Fisher J, Nevelos AB. Analysis of retrieved alumina ceramic components from Mittelmeier total hip prostheses. Biomaterials. 1999;20(19): 1833-40.

[35] Catelas I, Huk OL, Petit A, Zukor DJ, Marchand R, Yahia LH. Flow cytometric analysis of macrophage response to ceramic and polyethylene particles: Effects of size, concentration, and composition. J Biomed Mater Res. 1998;41(4):600-7.

[36] Bascarevic Z, Vukasinovic Z, Slavkovic N, Dulic B, Trajkovic G, Bascarevic V et al. Alumina-on-alumina ceramic versus metal-on-highly cross-linked polyethylene bearings in total hip arthroplasty: a comparative study. International Orthopaedics. 2010;34(8):1129-35. doi:10.1007/s00264-009-0899-6.

[37] Amanatullah DF, Landa J, Strauss EJ, Garino JP, Kim SH, Di Cesare PE. Comparison of Surgical Outcomes and Implant Wear Between Ceramic-Ceramic and Ceramic-Polyethylene Articulations in Total Hip Arthroplasty. J Arthroplast. 2011;26(6):72-7. doi:10.1016/j.arth.2011.04.032.

[38] Johansson HR, Johnson AJ, Zywiel MG, Naughton M, Mont MA, Bonutti PM. Does Acetabular Inclination Angle Affect Survivorship of Alumina-ceramic Articulations? Clin Orthop Rel Res. 2011;469(6):1560-6. doi:10.1007/s11999-010-1623-y.

[39] Nikolaou VS, Edwards MR, Bogoch E, Schemitsch EH, Waddell JP. A prospective randomised controlled trial comparing three alternative bearing surfaces in primary total hip replacement. J Bone Joint Surg-Br Vol. 2012;94B(4):459-65. doi: 10.1302/0301-620x.94b4.27735.

[40] Stafford GH, Ul Islam S, Witt JD. Early to mid-term results of ceramic-on-ceramic total hip replacement ANALYSIS OF BEARING-SURFACE-RELATED COMPLICATIONS. J Bone Joint Surg-Br Vol. 2011;93B(8):1017-20. doi:10.1302/0301-620x. 93b8.26505.

[41] Mesko JW, D'Antonio JA, Capello WN, Bierbaum BE, Naughton M. Ceramic-on-Ceramic Hip Outcome at a 5- to 10-Year Interval. J Arthroplast. 2011;26(2):172-7. doi: 10.1016/j.arth.2010.04.029.

[42] Yeung E, Bott PT, Chana R, Jackson MP, Holloway I, Walter WL et al. Mid-Term Results of Third-Generation Alumina-on-Alumina Ceramic Bearings in Cement less Total Hip Arthroplasty A Ten-Year Minimum Follow-up. J Bone Joint Surg-Am Vol. 2012;94A(2):138-44. doi:10.2106/jbjsj.00331.

[43] Capello WN, D'Antonio JA, Feinberg JR, Manley MT, Naughton M. Ceramic-on-Ceramic Total Hip Arthroplasty: Update. J Arthroplast. 2008;23(7):39-43. doi:10.1016/ j.arth.2008.06.003.

[44] Lee YK, Ha YC, Yoo JJ, Koo KH, Yoon KS, Kim HJ. Alumina-on-Alumina Total Hip Arthroplasty A Concise Follow-up, at a Minimum of Ten Years, of a Previous Report. J Bone Joint Surg-Am Vol. 2010;92A(8):1715-9. doi:10.2106/jbjs.i.01019.

[45] Hernigou P, Zilber S, Filippini P, Poignard A. Ceramic-Ceramic Bearing Decreases Osteolysis: A 20-year Study versus Ceramic-Polyethylene on the Contralateral Hip. Clin Orthop Rel Res. 2009;467(9):2274-80. doi:10.1007/s11999-009-0773-2.

[46] Petsatodis GE, Papadopoulos PP, Papavasiliou KA, Hatzokos IG, Agathangelidis FG, Christodoulou AG. Primary Cementless Total Hip Arthroplasty with an Alumina Ceramic-on-Ceramic Bearing Results After a Minimum of Twenty Years of Follow-up. J Bone Joint Surg-Am Vol. 2010;92A(3):639-44. doi:10.2106/jbjs.h.01829.

[47] Sugano N, Takao M, Sakai T, Nishii T, Miki H, Ohzono K. Eleven- to 14-year Follow-up Results of Cementless Total Hip Arthroplasty Using a Third-generation Alumina Ceramic-on-ceramic Bearing. J Arthroplast. 2012;27(5):736-41. doi:10.1016/j.arth.2011.08.017.

[48] Mai K, Hardwick ME, Walker RH, Copp SN, Ezzet KA, Colwell CW, Jr. Early dislocation rate in ceramic-on-ceramic total hip arthroplasty. Hss J. 2008;4(1):10-3.

[49] Garcia-Cimbrelo E, Garcia-Rey E, Murcia-Mazon A, Blanco-Pozo A, Marti E. Alumina-on-alumina in THA - A multicenter prospective study. Clin Orthop Rel Res. 2008;466(2):309-16. doi:10.1007/s11999-007-0042-1.

[50] Greene JW, Malkani AL, Kolisek FR, Jessup NM, Baker DL. Ceramic-on-Ceramic Total Hip Arthroplasty. J Arthroplast. 2009;24(6):15-8. doi:10.1016/j.arth.2009.04.029.

[51] Kim YH, Choi Y, Kim JS. Cementless total hip arthroplasty with ceramic-on-ceramic bearing in patients younger than 45 years with femoral-head osteonecrosis. International Orthopaedics. 2010;34(8):1123-7. doi:10.1007/s00264-009-0878-y.

[52] Jarrett CA, Ranawat AS, Bruzzone M, Blum YC, Rodriguez JA, Ranawat CS. The Squeaking Hip: A Phenomenon of Ceramic-on-Ceramic Total Hip Arthroplasty. J Bone Joint Surg-Am Vol. 2009;91A(6):1344-9. doi:10.2106/jbjs.f.00970.

[53] Colwell CW, Jr., Hozack WJ, Mesko JW, D'Antonio JA, Bierbaum BE, Capello WN et al. Ceramic-on-ceramic total hip arthroplasty early dislocation rate. Clin Orthop Relat Res. 2007;465:155-8.

[54] Lusty PJ, Watson A, Tuke MA, Walter WL, Walter WK, Zicat B. Orientation and wear of the acetabular component in third generation alumina-on-alumina ceramic bearings - An analysis of 33 retrievals. J Bone Joint Surg-Br Vol. 2007;89B(9):1158-64.

[55] D'Antonio J, Capello W, Manley M, Naughton M, Sutton K. Alumina ceramic bearings for total hip arthroplasty - Five-year results of a prospective randomized study. Clin Orthop Rel Res. 2005(436):164-71. doi:10.1097/01.blo.0000162995.50971.39.

[56] Lusty PJ, Tai CC, Sew-Hoy RP, Walter WL, Walter WK, Zicat BA. Third-generation alumina-on-alumina ceramic bearings in cementless total hip arthroplasty. J Bone Joint Surg-Am Vol. 2007;89A(12):2676-83. doi:10.2106/jbjs.f01466.

[57] Murphy SB, Ecker TM, Tannast M. Two- to 9-year clinical results of alumina ceramic-on-ceramic THA. Clin Orthop Rel Res. 2006(453):97-102. doi:10.1097/01.blo. 0000246532.59876.73.

[58] Chevillotte C, Pibarot V, Carret JP, Bejui-Hugues J, Guyen O. Nine years follow-up of 100 ceramic-on-ceramic total hip arthroplasty. International Orthopaedics. 2011;35(11):1599-604. doi:10.1007/s00264-010-1185-3.

[59] Salih S, Currall VA, Ward AJ, Chesser TJS. Survival of ceramic bearings in total hip replacement after high-energy trauma and periprosthetic acetabular fracture. J Bone Joint Surg-Br Vol. 2009;91B(11):1533-5. doi:10.1302/0301-620x.91b11.22737.

[60] Lewis PM, Al-Belooshi A, Olsen M, Schemitch EH, Waddell JP. Prospective Randomized Trial Comparing Alumina Ceramic-on-Ceramic With Ceramic-On-Conventional Polyethylene Bearings in Total Hip Arthroplasty. J Arthroplast. 2010;25(3):392-7. doi: 10.1016/j.arth.2009.01.013.

[61] Baek SH, Kim SY. Cementless total hip arthroplasty with alumina bearings in patients younger than fifty with femoral head osteonecrosis. J Bone Joint Surg-Am Vol. 2008;90A(6):1314-20. doi:10.2106/jbjs.g.00755.

[62] Yoo JJ, Kim YM, Yoon KS, Koo KH, Song WS, Kim HJ. Alumina-on-alumina total hip arthroplasty - A five-year minimum follow-up study. J Bone Joint Surg-Am Vol. 2005;87A(3):530-5. doi:10.2106/jbjs.d01753.

[63] Park YS, Hwang SK, Choy WS, Kim YS, Moon YW, Lim SJ. Ceramic failure after total hip arthroplasty with an alumina-on-alumina bearing. J Bone Joint Surg-Am Vol. 2006;88A(4):780-7. doi:10.2106/jbjs.e.00618.

[64] Hannouche D, Nich C, Bizot P, Meunier A, Nizard RM, Sedel L. Fractures of ceramic bearings - History and present status. Clin Orthop Rel Res. 2003(417):19-26. doi: 10.1097/01.blo.0000096806.78689.50.

[65] Byun J-W, Yoon T-R, Park K-S, Seon J-K. Third-generation ceramic-on-ceramic total hip arthroplasty in patients younger than 30 years with osteonecrosis of femoral head. The Journal of Arthroplasty. 2012;27(7):1337-43.

[66] Solarino G, Piazzolla A, Notarnicola A, Moretti L, Tafuri S, De Giorgi S et al. Long-term results of 32-mm alumina-on-alumina THA for avascular necrosis of the femoral head. Journal of orthopaedics and traumatology : official journal of the Italian Society of Orthopaedics and Traumatology. 2012;13(1):21-7.

[67] Savarino L, Baldini N, Ciapetti G, Pellacani A, Giunti A. Is wear debris responsible for failure in alumina-on-alumina implants? Acta Orthopaedica. 2009;80(2):162-7. doi:10.3109/17453670902876730.

[68] Nam KW, Yoo JJ, Kim YL, Kim YM, Lee MH, Kim HJ. Alumina-debris-induced osteolysis in contemporary alumina-on-alumina total hip arthroplasty - A case report. J Bone Joint Surg-Am Vol. 2007;89A(11):2499-503. doi:10.2106/jbjs.g.00130.

[69] Chang JD, Kamdar R, Yoo JH, Hur M, Lee SS. Third-Generation Ceramic-on-Ceramic Bearing Surfaces in Revision Total Hip Arthroplasty. J Arthroplast. 2009;24(8):1231-5. doi:10.1016/j.arth.2009.04.016.

[70] Mai K, Verioti C, Ezzet KA, Copp SN, Walker RH, Colwell CW, Jr. Incidence of 'squeaking' after ceramic-on-ceramic total hip arthroplasty. Clin Orthop Relat Res. 2010;468(2):413-7.

[71] Keurentjes JC, Kuipers RM, Wever DJ, Schreurs BW. High incidence of squeaking in THAs with alumina ceramic-on-ceramic bearings. Clin Orthop Rel Res. 2008;466(6): 1438-43. doi:10.1007/s11999-008-0177-8.

[72] Cogan A, Nizard R, Sedel L. Occurrence of noise in alumina-on-alumina total hip arthroplasty. A survey on 284 consecutive hips. Orthopaedics & Traumatology-Surgery & Research. 2011;97(2):206-10. doi:10.1016/j.otsr.2010.11.008.

[73] Chevillotte C, Pibarot V, Carret JP, Bejui-Hugues J, Guyen O. Hip Squeaking A 10-Year Follow-Up Study. J Arthroplast. 2012;27(6):1008-13. doi:10.1016/j.arth. 2011.11.024.

[74] Stanat SJC, Capozzi JD. Squeaking in Third- and Fourth-Generation Ceramic-on-Ceramic Total Hip Arthroplasty Meta-Analysis and Systematic Review. J Arthroplast. 2012;27(3):445-53. doi:10.1016/j.arth.2011.04.031.

[75] Sexton SA, Yeung E, Jackson MP, Rajaratnam S, Martell JM, Walter WL et al. The role of patient factors and implant position in squeaking of ceramic-on-ceramic total hip replacements. J Bone Joint Surg-Br Vol. 2011;93B(4):439-42. doi:10.1302/0301-620x. 93b4.25707.

[76] Restrepo C, Matar WY, Parvizi J, Rothman RH, Hozack WJ. Natural History of Squeaking after Total Hip Arthroplasty. Clin Orthop Rel Res. 2010;468(9):2340-5. doi: 10.1007/s11999-009-1223-x.

[77] Parvizi J, Adeli B, Wong JC, Restrepo C, Rothman RH. A Squeaky Reputation: The Problem May Be Design-dependent. Clin Orthop Rel Res. 2011;469(6):1598-605. doi: 10.1007/s11999-011-1777-2.

[78] Walter WL, Waters TS, Gillies M, Donohoo S, Kurtz SM, Ranawat AS et al. Squeaking Hips. J Bone Joint Surg-Am Vol. 2008;90A:102-11. doi:10.2106/jbjs.h.00867.

[79] Walter WL, O'Toole GC, Walter WK, Ellis A, Zicat BA. Squeaking in ceramic-on-ceramic hips - The importance of acetabular component orientation. J Arthroplast. 2007;22(4):496-503. doi:10.1016/j.arth.2006.06.018.

[80] Savarino L, Padovanni G, Ferretti M, Greco M, Cenni E, Perrone G et al. Serum Ion Levels after Ceramic-on-Ceramic and Metal-on-Metal Total Hip Arthroplasty: 8-Year Minimum Follow-up. J Orthop Res. 2008;26(12):1569-76. doi:10.1002/jor.20701.

[81] Swanson TV, Peterson DJ, Seethala R, Bliss RL, Spellmon CA. Influence of Prosthetic Design on Squeaking After Ceramic-on-Ceramic Total Hip Arthroplasty. J Arthroplast. 2010;25(6):36-42. doi:10.1016/j.arth.2010.04.032.

[82] Matar WY, Restrepo C, Parvizi J, Kurtz SM, Hozack WJ. Revision Hip Arthroplasty for Ceramic-on-Ceramic Squeaking Hips Does Not Compromise the Results. J Arthroplast. 2010;25(6):81-6. doi:10.1016/j.arth.2010.05.002.

[83] Taylor S, Manley MT, Sutton K. The role of stripe wear in causing acoustic emissions from alumina ceramic-on-ceramic bearings. J Arthroplast. 2007;22(7):47-51. doi: 10.1016/j.arth.2007.05.038.

[84] Hothan A, Huber G, Weiss C, Hoffmann N, Morlock M. The influence of component design, bearing clearance and axial load on the squeaking characteristics of ceramic hip articulations. J Biomech. 2011;44(5):837-41. doi:10.1016/j.jbiomech.2010.12.012.

[85] Sanders A, Tibbitts I, Brannon R. Concomitant evolution of wear and squeaking in dual-severity, lubricated wear testing of ceramic-on-ceramic hip prostheses. J Orthop Res. 2012;30(9):1377-83. doi:10.1002/jor.22080.

[86] Currier JH, Anderson DE, Van Citters DW. A proposed mechanism for squeaking of ceramic-on-ceramic hips. Wear. 2010;269(11-12):782-9. doi:10.1016/j.wear.2010.08.006.

[87] Walter WL, Kurtz SM, Esposito C, Hozack W, Holley KG, Garino JP et al. Retrieval analysis of squeaking alumina ceramic-on-ceramic bearings. J Bone Joint Surg-Br Vol. 2011;93B(12):1597-601. doi:10.1302/0301-620x.93b12.27529.

[88] Capello WN, Feinberg JR. Use of an alumina ceramic-on-alumina ceramic bearing surface in THA in a 13 year old with JIA--a single case study. Bull NYU Hosp Jt Dis. 2009;67(4):384-6.

[89] Nizard R, Pourreyron D, Raould A, Hannouche D, Sedel L. Alumina-on-alumina hip arthroplasty in patients younger than 30 years old. Clin Orthop Rel Res. 2008;466(2): 317-23. doi:10.1007/s11999-007-0068-4.

Permissions

The contributors of this book come from diverse backgrounds, making this book a truly international effort. This book will bring forth new frontiers with its revolutionizing research information and detailed analysis of the nascent developments around the world.

We would like to thank Rosario Pignatello, for lending his expertise to make the book truly unique. He has played a crucial role in the development of this book. Without his invaluable contribution this book wouldn't have been possible. He has made vital efforts to compile up to date information on the varied aspects of this subject to make this book a valuable addition to the collection of many professionals and students.

This book was conceptualized with the vision of imparting up-to-date information and advanced data in this field. To ensure the same, a matchless editorial board was set up. Every individual on the board went through rigorous rounds of assessment to prove their worth. After which they invested a large part of their time researching and compiling the most relevant data for our readers. Conferences and sessions were held from time to time between the editorial board and the contributing authors to present the data in the most comprehensible form. The editorial team has worked tirelessly to provide valuable and valid information to help people across the globe.

Every chapter published in this book has been scrutinized by our experts. Their significance has been extensively debated. The topics covered herein carry significant findings which will fuel the growth of the discipline. They may even be implemented as practical applications or may be referred to as a beginning point for another development. Chapters in this book were first published by InTech; hereby published with permission under the Creative Commons Attribution License or equivalent.

The editorial board has been involved in producing this book since its inception. They have spent rigorous hours researching and exploring the diverse topics which have resulted in the successful publishing of this book. They have passed on their knowledge of decades through this book. To expedite this challenging task, the publisher supported the team at every step. A small team of assistant editors was also appointed to further simplify the editing procedure and attain best results for the readers.

Our editorial team has been hand-picked from every corner of the world. Their multi-ethnicity adds dynamic inputs to the discussions which result in innovative outcomes. These outcomes are then further discussed with the researchers and contributors who give their valuable feedback and opinion regarding the same. The feedback is then collaborated with the researches and they are edited in a comprehensive manner to aid the understanding of the subject.

Apart from the editorial board, the designing team has also invested a significant amount of their time in understanding the subject and creating the most relevant covers. They scrutinized every image to scout for the most suitable representation of the subject and create an appropriate cover for the book.

The publishing team has been involved in this book since its early stages. They were actively engaged in every process, be it collecting the data, connecting with the contributors or procuring relevant information. The team has been an ardent support to the editorial, designing and production team. Their endless efforts to recruit the best for this project, has resulted in the accomplishment of this book. They are a veteran in the field of academics and their pool of knowledge is as vast as their experience in printing. Their expertise and guidance has proved useful at every step. Their uncompromising quality standards have made this book an exceptional effort. Their encouragement from time to time has been an inspiration for everyone.

The publisher and the editorial board hope that this book will prove to be a valuable piece of knowledge for researchers, students, practitioners and scholars across the globe.

List of Contributors

Juliana Lott Carvalho, Dawidson Assis Gomes and Alfredo Miranda de Goes
Department of Biochemistry and Immunology, Federal University of Minas Gerais, Belo Horizonte, Brazil

Pablo Herthel de Carvalho
Department of Veterinary Clinicals and Surgery of the Federal University of Minas Gerais, Belo Horizonte, Brazil

Tiago Pereira, Andrea Gärtner, Raquel Gomes, Miguel L. França, Ana Lúcia Luís and Ana Colette Maurício
Centro de Estudos de Ciência Animal (CECA), Instituto de Ciências e Tecnologias Agrárias e Agro - Alimentares (ICETA), Universidade do Porto (UP), Portugal
Instituto de Ciências Biomédicas Abel Salazar (ICBAS), Universidade do Porto (UP), Portugal

Irina Amorim
Instituto de Ciências Biomédicas Abel Salazar (ICBAS), Universidade do Porto (UP), Portugal

Paulo Armada-da-Silva and Cátia Pereira
Faculdade de Motricidade Humana (FMH), Universidade Técnica de Lisboa (UTL), Portugal

Diana M. Morais, Miguel A. Rodrigues, Maria A. Lopes and José D. Santos
CEMUC, Departamento de Engenharia Metalúrgica e Materiais, Faculdade de Engenharia, Universidade do Porto (FEUP), Portugal

Ning Zhu and Xiongbiao Chen
Division of Biomedical Engineering, University of Saskatchewan, Saskatoon, SK, Canada

François A. Auger and Lucie Germain
Laval University LOEX center, Tissue Engineering And Regenerative Medecine: LOEX – FRQS Research Center of the "Centre Hospitalier Affilié Universitaire de Québec", Canada
Department of Surgery, Faculty of Medicine, Laval University, Quebec, Canada

Jean-Michel Bourget
Laval University LOEX center, Tissue Engineering And Regenerative Medecine : LOEX – FRQS Research Center of the "Centre Hospitalier Affilié Universitaire de Québec", Canada
Department of Surgery, Faculty of Medicine, Laval University, Quebec, Canada
National Research Council Canada, Boucherville, PQ, Canada

Maxime Guillemette
Physics Department, Faculty of Science and Engineering, Laval University, and Medical Physics Unit, "Centre Hospitalier Universitaire de Québec", Québec, QC, Canada

Teodor Veres
Life Sciences Division, National Research Council Canada, Biomedical Engineering, McGill University, National Research Council Canada, Boucherville, PQ, Canada

Masaru Murata, Md Arafat Kabir and Yasuhito Minamida
Health Sciences University of Hokkaido, Japan

Toshiyuki Akazawa
Hokkaido Organization, Japan

Masaharu Mitsugi
Takamatsu Oral and Maxillofacial Surgery, Japan

In-Woong Um
Korea Tooth Bank Co. Ltd, Korea

Kyung-Wook Kim
Dankok University, Korea

Young-Kyun Kim
Seoul National University, Korea

Yao Sun
Harbin Medical University, China
Texas A&M Health Science Center Baylor College of Dentistry, USA

Chunlin Qin
Texas A&M Health Science Center Baylor College of Dentistry, USA

Xiaohong Wang
Business Innovation Technology (BIT) Research Centre, School of Science and Technology, Aalto University, Aalto, Finland
Key Laboratory for Advanced Materials Processing Technology, Ministry of Education & Center of Organ Manufacturing, Department of Mechanical Engineering, Tsinghua University, Beijing, P.R. China
State Key Laboratory of Materials Processing and Die & Mould Technology, Huazhong University of Science and Technology, Wuhan, P.R. China

Marjo Yliperttula
Division of Biopharmaceutics and Pharmacokinetics, Faculty of Pharmacy, University of Helsinki, Helsinki, Finland

Jukka Tuomi, Kaija-Stiina Paloheimo and Jouni Partanen
Business Innovation Technology (BIT) Research Centre, School of Science and Technology, Aalto University, Aalto, Finland

Antti A. Mäkitie
Business Innovation Technology (BIT) Research Centre, School of Science and Technology, Aalto University, Aalto, Finland
Department of Otolaryngology - Head & Neck Surgery, Helsinki University Hospital and University of Helsinki, Helsinki, Finland

Young-Kyun Kim
Department of Oral and Maxillofacial Surgery, Section of Dentistry, Seoul National University Bundang Hospital, Seongnam, Korea

Jeong Keun Lee
Department of Dentistry Oral & Maxillofacial Surgery, Ajou University School of Medicine, Suwon, Korea

Kyung-Wook Kim
Department of Oral and Maxillofacial Surgery, College of Dentistry, Dankook University, Cheonan, Korea

In-Woong Um
Director, Korea Tooth Bank, R&D Institute, Seoul, Korea

Masaru Murata
Division of Oral and Maxillofacial Surgery, University of Hokkaido, Hokkaido, Japan

Andrea Gärtner, Tiago Pereira, Raquel Gomes, Ana Lúcia Luís, Miguel Lacueva França and Ana Colette Maurício
Instituto de Ciências Biomédicas Abel Salazar (ICBAS), Universidade do Porto (UP), Portugal
Centro de Estudos de Ciência Animal (CECA), Instituto de Ciências e Tecnologias Agrárias e Agro-Alimentares (ICETA), Universidade do Porto (UP), Portugal

Stefano Geuna
Department of Clinical and Biological Sciences, University of Turin, Italy

Paulo Armada-da-Silva
Faculdade de Motricidade Humana (FMH), Universidade Técnica de Lisboa (UTL), Portugal

Junko Hieda, Mitsuo Niinomi, Masaaki Nakai and Ken Cho
Department of Biomaterials Science, Institute for Materials Research, Tohoku University, Katahira, Aoba-ku, Sendai, Japan

Michel Simonet
Veterinary hospital, Nuit Saint Georges, France

Nicole Rouquet and Patrick Frayssinet
Urodelia, St Lys, France

Susan C. Scholes and Thomas J. Joyce
School of Mechanical and Systems Engineering, Newcastle University, Newcastle-upon-Tyne, UK

9 781632